Andrea Gaggioli, Alois Ferscha, Giuseppe Riva, Stephen Dunne, Isabelle Viaud-Delmon

Human Computer Confluence

Transforming Human Experience Through Symbiotic Technologies

Andrea Gaggioli, Alois Ferscha, Giuseppe Riva,
Stephen Dunne, Isabelle Viaud-Delmon

Human Computer Confluence

Transforming Human Experience through Symbiotic Technologies

Managing Editor: Aneta Przepiórka
Associate Editor: Pietro Cipresso
Language Editor: Catherine Lau

DE GRUYTER
OPEN

ISBN 978-3-11-047112-0
e-ISBN (PDF) 978-3-11-047113-7
e-ISBN (EPUB) 978-3-11-047169-4

Library of Congress Cataloging-in-Publication Data
A CIP catalog record for this book has been applied for at the Library of Congress.

Published by De Gruyter Open Ltd, Warsaw/Berlin Part of Walter de Gruyter GmbH, Berlin/Boston
The book is published with open access at www.degruyter.com.

Managing Editor: Aneta Przepiórka
Associate Editor: Pietro Cipresso
Language Editor: Catherine Lau

www.degruyteropen.com

Cover illustration: © Thinkstock ra2studio

Contents

Section I: Conceptual Frameworks and Models

Section III: Applications

List of contributing authors

Alois Ferscha
Johannes Kepler University, Linz, Austia
Chapter 1

David Benyon
Edinburgh Napier University, UK
Chapter 2

Oli Mival
Edinburgh Napier University, UK
Chapter 2

Francesca Morganti
University of Bergamo, Italy
Chapter 3

Giuseppe Riva
Catholic University of Sacred Heart, Milan, Italy
Istituto Auxologico Italiano, Milan, Italy
Chapter 4

Bruno Herbelin
Ecole Polytechnique Fédérale de Lausanne, Switzerland
Chapter 5

Roy Salomon
Ecole Polytechnique Fédérale de Lausanne, Switzerland
Chapter 5

Andrea Serino
Università di Bologna, Italy
Ecole Polytechnique Fédérale de Lausanne, Switzerland
Chapter 5

Olaf Blanke
Ecole Polytechnique Fédérale de Lausanne, Switzerland
University Hospital, Geneva, Switzerland
Chapter 5

Andrea Gaggioli
Catholic University of Sacred Heart, Milan, Italy
Istituto Auxologico Italiano, Milan, Italy
Chapter 6

Frederic Bevilacqua
Ircam, CNRS, UPMC, Paris, France
Chapter 7

Norbert Schnell
Ircam, CNRS, UPMC, Paris, France
Chapter 7

Fivos Maniatakos
IRCAM-CentrePompidou, Paris, France
Chapter 8

Doron Friedman
Sammy Ofer School of Communications of Interdisciplinary Center Herzliya, Herzliya, Israel
Chapter 9

Béatrice S. Hasler
Sammy Ofer School of Communications of Interdisciplinary Center Herzliya, Herzliya, Israel
Chapter 9

Robert Leeb
École Polytechnique Fédérale de Lausanne
Switzerland
Chapter 10

Ricardo Chavarriaga
École Polytechnique Fédérale de Lausanne
Switzerland
Chapter 10

José d. R. Millán
École Polytechnique Fédérale de Lausanne
Switzerland
Chapter 10

Jonathan Freeman
Goldsmiths, University of London, UK
i2 media research ltd
Chapter 11

Andrea Miotto
Goldsmiths, University of London, UK
i2 media research ltd
Chapter 11

Jane Lessiter
Goldsmiths, University of London, UK
i2 media research ltd
Chapter 11

Paul Verschure
Universitat Pompeu Fabra, Barcelona, Spain
Institució Catalana de Recerca i Estudis Avançats (ICREA), Barcelona, Spain
Chapter 11

Pedro Omedas
Universitat Pompeu Fabra, Barcelona, Spain
Chapter 11

Anil K. Seth
University of Sussex, Falmer, Brighton, UK
Chapter 11

Georgios Th. Papadopoulos
Centre for Research and Technology Hellas/ Information Technologies Institute (CERTH/ITI), Greece
Chapter 11

Andrea Caria
Eberhard Karls Universität Tübingen, Germany
Chapter 11

Elisabeth André
Universität Augsburg, Germany
Chapter 11

Marc Cavazza
Teesside University, UK
Chapter 11

Luciano Gamberini
University of Padua, Italy
Chapter 11

Anna Spagnolli
University of Padua, Italy
Chapter 11

Jürgen Jost
Max Planck Institute for Mathematics in the Sciences, Leipzig, Germany
Chapter 11

Sid Kouider
CNRS and Ecole Normale Supérieure, Paris, France
Chapter 11

Barnabás Takács
Technical University of Budapest, Hungary
Chapter 11

Alberto Sanfeliu
Institut de Robotica i Informatica Industrial (CSIC-UPC), Barcelona, Spain
Chapter 11

Danilo De Rossi
University of Pisa, Italy
Chapter 11

Claudio Cenedese
Electrolux Global Technology Center, Udine, Italy
Chapter 11

John L. Bintliff
Universiteit Leiden, the Netherlands
Chapter 11

Giulio Jacucci
University of Helsinki, Finland
Aalto University, Finland
Chapter 11

Alessandro D'Ausilio
IIT – Italian Institute of Technology, Genova, Italy
Chapter 12

Katrin Solveig Lohan
HWU-Heriot-Watt University, Genova, Italy
Chapter 12

Leonardo Badino
IIT – Italian Institute of Technology, Genova, Italy
Chapter 12

Alessandra Sciutti
IIT – Italian Institute of Technology, Genova, Italy
Chapter 12

Joris Favié
Delft University of Technology,The Netherlands
Chapter 13

Vanessa Vakili
Delft University of Technology,The Netherlands
Chapter 13

Willem-Paul Brinkman
Delft University of Technology,The Netherlands
Chapter 13

Nexhmedin Morina
University of Amsterdam, The Netherlands
Chapter 13

Mark A. Neerincx
Delft University of Technology,The Netherlands
TNO Human Factors, Soesterberg, The Netherlands
Chapter 13

Monica Cameirao
Universidade da Madeira, Portugal
Polo Científico e Tecnológico da Madeira, Portugal
Chapter 14

Sergi Bermúdez i Badia
Universidade da Madeira, Portugal
Polo Científico e Tecnológico da Madeira, Portugal
Chapter 14

Pedro Gamito
Lusophone University, Lisbon, Portugal
Chapter 15

Jorge Oliveira
Lusophone University, Lisbon, Portugal
Chapter 15

Rodrigo Brito
Lusophone University, Lisbon, Portugal
Chapter 15

Diogo Morais
Lusophone University, Lisbon, Portugal
Chapter 15

Dimitris Giakoumis
Information Technologies Institute, Thessaloniki, Greece
Chapter 16

Georgios Papamakarios
Information Technologies Institute, Thessaloniki, Greece
Chapter 16

Manolis Vasileiadis
Information Technologies Institute, Thessaloniki, Greece
Chapter 16

Anastasios Drosou
Information Technologies Institute, Thessaloniki, Greece
Chapter 16

Dimitrios Tzovaras
Information Technologies Institute, Thessaloniki, Greece
Chapter 16

Myounghoon Jeon
Michigan Technological University, Houghton, USA
Chapter 17

Andreas Riener
Johannes Kepler University Linz, Austria
Chapter 17

Walter Van de Velde[1]

Foreword

The editors of this volume bring together a collection of papers that, taken together, provide an interesting snapshot of current research on Human Computer Confluence (HCC). HCC stands for a particular vision of how computing devices and human beings (users) can be fruitfully combined. The term was coined some 10 years ago in an attempt to make sense of the increasingly complex technological landscape that was emerging from different interrelated research strands in Information and Communication Technology (ICT). It was clear that computers could no longer be seen just as machines that execute algorithms for turning input into output data. This simply seemed to miss a lot of the ways in which computers were starting to be used, in which 'users' could interact with them and the multitudes of shapes they could take. After the era of 'desktop computing', the power of an application was no longer just residing in the sophistication of its algorithmic core, but also, or maybe even mainly, in the way it blends into the user's sensation of being engaged into some value-adding experience (for work, for health, for entertainment,...). Moreover, everything that had been learned about how to design good screen-based interfaces seemed useless for dealing with settings of, for instance, wearable or embedded computing. In order to capture all this there was a pressing need for new concepts, a new language, new ways of measuring and comparing things.

Human Computer Confluence became the name of a 'proactive initiative' (EC, 2014), funded by the European Commission's Future and Emerging Technologies (FET) programme under the Seventh Framework Programme for Research (FP7). In a nutshell, the mission of FET is to explore radically new technological paradigms that can become the future assets for a globally competitive Europe that is worth to live in. A FET proactive initiative aims to assemble a critical mass of research around such a technological paradigm in order to shape its distinct research agenda and to help building up the multi-disciplinary knowledge base from which the paradigm can be explored and further developed into a genuinely new line of technology.

Not all the work that is documented in this volume has been funded through FET. Many of its authors would not even say that they are doing their work under the umbrella of HCC. HCC is not a strictly defined school of thought. It is rather an undercurrent that permeates across many lines of contemporary research activities in information and communication technologies. In that sense, the concept of Human Computer Confluence is more like a road sign marking a direction in the socio/technological landscape, rather than a precise destination.

1 The views expressed are those of the author and not necessarily those of the European Commission

What's in a name? Why was there a need for a new term or concept such as Human Computer Confluence? After all, there was already 'ubiquitous computing' to capture the visionary idea of anywhere, anytime and contextualised computing. After all, there were already emerging areas like Presence research and Interaction Design, both with their essential focus on techniques to develop characterise and even measure the 'user experience', be it in virtual reality, augmented reality or embedded and ambient computing/settings. These areas of research are all very relevant for the emerging HCC research agenda, and it is at their intersection that the idea of HCC takes shape.

As should be obvious from the name, perhaps the most essential feature of HCC is that it is not just a technological research agenda. Somewhat retrospectively, one can argue that its whole *raison d'être* was to counterbalance the technology-dominated vision of ubiquitous computing that (with a detour through ambient intelligence) is now developing into Internet of Things. The whole human side of it that was initially very strong (especially in Disappearing Computing and Ambient Intelligence) got overpowered by the more pressing and concrete technological research agenda of components, systems, protocols and infrastructures. With the more fundamental questions of the human side of the equation temporarily side lined, there was an obvious need for longer term research such as funded by FET to do some groundwork on this. It is in this context that HCC both as a term and as an initiative was born. Ultimately, it will be in its contribution to turning Ubiquity and Internet of Things into something worth to have for Europe's citizens that its long-term impact should be measured.

It is worth mentioning the other big school of thought for a human/technology combination, namely the convergence research agenda of NBIC – Nano-Bio-Info-Cogno. This is a strongly reductionist vision of human engineerability, based on its reduction to elementary material and ultimately engineerable building blocks over which perfect control can be exercised. In its most radical versions it leads to Transhumanism where human nature itself gets inevitably replaced by a superior bio-techno hybrid nature. Human Computer Confluence points to an alternative approach of trying to understand and enhance the human sense and experience of technological augmentation by building technology that takes into account the full human nature of the 'user'. In that sense it is also a good illustration of what the European version of the NBIC convergence agenda could look like (HLEG, 2004).

HCC addresses what seems to be a paradox: how can we become more human through technology, instead of less?[2]

– Humans as equal part of the system to be studied: HCC cannot be reduced to a purely technological challenge. Whereas before the human was a factor to be

2 This list is based on the outcome of a panel discussion at the second HC2 Summer School, IRCAM, 2013 (HC2, 2013)

taken into account (for example for usability) it is now an equally important part of the study. This redefines the boundaries of the 'system', and hybridises the nature of it in a fundamental way. The old idea of interface as the fine line that cuts between system and user is no longer tenable. One rather has to think about how complex process on both side interact and intertwine, at different levels (for instance, physical, behavioural, cognitive) and based on a deep understanding of both.
- Empowerment rather than augmentation: HCC is not about augmentation of specific human capabilities (for example force, memory, concentration, perception, reasoning), but about empowering humans to use their abilities in new ways, themselves deciding when and what for.
- Social enhancement rather than individual superiority: it appears useful to anchor HCC in a networked view of computing, such as ubiquity or internet of things, in order to keep it focused on group, community and social dimensions, in addition to the individual user's view (Internet of Everything).
- Privacy and trust are essential for user's to engage into the experiences that HCC enables for them. HCC requires much more transparency on who or what is in control or has certain rights. It remains to be seen whether current trends in big data are going to provide a sufficient framework for this.
- Another emerging feature of the HCC idea is that users are creative actors. In HCC there is a sense that we put things together, more than that they are pre-packaged technology bundles. The active involvement of the human as the composer or bricoleur of its own technology-mediated experience is stronger, maybe even more essential then the automated adaptation of the technology to the user. In this sense HCC resonates well with current trends of 'makers', fablabs and social innovation. Will HCC bring everyday creativity and popular cultural expression to the heart of the research agenda, not just as a creative methodology to design new technologies but as an integral feature of any human/socio-technological system?

Looking at this list, it is clear that HCC has not been achieved yet in a significant way. The combination through technology of such features as personal empowerment, social enhancement, trust and user creativity has not yet been demonstrated in a strong way. It is not even clear what form such a demonstration would take. Beyond research, one can only speculate about the killer application that would demonstrate its power. Maybe it could be in sports, in gaming or in fashion, where playfulness and serious results can be combined and where wiling early adopters can be easily found. What would be its first big market: commerce, entertainment, the grey economy, education, the public sector or ecology? Or will it be and remain generic from the outset, leaving it entirely to the users as creative actors to invent what it can do?

As the chapters of this book illustrate, Human Computer Confluence is a fascinating vision in which a lot remains to be understood. Some of the choices mentioned above will need to be made more consciously in order to grow beyond the incidental flashes of insight to a genuinely new paradigm of information technology. It has the potential to create the opportunities for a distinct European approach to how humans and technology can be combined.

References

EC. (2014). FP7: Human computer confluence (HC-CO). Retrieved 21 May 2015, from http://cordis.europa.eu/fp7/ict/fet-proactive/hcco_en.html

HC2. (2013). Second HC2 Summer School, IRCAM, Paris. Retrieved 21 May 2015, from http://hcsquared.eu/summer-school-2013

HLEG. (2004). Converging Technologies – Shaping the Future of European Societies. Brussels: European Commission.

Section I: **Conceptual Frameworks and Models**

Alois Ferscha

1 A Research Agenda for Human Computer Confluence

Abstract: HCI research over three decades has shaped a wide spanning research area at the boundaries of computer science and behavioral science, with an impressive outreach to how humankind is experiencing information and communication technologies in literally every breath of an individual's life. The explosive growth of networks and communications, and at the same time radical miniaturization of ICT electronics have reversed the principles of human computer interaction. Up until now considered as the interaction concerns when humans approach ICT systems, more recent observations see systems approaching humans at the same time. Humans and ICT Systems apparently approach each other confluently.

This article identifies trends in research and technology that are indicative for the emerging symbiosis of society and technology. Fertilized by two diametrically opposed technology trends: (i) the miniaturization of information and communication electronics, and (ii) the exponential growth of global communication networks, HCC over it's more than two decades of evolution, the field has been undergoing three generations of research challenges: The first generation aiming towards autonomic systems and their adaptation was driven by the availability of technology to connect literally everything to everything (Connectedness, early to late nineties). The second generation inherited from the upcoming context recognition and knowledge processing technologies (Awareness, early twentyhundreds), e.g. context-awareness, self-awareness or resource-awareness. Finally, a third generation, building upon connectedness and awareness, attempts to exploit the (ontological) semantics of Pervasive / Ubiquitous Computing systems, services and interactions (i.e. giving meaning to situations and actions, and "intelligence" to systems) (Smartness, from the mid twentyhundreds). As of today we observe that modern ICT with explicit user input and output are becoming to be replaced by a computing landscape sensing the physical world via a huge variety of sensors, and controlling it via a plethora of actuators. The nature and appearance of computing devices is changing to be hidden in the fabric of everyday life, invisibly networked, and omnipresent, with applications greatly being based on the notions of context and knowledge. Interaction with such globe spanning, modern ICT systems will presumably be more implicit, at the periphery of human attention, rather than explicit, i.e. at the focus of human attention.

Keywords: Humans and Computers, Pervasive and Ubiquitous Computing, Human Computer Interaction, Ambient Intelligence, Socio-technical Systems

1.1 Introduction

Human Computer Confluence (HCC) has emerged out of European research initiatives over the past few years, aiming at fundamental and strategic research studying how the emerging symbiotic relation between humans and ICT (Information and Communication Technologies) can be based on radically new forms of sensing, perception, interaction and understanding. HCC has been identified as an instrument to engage an interdisciplinary field of research ranging from cognitive neuroscience, computational social sciences to computer science, particularly human computer interaction, pervasive and ubiquitous computing, artificial intelligence and computational perception.

The first definition of HCC resulted out of a research challenges identification process in the Beyond-The-Horizon (FET FP6) effort:

"Human computer confluence refers to an invisible, implicit, embodied or even implanted interaction between humans and system components. ... should provide the means to the user to interact and communicate with the surrounding environment in a transparent "human and natural" way involving all sense..."

A working group of more than 50 distinguished European researchers structured and consolidated the individual position statements into a strategic report. The key issue identified in this report addressed fundamental research: *"Human computer confluence refers to an invisible, implicit, embodied or even implanted interaction between humans and system components. New classes of user interfaces may evolve that make use of several sensors and are able to adapt their physical properties to the current situational context of users. In the near future visible displays will be available in all sizes and will compete for the limited attention of users. Examples include body worn displays, smart apparel, interactive rooms, large display walls, roads and architecture annotated with digital information – or displays delivering information to the periphery of the observers' perception. Recent advances have also brought input and output technology closer to the human, even connecting it directly with the human sensory and neural system in terms of in-body interaction and intelligent prosthetics, such as ocular video implants. Research in that area has to cover both technological and qualitative aspects, such as user experience and usability"* as well as societal and technological implications *"Researchers strive to broker a unified and seamless interactive framework that dynamically melds interaction across a range of modalities and devices, from interactive rooms and large display walls to near body interaction, wearable devices, in-body implants and direct neural input and stimulation"*.

Based on the suggestions delivered with the Beyond-The-Horizon report, a consultation meeting was called for "Human Computer Confluence" in November 2007, out which resulted the FET strategy to *"propose a program of research that seeks to employ progress in human computer interaction to create new abilities for sensing, perception, communication, interaction and understanding..."*, and consequently the implementation of the respective research funding instruments like (i) new forms of interactive media (Ubiquitous Display Surfaces, Interconnected Smart Objects, Wearable Computing, Brain-Computer Interfaces), (ii) new forms of sensing and sensory perception (New Sensory Channels, Cognitive and Perceptual Prosthetics), (iii) perception and assimilation of massive scale data (Massive-Scale Implicit Data Collection, Navigating in Massively Complex Information Spaces, Collaborative Sensing, Social Perception), and (iv) Distributed Intelligence (Collective Human Decision Making, The Noosphere).

1.2 Generations of Pervasive / Ubiquitous (P/U) ICT

The novel research fields beyond Personal Computing could be seen as the early 'seeds' of HCC. Preliminarily suffering from a plethora of unspecific, competitive terms like "Ubiquitous Computing" (Weiser et al., 1996), "Calm Computing" (Weiser et al., 1996), "Universal Computing" (Weiser, 1991), "Invisible Computing" (Esler et al., 1999), "Context Based Computing" (UCB, 1999), "Everyday Computing" (Abowd & Mynatt, 2000), "Autonomic Computing", (Horn, 2001), "Amorphous Computing" (Servat & Drogoul, 2002), "Ambient Intelligence" (Remagnino & Foresti, 2005), "Sentient Computing", "Post-Personal Computing", etc., the research communities consolidated and codified their scientific concerns in technical journals, conferences, workshops and textbooks (e.g. the journals IEEE Pervasive, IEEE Internet Computing, Personal and Ubiquitous Computing, Pervasive and Mobile Computing, Int. Journal of Pervasive Computing and Communications, or the annual conferences PERVASIVE (International Conference on Pervasive Computing), UBICOMP (International Conference on Ubiquitous Computing), MobiHoc (ACM International Symposium on Mobile Ad Hoc Networking and Computing), PerComp (IEEE Conference on Pervasive Computing and Communications), ICPCA (International Conference on Pervasive Computing and Applications), ISWC (International Symposium on Wearable Computing), ISWPC (International Symposium on Wireless Pervasive Computing), IWSAC (International Workshop on Smart Appliances and Wearable Computing), MOBIQUITOUS (Conference on Mobile and Ubiquitous Systems), UBICOMM (International Conference on Ubiquitous Computing, Systems, Services, and Technologies), WMCSA (IEEE Workshop on Mobile Computing Systems and Applications), AmI (European Conference on Ambient Intelligence), etc. This process of consolidation is by far not settled today, and more specialized research conferences are emerging, addressing focussed research issues e.g. in Agent Technologies and Middleware (PerWare, ARM, PICom), Privacy and Trust (STPSA, PSPT, TrustCom), Security (UCSS), Sensors (ISWPC, Sensors, PerSeNS, Seacube), Activity Recognition and Machine Learning (e.g. IEEE SMC), Health Care (PervasiveHealth, PSH, WiPH, IEEE IREHSS), Social Computing (SocialCom), Entertainment and Gaming or Learning (PerEL).

Weiser's seminal vision on the "Computer for the 21st Century" (Weiser, 1991) was groundbreaking, and still represents the corner stone for what might be referred to as a first generation of Pervasive/Ubiquitous Computing research, aiming towards embedded, hidden, invisible and autonomic, but networked information and communication technology (ICT) systems (Pervasive / Ubiquitous ICT, P/U ICT for short). This first generation definitely gained from the technological progress momentum (miniaturization of electronics, gate packaging), and was driven by the upcoming availability of technology to connect literally everything to everything (Connectedness, mid to late Nineties), like wireless communication standards and the exponentially growing Internet. Networks of P/U ICT systems emerged, forming communication clouds of miniaturized, cheap, fast, powerful, wirelessly connected, "always on" systems, enabled by the massive availability of miniaturized computing, storage, communication, and embedded systems technologies. Special purpose computing and information appliances, ready to spontaneously communicate with one another, sensor-actuator systems to invert the roles of interaction from human to machine (implicit interaction), and organism like capabilities (self-configuration, self-healing, self-optimizing, self-protecting) characterize this P/U ICT generation.

The second generation of P/U ICT inherited from the then upcoming sensor based recognition systems, as well as knowledge representation and processing technologies (Awareness, early Two Thousands), where research issues like e.g. context and situation awareness, self-awareness, future-awareness or resource-awareness reshaped the understanding of pervasive computing. Autonomy and adaptation in this generation was reframed to be based on knowledge, extracted from low level sensor data captured in a particular situation or over long periods of time. The respective "epoch" of research on "context aware" systems was stimulated by Schillit, Adams and Want (Schilit et al., 1994), and fertilized by the PhD work of Dey (Dey, 2001), redefining the term "context" as:

"...any information that can be used to characterize the situation of an entity. An entity is a person, place, or object that is considered relevant to the interaction between a user and an application, including the user and application themselves.".

One result out of this course of research are autonomic systems (Kephart & Chess, 2003). Later, 'autonomic elements' able to capture context, to build up, represent and carry knowledge, to self-describe, -manage, and -organize with respect to the environment, and to exhibit behavior grounded on knowledge based monitoring, analyzing, planning and executing were proposed, shaping ecologies of P/U ICT systems, built from collective autonomic elements interacting in spontaneous spatial/temporal contexts, based on proximity, priority, privileges, capabilities, interests, offerings, environmental conditions, etc.

Finally, a third generation of P/U ICT was observed (mid of the past decade), building upon connectedness and awareness, and attempting to exploit the (ontological) semantics of systems, services and interactions (i.e. giving meaning to situations and actions). Such systems are often referred to as highly complex, orchestrated, cooperative and coordinated "Ensembles of Digital Artifacts". An essential aspect of such an ensemble is its spontaneous configuration towards a complex system, i.e. a

"... dynamic network of many agents (which may represent cells, species, individuals, nations) acting in parallel, constantly acting and reacting to what the other agents are doing where the control tends to be highly dispersed and decentralized, and if there is to be any coherent behavior in the system, it has to arise from competition and cooperation among the agents, so that the overall behavior of the system is the result of a huge number of decisions made every moment by many individual agents" (Castellani & Hafferty, 2009).

1.3 Beyond P/U ICT: Socio-Technical Fabric

Ensembles of digital artifacts as compounds of huge numbers of possibly heterogeneous entities constitute a future generation of socially interactive ICT to which we refer to as Socio-Technical Fabric (late last decade until now), weaving social and technological phenomena into the 'fabric of technology-rich societies'. Indications of evidence for such large scale, complex, technology rich societal settings are facts like 10^{12} -10^{13} "things" or "goods" being traded in (electronic) markets today, 10^9 personal computer nodes and 10^9 mobile phones on the internet, 10^8 cars or 10^8 digital cameras with sophisticated embedded electronics – even for internet access on the go, etc. Todays megacities approach sizes of 10^7 citizens. Already today some 10^8 users are registered on Facebook, 10^8 videos have been uploaded to YouTube, like 10^7 music titles haven been labeled on last.fm, etc. Next generation research directions are thus going away from single user, or small user group P/U ICT as addressed in previous generations, and are heading more towards complex socio-technical systems, i.e. large scale to very large scale deployments of ICT to large scale collectives of user up to whole societies (Ferscha et al., 2012).

A yet underexplored impact of modern P/U ICT relates to services exploiting the "social context" of individuals towards the provision of quality-of-life technologies that aim for the wellbeing of individuals and the welfare of societies. The research community is concerned with the intersection of social behavior and modern ICT, creating or recreating social conventions and social contexts through the use of pervasive, omnipresent and participative technologies. An explosive growth of social computing applications such as blogs, email, instant messaging, social networking (Facebook, MySpace, Twitter, LinkedIn, etc.), wikis, and social bookmarking is observed, profoundly impacting social behavior and life style of human beings while at the same time pushing the boundaries of ICT simultaneously.

Research emerges aiming at understanding the principles of ICT enabled social interaction, and interface technologies appear implementing "social awareness", like social network platforms and social smartphone apps. Human environment interfaces are emerging, potentially allowing individuals and groups to sense, explore and understand their social context. Like the human biological senses (visual, auditory, tactile, olfactory, gustatory) and their role in perception and recognition, the human "social sense" which helps people to perceive the "social" aspects of the environment, and allowing to sense, explore and understand the social context is more and more becoming the subject of research.

Inspired by the capacity of human beings acting socially, in that shaping intelligent societies, the idea of making the principles of social interaction also the design, operational and behavioral principle of modern ICT recently has led to the term "socio-inspired" ICT (Ferscha et al., 2012). From both theoretical and technological perspectives, socio-inspired ICT moves beyond social information processing, towards emphasizing social intelligence. Among the challenges are issues of modeling and analyzing social behavior facilitated with modern ICT, the provision access opportunities and participative technologies, the reality mining of societal change induced by omnipresent ICT, the establishment of social norm and individual respect, as well as e.g. the means of collective choice and society controlled welfare.

1.4 Human Computer Confluence (HCC)

Human Computer Confluence (HCC) has emerged out of European research initiatives over the past few years, aiming at fundamental and strategic research studying how the emerging symbiotic relation between humans and ICT can be based on radically new forms of sensing, perception, interaction and understanding (Ferscha, 2011). HCC has been identified as an instrument to engage an interdisciplinary field of research ranging from cognitive neuroscience, computational social sciences to computer science, particularly human computer interaction, pervasive and ubiquitous computing, artificial intelligence and computational perception.

In order to further establish and promote the EU research priority on Human Computer Confluence, research road-mapping initiatives were started (see e.g. HCC Visions White Book, 2014), aiming to (i) identify and address the basic research problems and strategic research fields in HCC as seen by the scientific community, then (ii) bring together the most important scientific leaders and industrial/commercial stakeholders across disciplines and domains of applications to collect challenges and priorities for a research agenda and roadmap, i.e. the compilation of white-books identifying strengths, weaknesses, opportunities, synergies and complementarities of thematic research in HCC, and ultimately to (iii) negotiate and agree upon strategic joint basic research agendas together with their road-mapping, time sequencing and priorities, and maintain the research agenda in a timely and progressive style.

One of these initiatives created the HCC research agenda book entitled "Human Computer Confluence – The Next Generation Humans and Computers Research Agenda" (HCC Visions White Book, 2014). It has been published under the acronym "Th. Sc. Community" ("The Scientific Community"), standing for a representative blend of the top leading scientists worldwide in this field. More than two dozens of research challenge position statements solicited via a web-based solicitation portal are compiled into the book, which is publicly available to the whole scientific community for commenting, assessment and consensus finding. Some 200 researchers (European and international) have been actively involved in this process. In addition, the HCC Research Agenda and Roadmap is presented also in the format of a smartphone app, available in online ("The HCC Visions Book"-app). In the past 3 years (2010–2013), the HCC community has become a 650 strong group of researchers and companies working together to understand, not only the technological aspects of the emerging symbiosis between society and ICT, but also the social, industrial, commercial, and cultural impact of this confluence.

1.5 The HCC Research Agenda

The HCC research agenda as collected in "Human Computer Confluence – The Next Generation Humans and Computers Research Agenda" (HCC Visions White Book, 2014) can be structured along the following trails of future research:

1.5.1 Large Scale Socio-Technical Systems

A significant trail of research appears to be needed along the boundaries where ICT "meets" society, where technology and social systems interact. From the observation how successful ICT (smartphones, mobile internet, autonomous driver assistance systems, social networks, etc.) have radically transformed individual communication and social interaction, the scientific community claims for new foundations for large-scale Human-ICT organisms ("superorganisms") and their adaptive behaviors, also including lessons form applied psychology, sociology, and social anthropology, other than from systemic biology, ecology and complexity science. Self-organization and adaptation as ways of harnessing the dynamics and complexity of modern, networked, environment-aware ICT have become central research topics leading to a number of concepts such as autonomic, organic or elastic computing. Existing work on collective adaptive systems is another example considering features such as self-similarity, complexity, emergence, self-organization, and recent advances in the study of collective intelligence. Collective awareness is related to the notion of resilience, which means the systemic capability to anticipate, absorb, adapt to, and/or rapidly recover from a potentially disruptive event. Resilience has been subject to a number of studies in complex networks and social-ecological systems. By creating algorithms and computer systems that are modeled based on social principles, socio-inspired will find better ways of tackling complexity, while experimenting with these algorithms may generate new insights into social systems. In computer science and related subjects, people have started to explore socially inspired systems, e.g. in P2P networks, in robotics, in neuroscience, and in the area of agent systems. Despite this initial work, the overall field of socio-inspired system is still in an early stage of development, and it will be one of future research goals to demonstrate the great potential of social principles for operating large-scale complex ICT systems.

1.5.2 Ethics and Value Sensitive Design

ICT has become more sensitive to its environment: to users, to organizational and social context, and to society at large. While ICT has largely been the outcome of a technology-push focused on core computational functionality in the previous century in the first place, it later extended to the users needs, usability, and even social and psychological and organizational context of computer use. Nowadays we are approaching ICT developments, where the needs of human users, ethics, systems of value and moral norm, the values of citizens, and the big societal questions are in part driving research and development. The idea of making social and moral values central to the matrices, identity management tools) first originated in Computer Science at Stanford in the seventies. This approach is now referred to as 'Value Sensitive Design' or 'Values in Design'. Among the most prevalent, ubiquitously recognized, and meanwhile also socially pressing research agenda items relate to the concerns humans might have in using and trusting ICT. Well beyond the privacy and trust related research we see already today, the claim goes towards ethics and human value (privacy, respect, dignity, trust) sensitivity already at the design stage of modern ICT (value sensitive design), on how to integrate human value building processes into ICT, and how to cope with ignorance, disrespectful, offending and violating human values.

1.5.3 Augmenting Human Perception and Cognition

To escape the space and time boundaries of human perception (and cognition) via ICT (sensors, actuators) has been, and continues to be among the major HCC research challenges. Argued with the "Total Recall" prospect, the focused quests concern the richness of human experience, which results not only from the pure sensory impressions perceived via human receptors, but mostly from the process of identifying, interpreting, correlating and attaching "meaning" to those sensory impressions. This challenge is even posed to be prevalent over the next 50 years of HCC research. Dating back to the "As we may think" idea (Bush & Think, 1945), claiming ICT to support, augment or even replace intellectual work, new considerations for approaching the issue are spawned by the technological, as well as cognitive modelling advance in the context of brain computer interfaces. Understanding the operational principles (chemo-physical), but much more than that the foundational principles of the human brain at the convergence of ICT and biology poses a 21st century research challenge. The ability to build revolutionary new ICT as a "brain-like" technology, and at the same time the confluence of ICT with the biological brain mobilizes great science not only in Europe (see e.g. FTE flagship initiative HBP), but in neuroscience, medical and computing research worldwide.

1.5.4 Empathy and Emotion

Humans are emotional, and at the same time empathic beings. Emotion and empathy are not only expressed (and delivered via a subtle channel) when humans interact with humans, but also when humans interact with machines. The ability to capture and correlate emotional expressions by machines (ICT), as well as the ability of machines (ICT) to express emotions and empathic behavior themselves is considered a grand challenge of human computer confluence, while at the same time realism is expressed on the potential success ever being possible towards it.

1.5.5 Experience and Sharing

With novel ICT, particularly advanced communication systems and ubiquitous networking, radically new styles of human-to-human communication -taking into account body movements, expressions, physiological and brain signals- appear technologically feasible. With cognitive models about individuals, and digital representations of their engagements and experiences abstracted and aggregated from a combination of stimuli (e.g. visual, olfactory, acoustic, tactile, and neuro-stimulation), a new form of exchanging of these experiences and "thoughts" seem possible. Novel communication experiences which are subtle, i.e. unobtrusive, multisensory, and open for interpretation could build on expressions and indications of thoughts as captured and related to a cognitive model on the sending side, encoded and transmitted to a recipient through advanced communication media, and finally translated into multimodal stimuli to be exposed to the receiving individual, and by that induce mental and emotional states representing the "experience" of the sender.

1.5.6 Disappearing Interfaces

Seemingly in analogy to what was addressed at the turn of the century as the ICT research challenge "The Disappearing Computer" (EU FP4, FP5), articulated as (i) the physical disappearance of ICT, observed as the miniaturization of devices and their integration in other everyday artefacts as, e.g., in appliances, tools, clothing, etc. and (ii) mental disappearance, referring to the situation that artefacts with large physical appearance may not be perceived as computers because people discern them as (ICT also mentally move into the background) – appears to have come to a revival as far as notions of interfaces are concerned. As of today we observe that modern ICT with explicit user input and output is becoming to be replaced by a computing landscape sensing the physical world via a huge variety of sensors, and controlling it via a plethora of actuators. Since the nature and appearance of computing devices has widely changed to be hidden in the fabric of everyday life, invisibly networked, and omnipresent, "everything" has turned to become the interface: things and objects of everyday use, the human body, the human brain, the environment, or even the whole planet. Systems that happen to be perceived, understood and used explicitly and intently as the interface tend to disappear. Implicit interaction replaces explicit interaction.

1.6 Conclusion

Human computer confluence is a research area with the union of human brains and computers at its center. Its main goal is to develop the science and technologies necessary to ensure an effective, even transparent, bidirectional communication between humans and computers, which will in turn deliver a huge set of applications: from new senses, to new perceptive capabilities dealing with more abstract information spaces to the social impact of such communication enabling technologies. Inevitably, these technologies question the notion of interface between the human and the technological realm, and thus, also in a fundamental way, put into question the nature of both. The long-term implications can be profound and need to be considered from an ethical/societal point of view. Clearly, this is just a preliminary, yet evidenced classification of HCC research from the solicitation process so far. As this research roadmap aims to evolve continuously, some next steps of consolidation may possibly rephrase and reshape this agenda, as new considerations, arguments and assessments emerge.

References

Abowd, G. D., & Mynatt, E. D. (2000). Charting past, present, and future research in ubiquitous computing. *ACM Transactions on Computer-Human Interaction (TOCHI)*, *7*(1), 29–58.

Bush, V., & Think, A. W. M. (1945). The atlantic monthly. *As we may think,176*(1), 101–108.

Castellani, B., & Hafferty, F. W. (2009). *Sociology and complexity science: a new field of inquiry*: Springer Science & Business Media.

Dey, A. K. (2001). Understanding and using context. *Personal and ubiquitous computing, 5*(1), 4–7.

Esler, M., Hightower, J., Anderson, T., & Borriello, G. (1999, August). Next century challenges: data-centric networking for invisible computing: the Portolano project at the University of Washington. In *Proceedings of the 5th annual ACM/IEEE international conference on Mobile computing and networking* (pp. 256–262). ACM.

Ferscha, A. (2011). 20 Years Past Weiser: What's Next?. *IEEE Pervasive Computing*, (1), 52–61.

Ferscha, A., Farrahi, K., van den Hoven, J., Hales, D., Nowak, A., Lukowicz, P., & Helbing, D. (2012). Socio-inspired ICT. *The European Physical Journal Special Topics*, *214*(1), 401–434.

Ferscha, A., Lukowicz, P., & Pentland S. (2012). From Context Awareness to Social Awareness. *IEEE Pervasive Computing, 11(1),* 32–41.
HCC Visions White Book. http://www.pervasive.jku.at/hccvisions/book/#home, last accessed July 18, 2014.
Horn, P. (2001). Autonomic computing: IBM\'s Perspective on the State of Information Technology.
Kephart, J. O., & Chess, D. M. (2003). The vision of autonomic computing. *Computer, 36*(1), 41–50.
Remagnino, P., & Foresti, G. L. (2005). Ambient intelligence: A new multidisciplinary paradigm. *Systems, Man and Cybernetics, Part A: Systems and Humans, IEEE Transactions on, 35*(1), 1–6.
Schilit, B., Adams, N., & Want, R. (1994, December). Context-aware computing applications. In *Mobile Computing Systems and Applications, 1994. WMCSA 1994. First Workshop on* (pp. 85–90). IEEE.
Servat, D., & Drogoul, A. (2002, July). Combining amorphous computing and reactive agent-based systems: a paradigm for pervasive intelligence? In *Proceedings of the first international joint conference on Autonomous agents and multiagent systems: part 1* (pp. 441–448). ACM.
Streitz, N., & Nixon, P. (2005). The disappearing computer. *Communications of the ACM, 48*(3), 32–35
Weiser, M. (1991). The computer for the 21st century. *Scientific american,265*(3), 94–104.
Weiser, M., & Brown, J. S. (1996). Designing calm technology. *PowerGrid Journal, 1*(1), 75–85.

David Benyon and Oli Mival

2 Designing Blended Spaces for Collaboration

Abstract: In this paper, we reflect on our experiences of designing, developing, implementing and using a real world, functional multi-touch enabled interactive collaborative environment (ICE). The paper provides some background theory on blended spaces derived from work on blending theory, or conceptual integration. This is applied to the ICE and results in a focus on how to deal with the conceptualization that people have of new collaborative spaces such as the ICE. Five key themes have emerged from an analysis of two years of observations of the ICE is use. These provide a framework, TACIT, that focuses on Territoriality, Awareness, Control, Interaction and Transitions in ICE type environments. The paper concludes by bringing together the TACIT framework with the principles of blended spaces to highlight key areas for design so that people can conceptualize the opportunities for creative collaboration that the next generation of interactive blended spaces provide.

Keywords: Interaction Design, Collaboration, Multi-touch, Multi-surface Environment, Interactive Environments, Blended Spaces

2.1 Introduction

Blended spaces are spaces where a physical space is deliberately integrated in a close-knit way with a digital space. Blended spaces go beyond mixed reality (Milgram & Kishino, 1994) and conceptually are much closer to tangible interactions (Ishii & Ullmer, 1997) where the physical and digital are completely coupled. The concept of blending has been in existence for many years in the field of blended learning where the aim is to design a learning experience for students that blends the benefits of classroom learning with the benefits of distance, on-line learning, but more recently the concept of blending has been applied to spaces and to interaction.

O'Hara, Kjelsko and Paay (O'hara, Kjeldskov, & Paay, 2011) refer to the distributed spaces linked by very high quality video-conferencing systems such as Halo as blended spaces because of the apparently seamless joining of remote sites. In systems such as Halo, great attention is paid to the design of the physical conference rooms and to the angle and geometry of the video technologies in order to give the impression that two distant rooms are collocated. High-end video conferencing supports the collaborative activity of business discussions, but it does not deal well with shared information resources. O'Hara, et al. (O'hara et al., 2011) use the term blended interaction spaces for 'blended spaces in which the interactive groupware is incorporated in ways spatially consistent with the physical geometries of the video-mediated set-up'. Their paper explores the design of a blended interaction space that highlights the importance of the design of the physical space in terms of human spaces and the different proxemics (Hall, 1969) of personal spaces, intimate spaces and so on. They also draw on a theory of spaces proposed by Kendal (1990) that describes the interactional spaces that participants in collaborative activity share.

Jetter, Geyer, Schwarz and Reiterer (Jetter et al., 2012) also discuss blended interaction. They develop a framework for looking at the personal, social, workflow and collaborative aspects of blended interaction. Benyon and Mival (Benyon & Mival 2013, 2012) describe the design of their interactive collaborative environment (ICE, discussed later in this chapter) focusing on the close integration of hardware, software and room design to create new interactive spaces for creativity. A workshop at AVI 2012 conference on collaborative interactive spaces has led to a special issue of the journal Personal and Ubiquitous Computing and another workshop at the CHI2013 conference on blended interaction. In these meetings researchers are developing theories and examples of blended spaces and blended interactions in a variety of settings.

In addition to these examples of blended spaces and interaction in room environments, the idea of blended spaces has been applied to the domain of digital tourism (Benyon, Mival and Ayan, 2012). Here the emphasis is on providing appropriate digital content at appropriate physical places in order to provide a good user experience (UX) for tourists. The concept of blending has also been used for the design of ambient assisted living environments for older people (Hoshi, Öhberg, & Nyberg, 2011) and for the design of products including a blood taking machine (Markussen, 2007) and a table lamp (Wang, 2014).

A central feature about these latter examples is that they take as their theoretical basis the work of Fauconnier and Turner (Fauconnier, 1997; Fauconnier & Turner, 2002) on blending theory (BT), or conceptual integration. Originally developed as a theory of linguistics and language understanding, BT has been applied to a huge range of subject areas from mathematics to history to creativity (Turner, 2014) making it more a general theory of creativity than just a theory of language construction. BT is concerned with how people conceptualise new experiences and new ideas in terms of their prior knowledge. Imaz and Benyon (Imaz & Benyon, 2007) originally applied BT to Human-Computer Interaction (HCI) and Software Engineering (SE) looking at how the metaphors in HCI and SE have changed over the years and how this effects how these disciplines are perceived. In their book they analyse many examples of user interfaces and interactive systems and suggest how BT could be used to design interfaces and interactions.

The aim of this chapter is to develop the concept of blended spaces, in the context of multi-user, multi-device, collaborative environments and to see the contribution that BT can make to the design of multi-device collaborative spaces. We see the concept of a blended space as a clear example of human-computer confluence (HCC). Benyon (Benyon, 2014) discusses how blended spaces provide a new medium that enables new ways of doing things and of conceptualizing activities. He talks about the new sense of presence that comes from blended spaces (Benyon, 2012). Our view is that, in the days of blended spaces, designers need to design for interactions that exploit the synergy between the digital and the physical space.

The particular space that is the focus of this work is known as the Interactive Collaborative Environment (ICE). The concept of the ICE took shape through an interdisciplinary university project where the aim was to look at how the next generation of technologies would change people's ways of working. We envisaged a 'future meeting room' that would contain the latest multi-touch screens and surfaces, novel software and work with mobile and tangible technologies to create a new environment for meetings of all types including management meetings, research meetings, collaborative compositing for magazines, video-conferencing and creative brainstorming meetings. We negotiated a physical space for the meeting room and within a limited budget commissioned a multi-touch boardroom table and installed five multi-touch screens on three of the walls to produce a meeting room with an interactive boardroom table that can seat 10 people, interactive whiteboard walls and five wall mounted multi-touch screens (Figure 2.1).

During the last two years the ICE has been used for meetings of all kinds by people from all manner of disciplinary backgrounds. This activity has been observed and analyzed in a variety of different ways, resulting in a set of five generic themes that designers of such environments need to consider. These provide our framework for describing the design issues in ICE environments, TACIT, that stands for territoriality, awareness, control, interaction and transitions.

The chapter is organized as follows. Section 2 provides a background to the work on conceptual integration, or blending theory. Section 3 describes the design rationale for the ICE in the context of the design of the physical space and the design of the digital space. We discuss how physical and digital spaces are blended to create a new space with its own emergent properties. It is within this blended space that people must develop their conceptual understanding about the opportunities afforded by the blended space and how this can alter their ways of working. Section 4 provides an analysis of the ICE in use, drawing upon observations over a period of two years, a controlled study of the room being used and interviews with users of the ICE. This analysis highlights five key characteristics of cooperative spaces such as the ICE that reflect our own experiences and many of the issues raised elsewhere in the literature. In section 5 we see how these characteristics are reflected in the physical, digital and conceptual spaces that make up the blended space. Section 6 provides some conclusions for designing blended spaces such as the ICE.

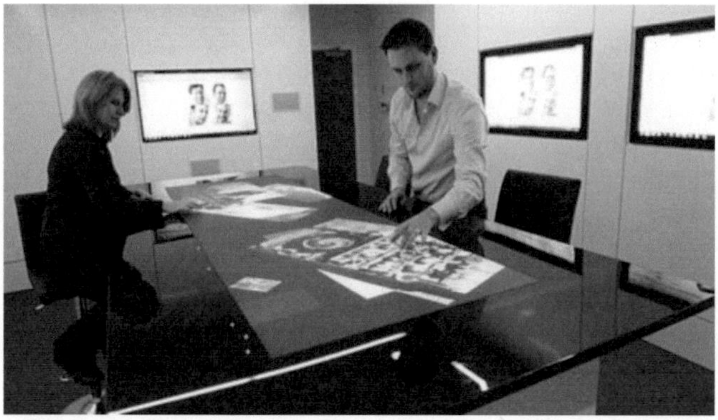

Figure 2.1: The Interactive Collaborative Environment (ICE)

2.2 Blending Theory

Fauconnier and Turner's book *The Way We Think* (Fauconnier & Turner, 2002) introduced their ideas on a creative process that they called conceptual integration or blending. They argued that cognition could be seen in terms of mental spaces, or domains. Cognition involves the projection of concepts from domains and their integration into new domains. Blending Theory (BT) develops and extends the ideas of Lakoff and Johnson on the importance of metaphor to thought (Lakoff & Johnson, 1980), (Lakoff & Johnson, 1999). Where metaphor is seen as a mapping between two domains, Fauconnier and Turner see blending in terms of four domains. They explain the simple but powerful process as follows (see Figure 2.2). Two input spaces (or domains) have something in common with a more generic space. Blending is an operation that is applied to these two input mental spaces which results in a new, blended space. The blend receives a partial structure from both input spaces but has an emergent structure of its own.

In linguistics blending theory is used to understand various constructs such as counterfactual statements, metaphors and how different concepts arise (Fauconnier, 1997). For example blending theory can be used to understand the difference between houseboat and boathouse by looking at the different ways in which the concepts of house and boat can be combined. There is now extensive work on blending theory applied to all manner of subjects that offer different insights into the way we think. Mark Turner's web site is a good starting place (Turner, 2014).

The main principles of blending are that the projections from the input spaces create new relationships in the blend that did not exist in the original inputs, and that our background knowledge in the form of cognitive and cultural models allow the composite structure to be experienced in a new way. The blend has its own emergent logic and this can be elaborated to produce new ideas and insights. This blended space may then go on to be blended with other mental spaces.

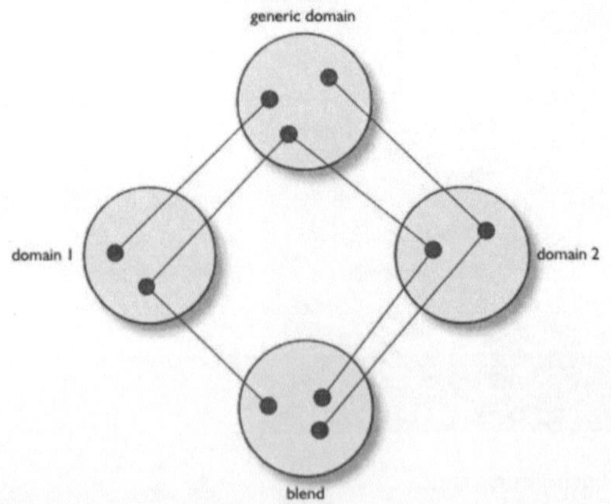

Figure 2.2: Concept of Blend

Fauconnier and Turner (Fauconnier & Turner, 2002) discuss different types of blend and provide guidance on what makes a good blend. Four types of blend are identified based on the way in which concepts from the input spaces are projected into the blended space, from simple one-to-one mappings to more complex 'double scope' blends that creatively merge concepts from the input domains to produce a new experience. Fauconnier and Turner see the process of blending as consisting of three main processes. Composition is the process of understanding the structure of the domains, completion is the process of bringing relevant background knowledge to the process and elaboration is the process of making inferences and gaining insight based on these relationships. They propose six guiding principles to support the development of blends. The first three, integration, web and unpacking, concern getting a blend that is coherent and in a form that people can understand where the blend has come from. The fourth, topology, concerns the correspondences between the input spaces. The fifth, 'good reason', captures the generic design principle that things should only be in the blend if there is a good reason for them to be there and the sixth, metonymic tightening, concerns achieving a blend that does not have superfluous items in it.

Imaz and Benyon (2007) have applied the ideas of conceptual blending to analyze developments in HCI and software engineering. They analyze a number of well-known examples of user interfaces, including the trash can icon and the device eject function in Mac OS and critical HCI concepts such as scenarios and use cases. One example they consider is the concept of a window in a computer operating system. This is a blend of one mental space – the concept of a window in a house – and another mental space, the concept of collecting some computer operations together. The generic space is the idea of being able to see a part of a large object; a window on the world if you like. The process of bringing these spaces together results in a new concept of 'window' that now includes things such as a scroll bar, a minimize button and so on that you would not associate with a window in a house. The blended space of a computer window has inherited some shared characteristics from the generic space of 'looking onto something', but now has its own characteristics and emergent properties. This can be illustrated as in Figure 2.3.

Imaz and Benyon argue that in interaction design, designers need to reflect and think hard about the concepts that they are using and how these concepts affect their designs. They emphasize the physical grounding of thought by arguing that designers need to find solutions to problems that are 'at a human scale'. Drawing upon the principles of blends suggested by Fauconnier and Turner they present a number of HCI design principles. When creating a new interface object, or new interactive product designers will often create a blend from existing designs. Designers should aim to preserve an appropriate topology for the blend, allowing people to unpack the blend so that they can understand where the new conceptual space has come from. There are principles for compressing the input spaces into the blend, aiming for a complete structure that can be understood as a whole (the integration principle) and for keeping the blend relevant and at a human scale.

They go on to present an abstract design method that shows how conceptual blending can be used during the analysis phase of systems development to understand the issues of a particular situation and how it can be used during the design stage to produce and critique design solutions. For example, they discuss the existence of the trashcan on the Windows desktop. Here the designers have chosen not to enforce the topology principle (which would suggest in this case that since trash cans normally go underneath a desk the trash can should not be on the desk top). Instead the designers have promoted the integration principle, keeping the main functions of the interface together in a 'desk top' metaphor.

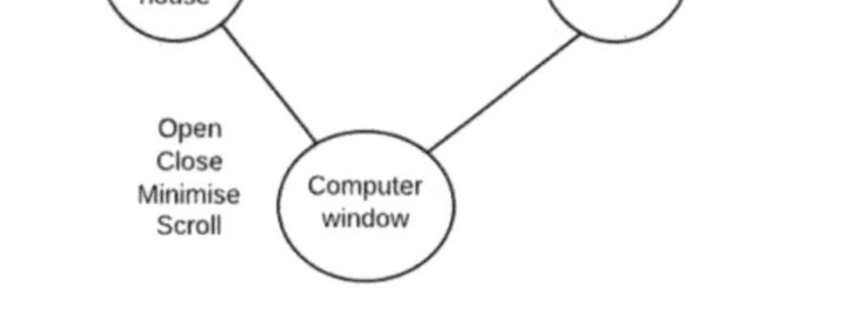

Figure 2.3: Blend for a computer window

The danger in presenting blending theory in such a short section is that it can seem trivial, when in fact it is a very powerful idea. Underlying BT are ideas about embodied cognition that go back to the roots of how human cognition starts with the bodily experiences that we have as human babies growing up in a three dimensional world. Lakoff and Johnson (1999) develop this 'philosophy of the flesh' from a conceptual perspective and Rohrer (2010) develops related ideas from a cognitive science and neurological perspective. People think the way they do because of their inherent physical and perceptual schemata that are blended to produce new concepts that in their turn are blended to form new concepts. Understanding this background helps designers to create experiences 'at a human scale'.

2.3 Blended Spaces

In looking at the sense of presence in mixed reality spaces, Benyon (Benyon, 2012) develops a view of digital and physical spaces in terms of four characteristics; ontology, topology, volatility and agency. These constitute the generic space structure that both physical and digital spaces share. Bringing blending theory together with the idea of physical and digital spaces leads to the position illustrated in Figure 2.4. He argues that for the purpose of designing mixed reality experiences, physical and digital space can be usefully conceptualized in terms of these four key characteristics.

The ontology of the spaces concerns the objects in the spaces. The topology of the spaces concerns how those objects are related to one another. The dynamics or volatility of the spaces concerns how elements in the spaces change over time. The agency in the spaces concerns the people in the spaces, the artificial agents and the opportunities for action in the spaces. By understanding these characteristics and looking at the correspondences between the physical and the digital spaces, designers will produce new blended spaces that have emergent properties. In these spaces, people will not be in a physical space with some digital content bolted on. People will be present in a blended space and this will give rise to new experiences and new ways of engaging with the world.

The conceptualization of blended spaces illustrated in Figure 2.4 relies on a generic way of talking about spaces – ontology, topology, volatility and agency. This is the generic space of spaces and places that is projected onto both the physical and the digital spaces. The correspondences between the physical and the digital are exploited in the design of the blended space. The job of the designer is to bring the spaces together in a natural, intuitive way to create a good user experience. The designer should design the blended space according to the principles of designing with blends such as drawing out the correspondences between the topology of the physical and digital spaces, using the integration principle to deliver a whole experience and designing at a human scale.

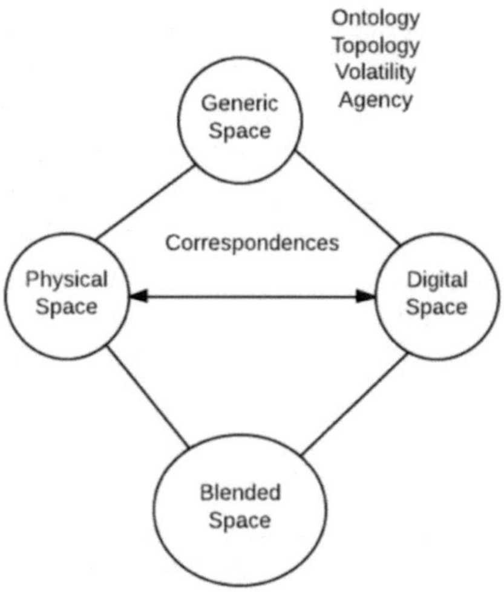

Figure 2.4: Conceptual blending in mixed reality spaces

Another consideration that is important in the design of blended spaces is that the physical and the digital spaces rarely co-exist. There are anchors, or touch points, where the physical is linked to the digital, but there are many places where the physical and the digital remain separate. QR codes or GPS are examples of anchor technologies that bring the physical and the digital together. In the context of an ICE type environment people will be collaborating through some physical activity such as talking to each other, but then may access the digital space to bring up some media to illustrate what they are saying. The conversation may then continue with shared access to the digital content. In the context of digital tourism we may observe someone walking through a physical space, accessing some digital content on an iPad and then continuing his or her physical movement. Thus, in blended spaces, people move between the physical, the digital and the blended spaces. This movement through and between spaces is an important part of the blended space concept and leads on to issues of navigation in physical, digital and blended spaces. It appears in Benford's work on spectator interfaces as the idea of a hybrid trajectory (Benford, Giannachi, Koleva, & Rodden, 2009). Related ideas from Yvonne Rogers on access points, or entry points are discussed later.

The blended space encompasses a conceptual space of understanding and making meaning and this is where the principles of designing with blends are so important. People need to be aware of both the physical and the digital spaces, what they contain and how they are linked together. People need to understand the opportunities afforded by the blended space and to be able to unpack the blend to see how and why the spaces are blended in a particular way. People need to be aware of the structure of the physical and the digital, so that there is a harmony; the correspondences between the objects in the spaces. The overall aim of blended spaces is to design for a great UX, at a human scale.

2.4 Designing the ICE

The aim of the project to develop the ICE was to provide a great experience for people and to give them an insight on what leading edge meeting spaces can be like. The aim is to generate enthusiasm and to get people to see how new spaces could be used by domain experts in very different areas and the impact that these spaces will have on their working practices.

As with all real-world projects, the ICE had to comply with a number of constraints such as the existence of a room and a budget. It was also to be a 'bring your own device' (BYOD) environment. The philosophy underlying the design focused on providing an environment that would help people within it fulfill their activities and do so in pleasurable intuitive ways. Wherever possible the aim is to remove function from the content of devices (screens, laptops, mobile devices) and instead consider these devices as portals onto function and content that is resident in a shared space. This should enable and facilitate real time, concurrent, remote collaboration. Another key aim is to enable the seamless mixing of digital and analogue media. People bring notebooks, pens and paper to meetings and we are keen that such analogue media should co-exist happily alongside the digital spaces.

2.4.1 The physical Space

The physical space that was available for the ICE was an empty office, so the design started with a room, a vision and a budget of €150,000 about a third of which went on technologies for the digital space, a third on room alterations and a third on necessary infrastructure. After extensive research into the options available we settled on the following technologies. A 46" n-point HD (1080p) multi touch LCD screen mounted on the end wall of the room. This screen uses the diffused illumination (DI) method for detecting multi-touch and is capable of detecting finger and hand orientation as well as distinguishing between different users' hands. A 108" n-point multi-touch rear projection boardroom table, also using DI is the centrepiece of the room. The table can recognize and interact with objects placed on its surface such as mobile phones, laptops or books using infrared fiducial markers. It has 2 patch panels on either side allowing the connection of USB peripherals and storage devices as well as any external DVI or VGA video source, such as a laptop or tablet, to any of the surfaces.

The table was designed specifically for the space available, which determined its dimensions and technical specification. Due to the requirement of using the table both when sitting and standing the surface is 900mm from the floor, the standard ergonomic height for worktops. Four 42" HD (1080p) dual point multi-touch LCD screens utilizing infrared overlays are mounted on the room's side walls. Each screen is driven by a dedicated Apple Mac Pro, which can triple boot into Mac OSX, Windows 7 and Linux. The room has 8-channel wireless audio recording for 8 wearable microphones as well as 2-channel recording for 2 room microphones. Each audio channel can be sent individually to any chosen destination (either a computer in the ICE or to an external storage via IP) or combined into a single audio stream. A webcam allows for high definition video (1080p) to be recorded locally or streamed over IP. The recording facility is used both as a means of archiving meetings (for example, each audio channel can record an individual participant) or for tele- and video conferencing activities. Any recordings made can be stored both locally and on an external cloud storage facility for remote access.

The walls are augmented with the Mimio™ system to serve as digital whiteboards, thus when something is written on the whiteboard it is automatically digitally captured. Importantly no application needs to be launched before capture begins, the process of contact between the pen and the wall initiates the digital capture.

2.4.2 The Digital Space

The ICE hardware has been selected to offer the widest range of development and design opportunities and as such we have remained platform agnostic. To achieve this, all the hardware runs on multiple operating systems (Mac OS X, Windows 7 & 8, Linux). Alongside the standard development environments are the emerging options for multi-touch, central to which is the Tangible User Interface Objects (TUIO) protocol, an open framework that defines a common protocol and API for tangible multi-touch surfaces. TUIO enables the transmission of an abstract description of interactive surfaces, touch events and tangible object states from a tracker application and sends it to a client application. All the hardware in the room is TUIO compliant. The TUIO streams generated by the screens and table in the ICE are passed to the computers via IP thus enabling the possibility for more extensive remote screen sharing. Indeed, if a remote participant has the capacity to generate a TUIO stream of their own, as is the capability with many modern laptop track-pads, they can collaborate with the ICE surfaces both through traditional point and click methods but also multi-touch gestures.

A key design issue for the software is that there is no complex software architecture required. All applications are available at the top level; the TUIO protocol means that any device running it can interact with other devices running it. This allows for easy integration of mobile devices into the room and sharing control across devices. Since everything in the room is interconnected through the Internet, the room demonstrates how such sharing of content and manipulation of content could be physically distributed.

In terms of software, the ICE makes extensive use of freely available applications such as Evernote™, Skype™, etc. A key design decision for the ICE is to keep it simple and leverage the power of robust 3rd party services. People need to be able to come into the room and understand it and to conceptualize the opportunities it offers for new ways of working. It is little use having applications buried away in a hierarchical menu system where they will not be found. Hence the design approach is to make the applications all available at the top level. One particularly important application is Dropbox™, which is used to enable the sharing of content across devices. Since the Dropbox™ service is available across most devices; any content put into one device is almost immediately available on another. For example, take a photo on an iPhone or Android Phone and it is immediately available on the table and wall screens. Essentially Dropbox™ works as the synching bridge across all the separate computers driving each surface, which enables a seamless "shared repository" experience for users. Any file they utilize on one surface is also available on any other, as well as remotely should the user have the appropriate access authority.

Of course things are constantly changing, but the aim is to keep this philosophy stable.

2.4.3 The Conceptual Space

The conceptual space concerns how people understand what the novel blend of physical and digital spaces allows them to do and how they frame their activities in the context of that understanding. There are a lot of novel concepts to be understood. For example, people need to understand that the screens on the walls are not computers, but are windows onto data content in the cloud. They will recognise the Internet Explorer icon on a screen and rightly conceptualise that this gives them Internet access, but they may not realise that they can save files to a shared Dropbox™ folder and hence enable files to be viewed through different screens. They need to conceptualise the wall screens as input and output zones that can show different views at different times. People who have used the ICE a few times come to understand that they can see an overview of some data set on one screen and the detail on another and that this is useful for particular activities. The wall screens can be easily configured to mirror each other, or to show separate content. The challenge for spaces such as the ICE is that people do not have a mental model, a conceptualization, of the space when they first arrive. It is up to the designers to present an informative, coherent image of the system that enables people to develop an appropriate conceptual understanding of the opportunities. For example we developed a control room map to help people conceptualise the interaction between the different screens and how any screen could be the source of an image displayed on any number of other screens. This is one example of an attempt to provide a way into the conceptual space. Restricting the functionality of the digital space and providing this through a few familiar icons is another.

2.4.4 The Blended Space

We can summarise the ICE through the lens of conceptual blending as illustrated in Figure 2.5.

2.5 The TACIT Framework

We have now had the opportunity to observe many meetings in the ICE. It is a space that encourages people to get up and move to one of the screens to demonstrate something, or use the whiteboard capabilities of the wall surface to illustrate ideas. The room is highly flexible in terms of lighting, audio and the use of the blinds. Thus the atmosphere can be quickly changed as required. The ability of people to easily join in the room using internet-based video-conferencing has proved an important feature.

The room certainly encourages collaboration and participation. With five screens it is very natural to have documents displayed on one or two, web searches on another and perhaps YouTube videos on another. However, it is also true that many people find it difficult to conceptualize what the room can do and how they can make it do things. This serious challenge for interaction design – how to get people to understand the opportunities afforded by novel interactive spaces – remains stubbornly difficult to solve.

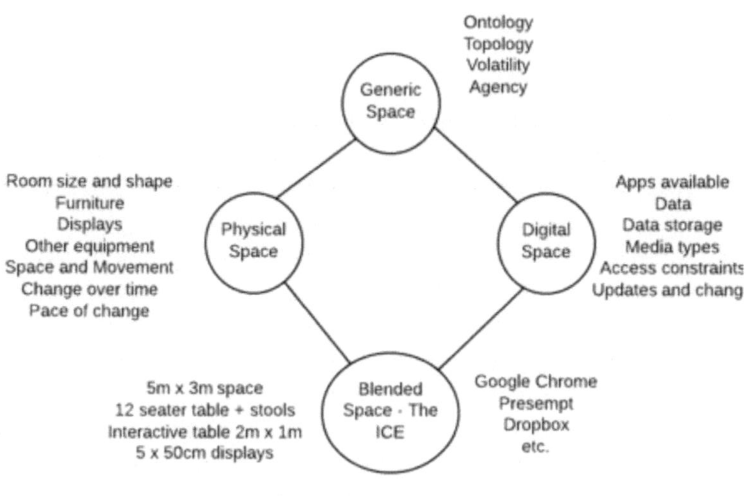

Figure 2.5: The ICE as a blended space

The meetings that we have observed have included conference organisation meetings, preparing research grant proposals, publicity preparation, teaching interaction design, remote viva voce examinations and numerous general business meetings. A controlled study of the ICE has been completed that included a grounded approach to analyzing video, interview and questionnaire data and a survey of user attitudes to the ICE has been completed. The results of this analysis of video, the interviews and the real-time observation have provided a rich picture of collaboration in the ICE.

Classic issues of computer supported cooperative work have been identified and described over the years (Ackerman, 2000). Against this background five themes have emerged from our analysis of the ICE in use that provide a way of structuring the issues that have arisen and that designers of room environments need to deal with. These reflect the main concerns identified in previous literature on collaborative environments. We discuss the issues in terms of territoriality, awareness, control, interaction and transitions between spaces: the TACIT framework.

2.5.1 Territoriality

Territoriality concerns spaces and the relationships between people and spaces. Scott and Carpendale (Scott & Carpendale, 2010) see territoriality as a key issue in the use of tabletops (both traditional and interactive) for cooperative work. They identify personal spaces, group spaces and storage spaces. They also point to the importance of orientation, positioning and proximity in addition to the partitioning of spaces into different regions. These all contribute to people's sense of territory and their relationships with their space. Territory is also important on large multiuser displays (Peltonen et al., 2008). There are many social and psychological characteristics of territories that designers need to consider such as proxemics (Hall, 1969), (Greenberg, Marquardt, Ballendat, Diaz-Marino, & Wang, 2011) and how comfortable people feel when they are physically close to others.

Issues of territoriality are central to working in the ICE and we have witnessed many examples of groups configuring and reconfiguring their spatial relations depending on the task. We have observed incidents where people cluster around a wall screen watching one person working and commenting on what is going on before going back to work individually. People have commented that being able to work in different places in the room helps collaboration and moving around in the room makes collaboration easier.

We have seen a number of incidents where the assignment of roles and tasks is influenced by location and proximity to a particular piece of technology. The role of penholder in brainstorming tasks may be assigned to the person sitting nearest to the whiteboard. Participants tend to use the wall-screen nearest to them and the person interacting with the tabletop applications at the table was the person sitting nearest the controls at the bottom edge of the screen. There is often a close connection between the control of physical space in the environment and the control of screen workspace, which in turn affects the assignment of roles and tasks.

The tabletop can be configured in different ways and there is one setting that has six individual places each with a digital keyboard and media browser. This allows people to have their personal space and then to move work into a public sphere when they are ready. Haller, et al., (2010) emphasise the importance of these different spaces in their NiCE environment. Personal spaces are provided through individual PCs and through personal sketching spaces. These can be shared with the group through a large wall display. In earlier contributions to collaborative spaces, Buxton (2009) describes media space in terms of the person space, task space and reference space and provides a number of design guidelines for ensuring quality spaces. It is the intersection of these and the ease of moving between them that is important.

2.5.2 Awareness

The issue of awareness is a common central theme running through the literature on cooperative work (e.g. (Tang, 1991)) and is a central issue for the ICE. The concept of awareness hides a large amount of complexity. Schmidt (Schmidt, 2002) lists seven common adjectives often attached to the word 'awareness' such as peripheral, background, passive, reciprocal and so on. He goes on to explore the concept in detail, finally arguing that "the term 'awareness' is being used to denote those practices through which actors tacitly and seamlessly align and integrate their distributed and yet interdependent activities". Awareness includes aspects of attention and focus, so explicit awareness of what others have done is also an important aspect. Awareness is much more than simple information, however. It is to do with the social aspects of how people align and integrate their activities. Awareness is an attribute of an activity that relates to many of the characteristics of a situation. Rogers and Rodden (Rogers & Rodden, 2003) also emphasise the importance of dealing with different types of awareness and with the transitions between them (see below).

In the ICE, different tasks invite different degrees of awareness. For example, brainstorming tasks require shared attention whereas an individual searching the web on a wall screen does not. Tasks that can be undertaken in parallel may need support to keep others aware of progress and when the task is completed. Several people have commented that a shared Dropbox™ folder is useful for maintaining awareness as it gives real time information on the progress of the work of the other participants; images dragged into Dropbox™ on a screen soon appear in Dropbox™ on the table.

Even during individual tasks there are frequent shifts between shared and divided attention with people participating in discussions in a group across the room and then turning their backs to individually search for images and information on the wall screens.

When collaborating in a shared physical environment like the ICE participants become aware of each other's activity through direct perception. People are able to see and hear each other as they work at the surfaces, moving around the room or talking to other participants. Writing on the whiteboards enhances awareness and collaboration and allows people to use gestures to refer to specific objects or the organisation of objects on the surfaces.

The various surfaces support collaboration through awareness differently. There have been instances where participants grew silent while working on the wall screens and focused on their own tasks loosing awareness of what was going on in the room behind them. Working around the table creates a higher degree of shared awareness; one of the advantages of table displays with respect to collaboration.

2.5.3 Control

Control refers both to the control of the software systems and to social control of the collaborative activity. Yuill and Rogers (Yuill & Rogers, 2012) highlight the importance of control in their discussion of collaborative systems. This is related to the concepts of access points (see below). Rogers and Lindley (Rogers & Lindley, 2004) also identify control as one of their factors describing collaborative environments along with awareness, interaction, resources, experience, progression, team and coordination.

In the ICE we have observed people taking turns to interact with the table with only one person touching it at a time in order to maintain control. However, some of the software on the table has a lack of support for multi user interaction and this creates issues with conflict of control. It is easy for one person to enlarge a display (often accidentally) so that it covers the whole of the tabletop and the whole workspace and all the objects on it are covered over. People have adapted to this by taking turns interacting with the table.

A common configuration of the input and output structure is to have two screens mirroring each other on opposite sides of the table. However, whilst this helps awareness, it can negatively impact control. One person may have started interacting with a screen without realising that another person was using the mirrored screen and hence takes over control of the pair of mirrored screens.

Often people sitting at the "bottom side" of the interface near the controls were also the ones who controlled and interacted with the application. However we also observed incidents where people are working at the table from both sides without regard to the orientation of the application. The location of the controls on the bottom edge at the lower left and right side of the screen demonstrated a "short arm problem". Due to the size of the table's screen, it is impossible for someone standing at the centre of an edge of the screen to reach the corners without actually moving his or her body to the left or right. This also gives rise to a mode of collaboration where the participant standing near to the controls would press buttons at appropriate times.

Control is a key component of Yuill and Rogers framework for collaboration. The locus of control is closely related to the access points provided by the technology. Their main focus is on aiming for equitable control in a collaborative setting and they emphasise that the location of access points and how people move between access points is critical.

Control, and people's understanding of what they can control is key to ideas of appropriation and 'tailoring culture'. People need to be encouraged to understand that tailoring is possible in an ICE organizationally, technically and socially. This tailoring, or customization is an essential part of the appropriation of technology and of spaces. People need to adapt, and shape the environment, the interactions, the content and the computational functions that are available to suit their ways of working. However, this is easier said than done. People have to be confident and capable to appropriate their technological spaces. They need a conceptual understanding of the digital and physical spaces so that they can change their ways of working, and designers need to design to support appropriation and the formation of an appropriate conceptualization of the space.

2.5.4 Interaction

This theme concerns how people interact with each other and how they interact with the activities they are undertaking. In collaborative tasks, articulation is concerned with how work is divided up and tasks are allocated between members of a group. How this happens is quite different with respect to how the surfaces of the room are used for the different tasks. The users' familiarity with the room, their experience with working on touch screens, their prior knowledge of each other and experience in working together are all factors in producing the different conceptualizations of the ICE and hence the best ways to interact. People do things in different ways and the variation in the use of the room and its facilities indicates that the environment effectively supports this variety.

The ICE supports articulation as it affords the distribution and execution of subtasks. The physical layout of the room gives easy access to workspace and this makes coordinating tasks easy. We have also seen numerous and at times very rapid shifts in the social organisation of work. For example, people will shift between working individually at the wall screens and turning around to communicate across the room as a group. Shifts also occur when people go to the wall screens to search web for information during a discussion or the execution of a task only to return to the group when information is found. Also while working at the table there is a variety of ways to organise the work. The parallel tasks of searching and sorting can be accelerated if the group divides itself into subgroups. This may be contrasted with serial tasks such as putting collaborative projects together.

We have observed tasks being distributed by negotiation through verbal communication, but also seen people spontaneously go to a surface and start doing a task. We also observed how roles and tasks were handed over simply by turning around workspace on the table surface.

Interaction is one of the four components in the model of collaboration discussed by O'Hara et al. (O'Hara et al., 2011) along with work, communication and service. They emphasise the importance of getting the granularity of the space right. The interplay between the spatial configuration, the social organisation and interaction is critical. O'Hara, et al. discuss their blended interaction space (BISi) as an example of workplace design, once again emphasising proxemics in design and the control and set up of work tools as an essential part of the interaction

Hurtienne and Israel (2013) offer sound design advice for designing ICE type environments with their PIBA-DIBA technique. PIBA-DIBA stands for 'physical is best at – digital is best at'. The aim is to identify where designers should allocate parts of the interaction to physical objects and where they should be allocated to digital objects. For example physical objects are perceived in 3D and are graspable whereas digital objects are easy to transfer and transform into other representations. The aim of PIBA-DIBA is to sensitize designers to the qualities of the different media in order to design for better interaction in blended spaces.

2.5.5 Transitions

Blended spaces are rarely completely integrated. Instead there are touch points where the digital and physical are brought together and where people transition from the digital to the physical or vice versa. In the context of digital tourism, for example, the global positioning system (GPS) is often used to link the physical world of a tourist location with some digital content that is relevant to that location. Quick Response (QR) codes also serve this purpose. In the context of blended spaces such as the ICE people transit from the physical to the digital and back again as they use personal and shared devices to access digital content and bring this into the physical world of displays and discussion.

Discussions with users of the ICE indicate that the physical layout of the room gives easy access to different workspaces. It seems to be less clear whether the individual platforms (whiteboard, wall screens or table) were easily accessible for all people. For example, the placement of the whiteboards at the corners of the room has been suggested as a problem limiting the physical access to the board, and others have argued that seeing objects from different perspectives when working at the table is a problem.

Transitions between spaces and between the physical and the digital are identified by Scott, Grant and Mandryk (Scott, Grant, & Mandryk, 2003) as a significant feature of tabletop interaction. Yvonne Rogers and her colleagues in a number of publications describe these transitions in terms of access points, or entry points. They find that people are excluded from equitable participation in collaborative activities because of difficulties in gaining access to the physical environment, or the digital environment or both, or in moving between the physical and the digital. In the Shared Information Space framework they offer advice on removing barriers to access and enabling entry points that provide a good overview of the space and the opportunities to move between locations in the spaces.

2.6 Discussion

People are aware of each other's actions because they can see and hear each other and they can sense what is going on in the room. People are able to move about and interact with physical and virtual objects and information in the room and on the surfaces. They are aware of each other as human beings and react to each other and the physical environment according to norms and habits they find appropriate for the situation. The physical and social interactions are intricately intertwined.

Visibility of information and objects in the environment – often referred to as the information and interaction resources – is another key finding. Different surfaces offer different opportunities for reference. People check notes on the whiteboards or use file browser windows to follow the progress of work or to recapture information needed for the work being done. These notes and traces of work were important tools in the collaborative work as they serve as external memory and a representation of common ground (Monk, 2003).

The shifts in social organisation of work are important. We have observed constant fluctuations of groups of participants being formed and broken up to work on tasks, communicate or just to observe the progress of a task. There are shifts between working collaboratively in groups and working alone on subtasks. The fluency in the social organisation of work reflects the way participants move around in the physical environment and take control of physical and interactional resources.

2.6.1 Designing the Physical Space

The design of physical space draws upon the disciplines of architecture and interior design and an understanding of social psychology. The physical space comes with the social expectations of people concerning behaviours and at the same time the physical space will help to shape those behaviours. The physical space allows for interaction between people through touch, proximity, hearing and visual perception. The physical space influences many aspects of the interaction such as territory, position, control, and orientation. Orientation is an issue on flat surfaces and occlusion needs to be avoided.

2.6.2 Designing the Digital Space

The digital space concerns data and how it is structured and stored. It concerns the content that is available and the software that is available to manipulate the content. The digital space is the medium through which people engage with content. Digital tools need to be appropriate for the physical space and for the characteristics of the devices that interface with the digital space. Gestures, touch and other forms of physical interaction provide a direct engagement between the physical and the digital. With no standards for gestures on multi-touch surfaces, designers need to attend to facilitating learning and minimizing mistakes.

2.6.3 Designing the Conceptual Space

In a blended space such as the ICE, designers bring together the digital and the physical to produce a new space. In the case of the ICE the aim was to create a space that would support collaborative activities such as meetings of various sorts. The conceptual space is where people produce meanings and understand where they can go and what they can do. People need to understand the relationships between the physical and digital spaces, their organization and structure, so that they can navigate these spaces. Conceptually these spaces are not easy to understand. It is through, or in, the conceptual space that people work out roles, task allocation and the social organisation of their work. This is where they figure out what they need to do and how best to do it conceptualizing the opportunities and reacting to the physical and digital constraints.

2.6.4 Designing the Blended Space

By thinking about the three spaces – conceptual, physical and digital – that make up the spaces of interaction, and the five themes that emerged from our reflections, we can sensitize designers to the bigger issues. Interaction designers need to design for space and movement as well as interaction with technology. They need to consider the devices that people will bring with them and how these can be integrated into the whole experience of being in, and working in rooms and other interactive spaces. They need to consider how to keep people connected to their personal digital spaces whilst working and collaborating in shared spaces.

Analogue and digital media are mixed in different ways and need to be managed and interchanged. There are multiple digital territories and physical spaces to manage. There are public, private and shared spaces, storage spaces, historical spaces and different types of content that exist in those spaces. Moving content between them, easily and naturally, is critical to providing the seamless experience of sharing. The physical space, seating, lighting and general ambience need to be well designed to enhance the quality of experience.

There is also a lot of design needed to deal with meta-level, conceptual issues in these new collaborative spaces. People need to know what the space can do, what applications there are and what they do. The design principle of consistency is not possible in an environment that exploits cloud-based applications from different providers, so designers need to provide guidance on how to transfer content from one view to another, how to link views and how to switch media.

Designing blended spaces for collaboration means thinking about the five themes and how the proposed blend of physical and digital spaces have new properties providing new opportunities. Design to support the different territories of interaction, both physical and digital. Design for physical and digital awareness of what others are doing and what they have done. Design for equitable control of spaces and resources. Design for flexible task allocation and execution and interaction. Design for transitions in the physical and digital and between the physical and digital.

2.7 Conclusions

Conceptual blending as extended here into ideas of blended spaces for collaborative interaction provides designers with a way of thinking about design issues involved in the design of room environments. The TACIT framework – derived from our own experiences and those of other researchers and designers – orientates designers to the key issues that need to be considered in ICEs; territoriality, awareness, control, interaction and transitions.

Our own design methodology (Mival & Benyon, 2013) reflects the fact that every use case for an ICE is different. One reason for applying blending theory and the TACIT framework to the design of ICEs is to help designers deal with the variety of physical and digital spaces that they will be dealing with. Five general steps are needed: identify and understand the purpose of the ICE; examine the current practice; determine the project constraints; determine appropriate technologies for the space (the digital space); model and map the physical space including layout, furniture and lighting and environment control. Understand the main objects in the spaces (the ontology) and how they are to be related to one another (the topology). Understand how things change within the spaces (the volatility) and understand what people need to do (the agency). Develop the space utilizing the concepts in designing with blends, aiming for an integrated blended space that deals with the known issues of collaborative environments of territories, awareness, control, interactions and transitions (TACIT). Recognize that your users will use conceptual blending when they come to use the ICE, bringing their background knowledge of computers, multi-touch domestic devices, domestic media players and naïve networking knowledge. Provide information in the conceptual space to help people understand the opportunities afforded by the new blended space.

Acknowledgments: Grateful acknowledgements are extended to all those who have worked on and in the ICE.

References

Ackerman, M. (2000). The intellectual challenge of CSCW: the gap between social requirements and technical feasibility *Human-Computer Interaction* vol. 15, nos. 2–3, 2000 pp. 181–205.

Benford, S., Giannachi, G., Kolva, B., Rodden, T. (2009). From interaction to trajectories: designing coherent journeys through user experiences. In *CHI '09 Proceedings of the SIGCHI Conference on Human Factors in Computing Systems*. ACM Press pp. 709–718.

Benyon, D., Mlval, O. (2012). Designing Blended Spaces. In *Proceedings of Designing Collaborative interactive Spaces*. AVI Workshop, Capri, May. Available at http://hci.uni-konstanz.de/dcis/ retrieved 12.12.14.

Benyon, D., Mival, R., Ayan, S.A. (2012). Designing Blended Spaces. *In HCI2012 – People & Computers XXVI Proceedings of HCI 2012 The 26th BCS Conference on Human Computer Interaction.*

Benyon, D. (2014). *Spaces of Interaction, Places for Experience*. Morgan and Claypool.

Benyon, D. (2012). Presence in Blended Spaces *Interacting with Computers* vol. 24 n. 4, pp. 219–226.

Buxton, B. (2009). Mediaspace – Meaningspace – Meetingspace in S. Harrison, (ed) *Media Spaces: 20+ years of mediated Life.* New York, NY: Springer.

Fauconniet, G., Turner, M. (2002). *The Way We Think*. New York: NY, Basic Books.

Fauconnier, G. (1997). *Mappings in Thought and Language*. Cambridge, UK: Cambridge University Press.

Greenberg, S.(2011). Proxemics Interactions: The New Ubicomp? In *Interactions* vol 18 no. 1, January + February, pp. 42–50.

Hall, E.T. (1966). *The Hidden Dimension*, New York, NY: Doubleday.

Haller, M., Leitner, J., Selfried, T., Wallace, J., Scot, S., Richter, C., Brandl, P., Gokcezade, A., Hunter, S. (2010). The NiCE Discussion Room: Integrating Paper and Digital Media to Support Co-Located Group Meetings. *In CHI '10 Proceedings of the SIGCHI Conference on Human Factors in Computing Systems.* pp 609–618.

Hoshi, K., Waterworth, J. (2009). Tangible Presence in Blended Reality Space. *Proceedings of Presence 2009* conference. Available t http://ispr.info/presence-conferences/previous-conferences/presence-2009/.

Hutlenne, J., Israel, J. (2013). PIBA-DIBA or How to blend the digital with the physical. Proceedings of CHI workshop on Blended Spaces for interaction. Available at http://hci.uni-konstanz.de/blendedinteraction2013/ retrieved 12.12.14.

Imaz, M., Benyon, D. (2007). *Designing with Blends* Cambridge, MA: MIT Press.

Ishii, H., Ulmer, B. (1997). Tangible Bits: towards seamless interfaces between people, bits and atoms. *Proceedings CHI '97 SIGCHI Conference on Human Factors in Computing Systems* 234–241.

Hans-Christian, J,, Dachselt, R., Reiterer, H., Quigley, A., Benyon, D., Haller, M. (2013). Blended interaction: envisioning future collaborative interactive spaces. In *Proceedings CHI EA '13 CHI '13 Extended Abstracts on Human Factors in Computing Systems* pp. 3271–3274. See also http://hci.uni-konstanz.de/blendedinteraction2013/ retrieved 12.12.14.

Hans-Christian, J., Geyer, F., Schwarz, T., Reiterer, H. (2012). Blended Interaction – Toward a Framework for the Design of Interactive Spaces In *Proceedings of Designing Collaborative interactive Spaces*. AVI Workshop, Capri, May. Available at http://hci.uni-konstanz.de/dcis/ retrieved 12.12.14.

Kendal, A. (1990). Spatial organization in social encounters: The F-formation system. In , A. Kendon Ed., *Conducting Interaction: Patterns of Behavior in Focused Encounters Cambridge, UK:* Cambridge University Press, pp. 209–237.

Lakoff, G., Johnson, M. (1980). *Metaphors we live by.* Chicago University Press.

Lakoff, G., Johnson, M. (1999). *The Philosophy of the Flesh*. Bradford Books.

Markussen, T. (2009). Bloody Robots and Emotional Design: How emotional structure my change expectations of use in hospitals. *International Journal of Design* vol. 3, no.2, pp. 27–39

Milgram, P., Kishino, F. (1994). A Taxonomy of Mixed Reality Visual Displays. *Journal E77-D* (12) 1321–1329.

Mlval, O., Benyon, D. (2013). A methodology for designing Blended Spaces. In *Proceedings of Blended Spaces for Collaborative Spaces. CHI2013 Workshop, Paris, May 2013.* Available at http://hci.uni-konstanz.de/blendedinteraction2013/ retrieved 12.12.14.

Monk, A. (2003). *Common Ground in Electronically Mediated Communication: Clark's Theory of Language Use*. Elsevier.

O'Hara, K., Kjelsko, J., Paay, J. (2011). Blended Interaction Spaces for Distributed Team Collaboration *ACM Transactions on Computer-Human Interaction, Vol. 18, No. 1, article 3.*

Peltonen, P., Kurvinen, E., Salovaara, A., Jacucci, G., Ilmonen, T., Evans, J., Oulasvirta, A., Saarikko, P. (2008). "It's mine, don't touch": Interactions at a large multi-touch display in a city center. *In CHI '10 Proceedings of the SIGCHI Conference on Human Factors in Computing Systems*. pp 1285–1294.

Rogers, Y., Rodden, T. (2003). Configuring spaces and surfaces to support collaborative interaction. In , K. O'Hara, ed., *Public and situated displays: social and interactional aspects of shared display technologies London, UK:* Springer.

Rogers, Y., Lindley, S. (2004). Collaborating around vertical and horizontal large displays: Which way is best to meet? *Interacting with Computers*, vol. 16. No 6. pp. 1133–1152.

Rohrer, T. (2010). Embodiment and Experientialism. In D. Geeraerts and H. Cuckyens *The Handbook of Cognitive Linguistics*, CUP.

Schmidt, K. (2002). The Problem with Awareness. *Journal Computer Supported Cooperative Work*, Vol. 11, nos. 3–4, pp 285–298.

Scott, S., Grant, K., Mandryk, R. (2003). System guidelines for co-located, collaborative work on a tabletop display. In *ECSCW'03 Proceedings of the eighth conference on European Conference on Computer Supported Cooperative Work.* 159–178.

Scott, S., Carpendale, S. (2010). Theory of Tabletop Territoriality. In C. Müller- Tomfelde (Ed.) *Tabletops – Horizontal Interactive Displays*, London, UK: Springer, , pp. 375–406

Steven, S., Wixon, D., MacKenzie, S., Jacucci, G., Morrison, A., Wilson, A. (2009). Multi-touch and surface computing In *Proceedings CHI EA '06 CHI '06 Extended Abstracts on Human Factors in Computing Systems* pp 4767–4770.

Tang, J. C. (1991). Findings from observational studies of collaborative work. *International Journal of Man-Machine Studies*, vol. 34, pp. 143–160.

Turner, M. (2014). http://markturner.org/blending.html#BOOKS retrieved 14.03.14

Wang, H-H (2013). A case study on design with conceptual blending. *International Journal of Design Creativity*. Vol. 1 pp. 109–122.

Francesca Morganti

3 "Being There" in a Virtual World: an Enactive Perspective on Presence and its Implications for Neuropsychological Assessment and Rehabilitation

Abstract: The most recent advances in neuroscience have shown that there is an increasing necessity of resuming the embodied vision of cognition and how it could produce a significant impact on research in neuropsychology. Moreover, from the enactive cognition perspective the ability of humans to acquire knowledge from environment can be conceived as the product of continuous cycles of embodied perception and action in which the mind and the world are constantly and mutually involved. This reciprocal relationship is fairly easy to understand when an agent is interacting within a not simulated complex space. It is rather more difficult to understand if the agent has a neurological disease that affects the ability to manage her everyday environment. The introduction of Human Computer Confluence (HCC) approach and its possible digital scenarios (such as virtual environments) has proposed new challenges for enactive cognition research because it provides atypical patterns of interaction that, through the emergence of a sense of presence, influence cognitive representations and meaningful experiences. In this chapter the agents' sense of presence in a virtual environment and its implications for the ability to catch appropriate affordances for action in space will be discussed. With the aim to clarify the similarities and differences between natural and HCC environments, the chapter starts from the explanation of the enactive cognition approach and will present a recent research approach on this topic in neuropsychology. At last, the implications for the assessment and rehabilitation of high level cognitive functions in elderly population and neurological patients will be provided.

Keywords: Embodiment, Enactive Cognition, Neuropsychology, Virtual Environments, Presence

3.1 Introduction

In the last century the human processes involved in interacting with technology were mainly characterized from the Model Human Processor described by Card, Moran and Newell in 1983. This model includes the perceptual, the motor and the cognitive systems as the modules through which Human Computer Interaction (HCI) makes possible (Card, Moran, Newell, 1983). The HCI has influenced the majority of the technological applications that are still widely in use and it also has extensively influenced the classical paradigms of cognitive science.

At present, with the upcoming pervasive and ubiquitous computing era, technologies become embedded, operating with its complete physical environment as interface and supporting a more implicit interaction that involves all human senses. The explosive growth of web-based communications and, at the same time, the radical miniaturization of technologies have reversed the principles of human computer interaction. Instead of text-based commands and generic interaction devices (such as keyboards and joypads), in fact, human body actions directly features a intuitive way to interact with objects in a technology-based environment. Up until now considered as the interaction concerns when humans approach technology, more recent observations see humans and technology apparently approach each other confluently. Thus, by "manipulating" technologies, by simultaneously involving different human senses, and by considering interaction related to the physical and psychological situation in which it occurs, the traditional understanding of having an interface among humans and computers expires. Accordingly, Human Computer Confluence (HCC) that proposes human and computer activity at a confluence appears to be a more adequate definition (Ferscha, Resmerita, Holzmann, 2007).

The first definition of HCC refers to an implicit or even embedded interaction between humans and technology system components that provides the means to interact with the surrounding environment in a transparent natural and pervasive way. Among some of the main features proposed by the HCC paradigm there is the idea of technologies self-organization and interoperation. It underlines the possibility of detecting and interpreting the overall environmental situation and consequently differentially adapt the support they provide to specific user needs during her interaction with those technologies (e.g. by including the interface auto-calibration or the coordination among different technological tools). Accordingly, new classes of devices evolve and become able to adapt their physical properties to users' current situational context. Examples might include body worn displays, smart apparel, interactive large display walls, and architecture annotated with digital information. More recent advances have also introduced innovative technology able to directly connect itself with the human sensory and neural system in terms of in-body experiential interactions.

Moreover the ability to capture and correlate human experiences by technology, as well as the ability of technology to provide meaningful experiences to end-users could be considered one of the main challenge of HCC. Through innovative communication systems and ubiquitous networked sensors – able to taking into account body movements, facial expressions, event-related physiological and brain activity – in fact, it could be feasible to introduce a radically new styles of human-to-technology communication. Moreover with the introduction of a technology-based representations of human engagements and experiences, derived from the combination of multimodal perceptual stimuli with the human cognitive model, a new challenge of experiences and emotions attunement and sharing between man and machine seems to be possible.

Thus, HCC paradigm seems to provide a more intuitive meaning of interaction and appears to have several contact points with the so-called enactive cognition perspective that is closely based on a peculiar definition of interaction named embodied interaction. As Francisco Varela, Evan Thompson and Eleanor Rosch stated, in fact, enactivism relies on a fundamental concept: cognition and environment are inseparable, and organisms bodily enact with each other from which they acquire knowledge (Varela, Thompson, Rosch, 1991). Accordingly, the interaction with a context is a continuous developing process not simply guided by agent goals or motor actions; rather it is agent's ways of experiencing the context in which she is included that involves sensorimotor processes and perpetually "welds" together perceptions and actions. Moreover, one of the ground concept of enactivism is co-emergence. It focuses on the idea that the change of both an agent and its environment depends on the interaction between this agent and the specific environment. When agent and environment interact, they are structurally coupled and they co-emerge.

In this paper I will explore the enactive cognition approach and its link with the sense of presence possible within virtual environments, I would like to clarify how, with respect to the traditional interaction concept provided by HCI – that considers the interface as the main link among humans and computers – it is rather the confluence concept among embodied activity and an experiential technology-based environments presented by HCC that best defines the relation among humans and computers. The second part of this contribution aims in determine how this theoretical bridge could be suitable for applied neuroscience.

3.2 Enactive Cognition

In the last decade, following the input derived from mirror neuron discovery – that suggests the strong linkage between perception and action – the classical approach to the study of cognition would have to be replaced by an enactive one. This approach considers living beings as autonomous agents that actively generate and maintain their own coherent and meaningful patterns of activity. Within this situated view of the mind, cognition is not the result of aggregation and organisation of noteworthy information from the outside world; rather it is the product of perception-action cycles where mind and world are constantly at play. This shift also reshaped the concept of interaction: the dynamic building up of meaning through the cognitive and affectively charged experience of self and not-self (e.g. the environment, an object or other agents).

A good description of this perspective may be found in studies on embodied cognition (Varela, Thompson, Rosch, 1991). Within the embodied cognition, the body becomes an interface between the mind and the world, not so much as a collector of stimuli, rather providing it as a stage for the enactment of a drama, an interface allowing a merger between thought and the specific surrounding space. The sensorimotor coupling between the organisms and the environment in which they are living determines recurrent patterns of perception and action that allow experience and knowledge acquisition. Thus, enactive knowledge unfolds through action and it is stored in the form of motor responses and acquired by the act of doing. The human mind is embodied in our organism and it is not reducible to structures inside the head, but it is embedded in the world we are enactively interacting with (Thompson, Varela, 2001).

According to this perspective it is reasonable to accept the suggestion, originally advanced from ecological psychology (Gibson, 1977), that an individual perceives the world not in terms of objective and abstract features, but directly in terms of spaces of possible actions: "affordances". An affordance is a relational notion. The possibilities for action depend on the encounter of the characteristics of the two poles of the interaction, and are shaped by the overarching activity in which the agent is involved. Therefore, in exploring a an environment an individual will take embodied opportunities for action (affordances) that are granted to the agent. Such affordances are not an intrinsic property of the environment alone, but a property of the interaction between the agent and the environment. The availability of the affordances depends on the activities in which the agent is participating at each moment.

Within this perspective cognition becomes a complex co-evolving interactional process of systems mutually affecting each other and influencing the environment they are immersed in. Consequently cognition can't be described as in some sense a passive information elaboration process, rather it is an active biological, social and situated phenomena. In one definition it is enactive. Every living system engages in cognition by a action-feedback-reward system through which she learns from and adapts to her environment. At the same time, this system also co-emerges with the world it lives in because her activity is a domain of possibilities (affordances) and emerges from a sequence of "structured coupling" where every change causes responses in the dynamics of an ever-evolving world (Varela, Thompson, Rosch, 1991). Thus, environment doesn't direct agent's decision but unfolds in events that evoke these particular possibilities of action. By this way agent is believed to be an integral part of the environment itself.

Knowledge acquisition therefore, is embedded in action and it is not about creating abstract representation of the context; rather it is an ongoing exploration of possibilities (that includes the self and the environment) during interaction in order to adapt to the evolving situation. Consequently, a meaningful experience is not basically a collection of selected events but it constitutes every intuition, emotional fluctuation, imaginative aspect that emerges from any visible and invisible action, even those that are at the backdrop of our attention. This approach has been some specific implications for neuroscience research.

3.3 Enactive Neuroscience

Embodied cognition has been recently described as a spectre who is haunting the research laboratories (Goldman, De Vigemont, 2009). From the neuroscientific perspective, after the mirror neuron discovery, the term embodied generally means that body structure and bodily actions play a crucial role in cognition. This vision emphasizes the central role of representations mapped on body for knowledge acquisition. Representations in these terms are characterized as a distinctive class of mental states by virtue of their specific format rather than their general content. Mental states are embodied because of their peculiar bodily format and might have partly overlapping contents with other states while differing from one another in their format. Thus, the body of a cognitive representation bind what a cognitive representation can stand for (Gallese, Sinigaglia, 2011). For instance, and agent who intend to use an object has to plan and execute a motor act according to her own body characteristics (such as height, posture and physical strength). It is this embodied format that constrains the representation not only of a single motor goal, but also of a sequence of behaviours in a complex space. This defines an act as every time different from a pure a-priori propositional representation of a generic motor act. From these statements connections with the concept of affordance and the enactive approach to cognition appears to be getting more clearly defined.

In spatial orientation, for example, by using affordances during an environment exploration an agent is capable of creating relationships between landmarks and, at the same time, of entertaining high-level spatial maps. Obtain a high level spatial map allows an agent to draw spatial inferences while she is engaged in an embodied egocentric exploration. Recent fMRI studies supports this enactive perspective of spatial cognition, showing how specific brain regions (e.g. the retrosplenial cortex) have a key role in translating the high level spatial information in egocentric spatial input during wayfinding. This suggests that the acquisition of knowledge is inseparable from the egocentric/embodied perspective and from action (Byrne, Becker, Burgess, 2007).

Despite neuroscience evidence of enactive cognition, neuropsychological assessment has been largely utilising tests that provide subjects with stimuli mainly based only on the not embodied cognition approach (Lezak, 2004). Generally in fact, the Mini Mental Evaluation Exam (Folstein et al., 1975) is used for general cognitive level evaluation, the Corsi's Block-tapping test (Kessels et al., 2000) is utilised to assess spatial memory, the Tower of London task (Shallice, 1982) is used for planning ability evaluation. All the above tests indubitably constitute an important vehicle through which the different aspects of cognition can be evaluated, but they do not allow the assessment of the active and body-centred interaction with the environment from which an agent acquire knowledge. This aspect results in an important bias for the neuropsychological evaluation because it requires subjects to use abstract simulations of tasks and to infer how the test stimuli could be like from a situated perspective.

In the last decades one of the main vision of HCC is to consider technology as a cognitive extension, able to develop new forms of knowledge and amplify humans' cognitive abilities. Technology-based environments, in facts, integrate so closely with agents that they will become a part of their extended minds in building internal models of the world and providing control functions. Accordingly, a large amount of literature supports the evidence that knowledge obtainable from 3D computer simulated environments (such as virtual environments) is largely comparable to the one obtainable from the active interaction with not simulated environments. It is due to the sense of presence experienced in virtual reality simulations. Presence is commonly defined as the subjective feeling of "being there" (Riva, Davide, Ijsselsteijn, 2003). It's largely agreed that during the exploration of a virtual environment agents create cognitive representation of it and obtain from it a meaningful experience. According to those evidences, in fact, virtual environments have been introduced in neuroscience and experimental psychology for the study of cognition (Morganti, 2003; 2004).

I would like to underline here that a full understanding of the great opportunity provided from virtual environments for neuroscience requires a multidisciplinary perspective that involves not only neurological research but also cognitive psychology and information communication technology. The great challenge, in fact, is to clarify what could be the role of emerging technologies in such process and how can it support us in delineating innovative and plausible scenarios for the future clinical work. In doing that the HCC perspective could help us defining long-term clinical goals and in understanding how the new technology is going to support neurological population on cognitive and social level, and in how it will change patients' perception and models of reality.

While agreeing with the HCC vision, there is the necessity to deepen some aspects about the experiential differences derived from the interaction with a simulated and a not simulated environment. By adopting an embodied approach to sensing people's state, in fact, virtual reality systems provide not just passive motion sensors but introduce also new challenges in implementing real-time and dynamic action possibilities. This mechanisms is able to create innovative fully interactive applications that enactively adapt theirselves according with users activities, providing users with a sense of action ownership that results in a presence feeling within the simulated environment. Before to largely use it in neuro-cognitive research, it become necessary to determine how this "being there" experience could influence cognition and can evidence differences between healthy subjects and neurological patients.

3.4 Enactive Presence in Virtual Reality

Several authors considered the *sense of presence* as mainly deriving from the result of subjective involvement in a highly interactive virtual environment (Slater, Wilbur, 1997). Presence, in fact, would be strong inasmuch as the virtual system enables an inclusive, extensive, surrounding and vivid illusion. The immersive quality of virtual reality would be enhanced by the perceptive features and the proprioceptive feedback provided by the technology. Accordingly in the last years research on presence has emphasized the role that activity plays in directing attention within complex interactive situations. The specific role of interaction with technology in creating presence was firstly considered by Lombard and Ditton (1997), who defined presence as the "perceptual illusion of non-mediation". In this perspective, presence occurs when a person misperceives an experience mediated by technology as if it were a direct (that is, non-mediated) one. Presence, thus, would not be a property of technology, rather it could vary depending on how much the user acknowledges the role of technology and could therefore be yielded by different kind of technologies. Thus, not only highly immersive technological solutions are needed to experience presence but also subjective involvement plays an important role. Sanchez-Vivez and Slater (2005) claim that visual realism does not strongly contribute to presence and that of particular importance is the degree to which simulated sensory data matches proprioception during a virtual environment exploration. Experiencing presence does not merely depend on appearances but is rather a function of the interaction between the subject and the environment. It suggests that it is the role of the subject's own body in eliciting presence. The sense of agency ownership could be provided not only by the visual reference of the agent body in the virtual environment, rather, what counts is the dynamic of the interactions between the body and the world that a virtual reality is able to support through a continuous coupling between perception and action.

Concordant with this theoretical position the definition of presence can be integrated within the enactive perspective described in the previous paragraphs and can be addressed to the various combination of physical and digital spaces today available. At present, for example, it is possible to augment a physical space with video observed through a mobile screen or interact with a digital space through some physical device or wearable movement sensors. Thus, the physical and the digital become woven together into hybrid spaces with their own properties. In cognitive science the term to define this kind of mixed space is 'blended' and it refers to a cross domain mappings and conceptual integration to thought process that are grounded in physically-based spatial schemas. A blend is defined as a cognitive structure that emerges when putting together two or more input spaces – mental spaces derived from different domains of knowledge (Fauconnier, Turner, 2003). They are defined as temporary cognitive models engaged in thinking, talking and planning subsequent actions. There are minimum four mental spaces involved in a blending process: the two input spaces (for example the physical and digital), one generic space containing the elements that are shared by the two input spaces and, finally, the blend – the emerging mental space possessing meanings extracted from the generic space but also new, emergent qualities that neither the input spaces nor the generic space possessed before entering the blending process. The blended space will be more effective if the physical and digital spaces have some recognizable and understandable correspondences.

The concept of blended spaces supports us in understanding how virtual reality experiences could be interpreted as the next level of enactive cognition. People will move through these spaces, following trajectories that weave in and out of physical and digital space, and will fell present within it. To be in this kind of space, in fact, depends on a suitable integration of aspects relevant to an agent's movement and perception, to her actions, and to her conception of the overall situation in which she finds herself, as well as on how these aspects mesh with the possibilities for action afforded in the interaction with the virtual environment (Carassa, Morganti, Tirassa, 2004; 2005). According to this vision, during the interaction with a digital environment an agent will choose and perform specific actions whose goals are part of a broader situation, which she represents as the weave of activities that she participates moment by moment. These activities are, in their turn, supported by goals, opportunities for action, and previous knowledge, that give them meaningful experiences. Therefore, in exploring a virtual environment an individual will take embodied opportunities for action that are granted to the agent, and such affordances are not an intrinsic property of the environment alone, but a property of the interaction between the agent and the environment. The availability of the affordances depend on the activities in which the agent is participating at each moment. In supporting the representation of herself as an agent, who carries on a narrative about herself in the world, the environment (even a virtual one) has always a subjective rather than objective nature. Finally, the degree to which people will feel really present in this kind of space is a measure of the quality of the user experience, of the naturalness of the medium interaction and of the appropriateness of digital content to the characteristics of the physical space.

Following the enactive interpretation of presence I am proposing that the differences between the action (as in the real world) and the simulation of an action (as in virtual reality) reflects a distinction between ability to anticipate the results of changing one's frame of reference with respect to the environment and the ability to imagine the results of changing the position of an object in the environment while maintaining one's current orientation in the physical environment. Specifically interaction ability with a virtual environment depends on the "cognitive anticipation" of agent behaviour in a particular place with a specific frame of reference. Consequently, embodied interaction ability creates an expectation/simulation of movement that in virtual reality was more manageable with a high level of presence.

At present the main open question is on how experiential differences derived from the interaction with a simulated and not simulated environment could influence cognitive representations. Moreover, as defined before, according with the technology they are using people will be differently present in the blended space, moving between and within them and moving up and down the layers of experience. The next paragraph aims in underline which are the critical difference between these two conditions and how the sense of presence can efficaciously support interaction and knowledge acquisition. I propose this point constitutes, in fact, the key factor for the use of virtual reality in neuropsychology not only for assessment, but also for the rehabilitation of cognitively impaired people.

3.5 Enactive Technologies in Neuropsychology

Although it has therefore been discussed about the importance of the enactive cognition approach and about its implication for the sense of presence for knowledge acquisition in digital spaces, how to use HCC technological solutions to assess specific cognitive functions it remains still widely unexplored. A key requirement for all HCC applications, in fact, is to recognize complex human activities in real-world environments over long time periods and in unconstrained environments and to provide users with a congruent support in choosing new opportunity for action in everyday life. This approach implies a number of consequences which are problematic when dealing with complex activities over different time periods in blended environments. In this case HCC technology must enactively adapt to new, likely unforeseen, situations encountered at run-time, by continuously tracking changes in the way user's activities map to sensor signals, and by being able to adapt itself to the way a user executes activities.

For how concerns one of the main challenge everyday space provide us, such as spatial orientation, for example, the reciprocal relationship between perception and action that underlies this ability is quite easy to understand when an agent is placed in a natural place, such as her house or a city square. However, this link is more difficult to understand when the agent is provided with a simulated space, such as a map that provides the agent with an allocentric perspective, or when she is placed in a virtual environment that provides the agent with an egocentric perspective. In the last decade, together with paper and pencil spatial grids and sketched maps, virtual reality environments were widely used in cognitive neuropsychology to study spatial orientation (Morganti, 2004). At present the great challenge in spatial cognition assessment is to determine if the orientation obtainable from a digital interactive environment might differ from the spatial orientation obtainable from a simulation of the same environment based on an analogical simulation (e.g. a sketched map). In the first type of simulation, in fact, an agent has an egocentric perspective on the environment and she can move within it, while in the second type of simulation, an agent has an allocentric perspective on the environment that requires a mental imagery effort to be translated in action. I claim that both perspectives are essential for spatial orientation in a complex environment and the linkage between them needs to be further investigated in order to obtain an effective HCC solution to support agents in exploring the surrounded everyday space. It could be essential not just to improve the use of complex spaces in daily activities, but it could be even more crucial for supporting the daily activities in people who have suffered neurological damage and which are no longer able to manage the surrounding spaces.

At this regard, for example, in the last years a virtual version of the Money's Road Map test was developed (VR-RMT; Morganti et al., 2009). Whereas the classical version of the test requires a mental imagery right/left turning to explore a stylized city provided to the subject in a allocentric perspective, the VR-MRT is a 3D version of the same environment in which participants can navigate by actively choosing right/left directions in a egocentric perspective. The introduction of this virtual version of the test provides the opportunity to observe several implications according to the enactive approach to cognition. From an enactive perspective, in fact, there is a difference in imaging a turn, as in classical version of the test, and actively performing a turn in order to obtain a spatial perspective from the virtual world as in the VR-RMT. Accordingly these two different spatial tasks, as they provide different embodied affordances, results in different orientation outcomes. Specifically, it might be argued that, by providing an external representation of the route perspective, these differences are underlined by the type of right/left turns and by their increasing complexity. This example could give us the possibility to understand how a HCC technological solution, such as virtual reality, supports perspective taking and could provide different performances in spatial cognition.

From a work of Gray and Fu (2004), we know that, when a computer-based interface is well designed, it supports the possibility of placing knowledge in-the-world instead of retrieving it from-in-the-head, in order to have it readily available when an agent needs it. Accordingly agents might prefer perfect knowledge in the world to imperfect knowledge in the head. Offloading cognitive work onto the environment (Wilson, 2002) could constitute one of the main advantages of the active interaction supported by a HCC system: it allows guiding orientation by obtaining spatial perspectives from in the world (the different spatial snapshots encountered by the agent after a right/left turn in virtual world) rather than retrieving it from in the head (the different inferences on how a perspective would be after a right/left turn) and could provide agent with new affordance for wayfinding. On this subject Schultz (1991) underlined how to plan in advance a wayfinding in a natural place could be done primarily by imagining egocentric spatial transformations. Thus and agent involved in this task have to imagine how to move on the body axis and finally obtain (and retain) the spatial perspective derived from the turn, whereas in a digital space an agent act the turn on the body axis and finally perceive in the simulated world the spatial perspective derived from that turn. In this case an HCC technology, such as virtual reality, does not require the agents to find their current place each time and the keeping track of each perspective does not require an additional cognitive effort. But, as pointed out by Tversky (2008), our own body is experienced from inside, and the space around our body does not depend on the physical situation per se. In a digital space, such as in the VR-RMT, there could be a dissociation between perspective taking and mental rotation (Hegarthy, Waller, 2004). Perspective taking involves imagining the results of changing one's egocentric frame of reference with respect to the environment, while mental rotation involves imagining the results of changing the positions of objects and maintaining one's current orientation in the environment. In accord with Keehner and colleagues (Keehner, Hegarthy, Cohen, Khooshabeh, Montello, 2008), I hypothesize that in the VR-MRT task participants must create a blended space and will be able to use it in order to manage a efficient wayfinding. In doing that they match the perspective that the virtual scenario is providing them to their right/left turn intentions in order to match the obtained perspective with the results of each turn, and this matching has to be tightly coupled with internal cognitive processes. In conclusion the option to offload cognition onto the external visualization provided by this kind of HCC (by observing the perspective resulting from a right/left turn) may require a cognitive effort mainly based on an embodied cognitive process.

3.6 Enactive Knowledge and Human Computer Confluence

As Maturana and Varela stated, stressing embodied action, "all doing is knowing and all knowing is doing" (Maturana, Varela, 1987; p. 27). In this contribution we have discussed on how an agent and the environment, both natural and artificial, are mutually specifying and how cognition is a co-emerging process of enactment of a world and our mind.

In the last paper Francisco Varela wrote before his death Gallagher, Varela, 2001), in order to understand the nature of human experience, several open questions were proposed, such as: How do humans perceive a space? How this perception is different from imagination or memory? Is memory stored in form of linguistic or image codification? Can consciousness exist independently from its context? Are my voluntary movements independent from my body awareness? All these questions were partially answered through investigating the sense of agency as intrinsic and indistinguishable to the action itself. There is, in fact, an intrinsic sense of ownership of the action, essentially based on the anticipation of action goals, that exists prior to the physical execution of the specific action (Georgieff, Jeannerod, 1998; Gallagher, Marcel, 1999). It is this anticipatory mechanism that entangled embodied actions to the context in which they are planned to be executed. Moreover, it is the same functional mechanism that allow to reorganize actions according to contextual changes that might occurs during the execution of actions or to the contextual changes that are yet to happen (Berthoz, 2000). At present, the theoretical questions proposed by Gallagher and Varela appear to be still unresolved if we consider the HCC approach. In a recent paper, Froese and Zimke (2009) argued that technologies can be considered as an opportunity to create hypothetical variations of a particular natural phenomenon by externalizing a crucial part of the imaginative process in what they defined 'technological supplementation'. I proposed here that the main difference between HCC experiential environments and non-technology-based contexts lies in the fact that the first extended by technology the cognitive phenomenon we would like to observe.

Specifically in this contribution I want to introduce how enactive technologies could be used in cognitive neuroscience in order to observe the types of representations an agent is able to obtain in order to adaptively interact with a simulated environment within a given activity. For neuropsychological assessment, in fact, a particular type of HCC technological solution, as virtual environments, seems able to maintain the sensorimotor dynamics of embodied agency – that is the locus of selfhood in the not simulated world – and provides us with the possibility to evaluate agent's spatial ability in a situated way. The introduction of such kind of simulation, that supports the sense of being in another place than the physical one, makes it possible to overcome some limitations of current neuropsychological evaluation: the confliction between the need to study cognition in conditions that allow a high methodological control and the need to create situations that have a high ecological validity. Virtual reality, in fact, allows the creation of flexible simulations in which humans can actively perform 'real-life' explorative behaviours in a daily environment. It might be important if the assessment requires a functional localisation of the brain areas involved in a specific kind of interaction while subjects are not allowed to physically move in the environment (such as in fMRI studies). Moreover, rather than lesion localisation the main purpose of the neuropsychological assessment should be to draw conclusions from assessments regarding patients' ability to live independently or return to a previous occupation (Troster, 2000). This issue is extremely important especially in the cognitive assessment of the elderly population, where we can find several "borderline" situations not always detectable with a classical neuropsychological assessment. Specifically it is important to gain a greater understanding of the nature of age-related cognitive impairment mainly because the age-associated limitations could potentially lead to restrictions in daily activities, especially if they are performed in new environments.

Despite this evidence, cognitive decline in healthy elderly population and its role in the difficulties experienced by neurological patients are grossly underestimated. As neurological patients are generally at high risk for cognitive impairments that could have a detrimental impact on everyday performance, they require a specifically contextualized user-centred intervention (Katz, 2005). At present, conventional neuropsychological evaluation and rehabilitation plan still present limited ecological validity and do not fully address the functional implications of cognitive deficits (Burgess et al., 2006). The more valuable solution to this gap could be to introduce new tools for the measurements of cognitive ability "in action", extremely important to individuate a possible rehabilitation plan focussed on patient's instrumental activities of daily living (Hartman-Maeir, Katz, & Baum, 2009). The HCC approach seems to provide us with a great challenge on this issue. There are, however, some considerations that have to be clearly identified in introducing HCC in neuroscience. Several parameters might interfere with HCC-based neuropsychological assessment (e.g. age-related vision lowering and motor slowing), that may differentiate performance between older and younger adults and may affect interpretation of data findings. It become, for example, strictly necessary to evaluate age differences in experience using computers and playing 3D video games that might influence navigational expertise in a virtual environment (Moffat, 2009). In order to overcome these interfering variables, researchers have either to find new ideas for supporting enactive interaction with technology and specifically provide older subjects with extensive training sections in order to give them the possibility to familiarize with the HCC devices interaction practices.

Several objections about equivalence between natural and digital environment can be moved from the use of such HCC solutions in the cognitive domains. I consider them essentials if we would like to maintain an idea of cognition strictly based on behaviour-representation-feedback model (such as the notion of interaction in HCI approach). From this perspective we need to stress the obvious physical difference between natural and simulated environments in terms of perception, possibility of physical interactions, proprioceptive and vestibular feedbacks, and so on. Contrariwise, I would like to endorse a more enactive view of cognition in which what an agent do during the human computer confluence with technology-based simulations is to maintain her self-identity (through her action ownership) and to treat the context modification she encounters with the anticipation of her action goals (that is not intrinsic to the context itself). From this perspective the artificial-natural reality equivalence problem disappears and the cognitive representation of a context is not determined by the mere perceptual contest but it is based on a co-determination of embodied representation and affordable context in a blended space. It is the co-determination, in the enactive sense, that constitutes sense-making generation in relation to the embodied and intentional perspective of the agent. This disappearing of the boundaries between the affordable situation and agents goals is the enaction of a meaningful world for the agent. Thus, knowledge is acquired in relation to the "being there" sensation an agent experiences both within a natural, a simulated environment or a blended one. It is the presence experience, possible in a human computer confluence, that supports agent's ongoing identity and the active creation of the overall context meaning possible even in a simulated situation. What makes the world is the significance that is continuously brought forth by the endogenous activity of the agent, as it appears from her affordance perspectives. It is distinct from the pure physical characteristics', instead depends on the specific mode of co-determination that each agent realizes with its context according to different modes of structural coupling that give rise to different meanings.

At last, HCC paradigm results in an interesting opportunity not only for the more situated clinical neuropsycology evaluation and rehabilitation, but also for providing a test bed for the enactive cognition approach.

Aknowledgements: This contribution originates from several "neverending" discussions with Andrea Gaggioli, Giuseppe Riva, Maurizio Tirassa and Antonella Carassa. I would like to thanks them for the suggestions and the criticisms provided to my research topics during these years.

This work was funded by the Department of Human Science, University of Bergamo (MIUR -Fondi di Ricerca di Ateneo 2012).

References

Berthoz, A. (2000). *The Brain's Sense of Movement.* Harvard University Press.

Burgess, N. (2006). Spatial memory: how egocentric and allocentric combine. *Trends in Cognitive Sciences*, 10, 551–557.

Byrne, P., Becker, S., Burgess N. (2007). Remembering the past and imagining the future: a neural model of spatial memory and imagery. *Psychological Review*, 114(2), 340–375.

Carassa, A., Morganti, F., Tirassa, M (2004). Movement, Action, and Situation: Presence in Virtual Environments. *Presence 2004*, UPV Edition, Valencia, p. 3–10.

Carassa, A., Morganti, F., Tirassa, M. (2005). A situated cognition perspective on presence. In B. Bara, L. W. Barsalou & M. Bucciarelli (Eds), *XXVII Annual Conference of the Cognitive Science Society* (pp. 384–389). Alpha, NJ: Sheridan Printing.

Card, S., Moran, T., Newell, A. (1983). *The psychology of human-computer interaction.* Hillsdale, NJ: Lawrence Erlbaum Associates

Fauconnier, G., Turner, M., (2003). *The Way We Think: Conceptual Blending and the Mind's Hidden Complexities.* New York: Basic Book.

Ferscha, A., Resmerita, S., & Holzmann, C. (2007). Human computer confluence. In *Universal Access in Ambient Intelligence Environments* (pp. 14–27). Springer Berlin Heidelberg.

Folstein, M. F., Folstein, S.E., McHugh, P.R. (1975). "Mini-mental state". A practical method for grading the cognitive state of patients for the clinician. *Journal of Psychiatric Research*, 12, 189–198.

Froese,T., Zimke, T. (2009). Enactive Artificial Intelligence: Investigating the systemic organization of life and mind Journal of Artificial Intelligence, 173, 466–500.

Gallagher, S., Marcel, A. (1999). The self in contextualized action. *Journal of consciousness studies*, 6, 4–30.

Gallagher, S., Varela, F. (2001). Redrawing the map and resetting the time: Phenomenology and the cognitive sciences, in Crowell, Embree and Julian (Eds.), *The reach of Reflection: Issues for Phenomenology's Second Century, Center for Advanced Research in Phenomenology*. pp.17–43.

Gallese, V., Sinigaglia, C. (2011). What is so special about embodied simulation? *Trends in Cognitive Sciences*, 15 (11), 512–519.

Georgieff, N., Jeannerod, M. (1998). Beyond consciousness of external reality: A ''who'' system for consciousness of action and self-consciousness. *Consciousness and Cognition* 7 (3),465–477.

Gibson, J.J. (1977). The theory of affordances. In R. Shaw & J. Bransford (eds.), *Perceiving, Acting and Knowing.* Hillsdale, NJ: Erlbaum.

Goldman, A., de Vignemont, F. (2009). Is social cognition embodied? *Trends in Cognitive Sciences*, 13, 154–159.

Gray, W. D., Fu, W. T. (2004). Soft constraints in interactive behavior: The case of ignoring perfect knowledge in-the-world for imperfect knowledge in-the-head. *Cognitive Science*, 28, 359–382.

Hartman-Maeir, A., Katz, N., Baum, C. (2009). Cognitive-Functional Evaluation (CFE) for individuals with suspected cognitive disabilities. *Occupational Therapy in Health Care*, 23, 1–23.

Hegarty, M., Waller, D. (2004). A dissociation between mental rotation and perspective-taking spatial abilities. *Intelligence*, 32, 175–191.

Katz, N. (2005). *Cognition and occupation across the life span: Models for intervention in occupational therapy.* Bethesda, MD: AOTA Press.

Keehner, M., Hegarty, M., Cohen, C. A., Khooshabeh, P., Montello, D. R. (2008). Spatial reasoning with external visualizations: What matters is what you see, not whether you interact. *Cognitive Science*, 32, 1099–1132.

Kessels, R. P. C., van Zandvoort, M. J. E., Postma, A., Kappelle, L. J., & de Haan, E. H. F. (2000). The Corsi Block-Tapping Task: Standardization and Normative Data. *Applied Neuropsychology*, 7(4), 252–258.

Lezak, M.D. (2004). *Neuropsychological assessment.* Oxford University Press.

Lombard, M., Ditton, V. (1997). At the heart of it all: The concept of presence. *Journal of Computer-Mediated Communication*, 3, 2.

Maturana, H.R., Varela, F.J. (1987). *The tree of Knowledge: The biological roots of human understanding.* Boston: New Science Library

Moffat, S. D. (2009). Aging and spatial navigation: What do we know and where do we go? *Neuropsychology Review*, 19, 478–489.

Morganti, F., Marrakchi, S., Urban, P.P., Iannoccari, G.A., Riva G. (2009). A virtual reality based tools for the assessment of "survey to route" spatial organization ability in elderly population: Preliminary data. *Cognitive Processing*, 10, 257–259.

Morganti, F. (2003). Spatial cognition and virtual environments: how the interaction with 3D computer based environments could support the study of spatial abilities. *Ricerche di Psicologia*, 26 (4), 105–149.

Morganti, F. (2004). Virtual interaction in cognitive neuropsychology. *Studies in Health Technology and Informatics*, 99, 55–70.

Riva, G., Davide, F., Ijsselsteijn, W.A. (2003). *Being There: Concepts, Effects and Measurements of User Presence in Synthetic Environments*. IOS Press.

Sanchez-Vives, M.V., Slater, M. (2005). From presence to consciousness through virtual reality. *Nature Reviews Neuroscience*, 6, 332–339.

Schultz, K. (1991). The contribution of solution strategy to spatial performance. *Canadian Journal of Psychology*, 45 ,474–491.

Shallice, T. (1982). "Specific impairments of planning". Philosophical Transactions of the Royal Society of London. Series B, *Biological Sciences* 298, 199–209.

Slater, M., Wilbur, S. (1997). A framework for immersive virtual environments (FIVE): Speculations on the role of presence in virtual environments. *Presence*, 6, 603–616.

Thompson, E., Varela, F.J. (2001). Radical embodiment: Neural dynamics and consciousness, *Trends in Cognitive Sciences*, 5, 418–425.

Troster, A. I. (2000). Clinical neuropsychology, functional neurosurgery, and restorative neurology in the next millennium: Beyond secondary outcome measures. *Brain and Cognition*, 42, 117–119.

Tversky, B. (2008). Spatial Cognition: Embodied and Situated. In P. Robbins & M. Aydede (Eds), *The Cambridge Handbook of Situated Cognition.* (pp. 201–216). New York: Cambridge University Press

Varela, F.J., Thompson, E., Rosch, E. (1991). *The Embodied Mind. Cognitive Science and Human Experience.* MIT Press.

Wilson, M. (2002). Six views of embodied cognition. *Psychonomic Bulletin and Review*, 9, 625–636.

Giuseppe Riva

4 Embodied Medicine: What Human-Computer Confluence Can Offer to Health Care

Abstract: In this chapter we claim that the structuration, augmentation and replacement of bodily self-consciousness is at the heart of the research in Human Computer Confluence, requiring knowledge from both cognitive/social sciences and advanced technologies. More, the chapter suggests that this research has a huge societal potential: it is possible to use different technological tools to modify the characteristics of bodily self-consciousness with the specific goal of improving the person's level of well-being. The chapter, after discussing the characteristics of bodily self-consciousness, suggests that different disorders – including PTSD, eating disorders, depression, chronic pain, phantom limb pain, autism, schizophrenia, Parkinson's and Alzheimer's – may be related to an abnormal interaction between perceptual and schematic contents in memory (both encoding and retrieval) and/or prospection altering on one or more layers of the bodily self-experience of the subjects. A critical feature of the resulting abnormal representations is that, in most situations, they are not accessible to consciousness and cannot be directly altered. If this happens, the only working approach is to create or strengthen alternative ones. The chapter suggests and discusses the possible use of technology for a direct modification of bodily self-consciousness. More, it presents three different strategies: the structuration of bodily self-consciousness through the focus and reorganization of its contents (Mindful Embodiment); the augmentation of bodily self-consciousness to achieve enhanced and extended experiences (Augmented Embodiment); the replacement of bodily self-consciousness with a synthetic one (Synthetic Embodiment).

Keywords: Bodily self-consciousness, Human Computer Confluence, Virtual Reality, Interreality, Positive Technology

4.1 Introduction

The term "Human Computer Confluence – HCC" refers to (Ferscha, 2013)

> "An invisible, implicit, embodied or even implanted interaction between humans and system components... Researchers strive to broker a unified and seamless interactive framework that dynamically melds interaction across a range of modalities and devices, from interactive rooms and large display walls to near body interaction, wearable devices, in-body implants and direct neural input and stimulation" (p. 5).

The work of different European research initiatives is currently shaping human computer confluence. In particular these initiatives are exploring how the emerging

symbiotic relation between humans and information and communication technologies – including virtual and augmented realities – can be based on radically new forms of sensing, perception, interaction and understanding (Ferscha, 2013). Specifically, the EU funded HC2 CSA (www.hcsquared.eu) identified the following key research areas in human computer confluence are:
- HCC DATA: new methods to stimulate and use human sensory perception and cognition to interpret massive volumes of data in real time;
- HCC TRANSIT: new methods and concepts towards unobtrusive mixed or virtual reality environment;
- HCC SENSE: new forms of perception and action in virtual world.

Within these research areas, a critical research object is "*bodily self-consciousness*" – the feeling of being in a body (Blanke, 2012; Lenggenhager, Tadi, Metzinger, & Blanke, 2007; Tsakiris, Hesse, Boy, Haggard, & Fink, 2007).

On one side, different researches demonstrated the possibility of using technology – in particular virtual reality (VR) – to develop virtual bodies (avatars) able to induce bodily self-consciousness (see (Riva & Waterworth, 2014; Riva, Waterworth, & Murray, 2014) and the chapter by Herbelin and colleagues in this book for an in-depth description of this possibility).

On the other side, bodily self-consciousness plays a central role in structuring cognition and the self. First, according to the influential Somatic Marker Hypothesis, modifications in bodily arousal influence cognitive processes themselves. As underlined by Damasio (Damasio, 1996):

> "Somatic markers" – biasing signals from the body – "influence the processes of response to stimuli, at multiple levels of operation, some of which occur overtly (consciously, 'in mind') and some of which occur covertly (non-consciously, in a non-minded manner)." (p. 1413).

Furthermore, it is through the development of their own bodily self-consciousness that subjects define their boundaries within a spatial and social space (Bermúdez, Marcel, & Eilan, 1995; Brugger, Lenggenhager, & Giummarra, 2013; Riva, 2014). According to Damasio (1999) the autobiographical self emerges only when – to quote the book's title – self comes to mind, so that in key brain regions, the encoded experiences of past intersect with the representational maps of whole-body sensory experience.

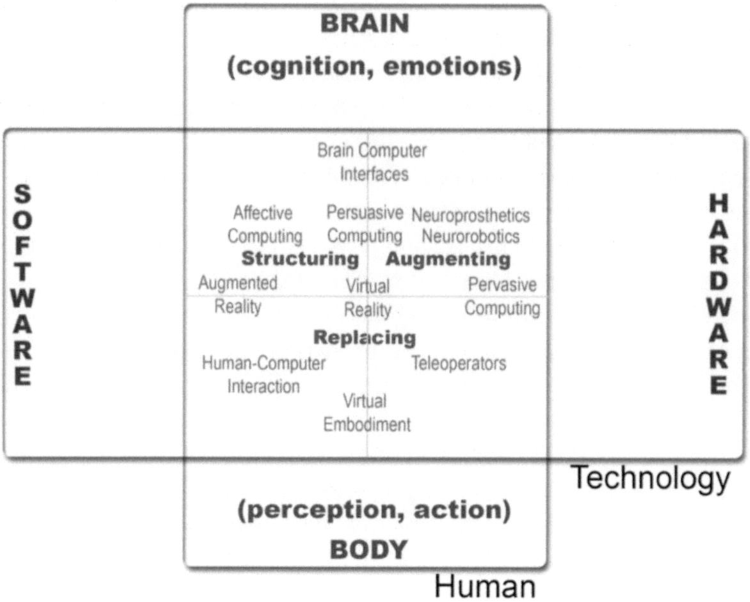

Figure 4.1: The role of bodily self-consciousness in Human Computer Confluence.

Starting from the above concepts, the chapter claims that the structuration, augmentation and replacement of bodily self-consciousness is at the heart of the research in Human Computer Confluence, requiring knowledge from both cognitive/social sciences and advanced technologies (see Figure 4.1). Furthermore, the chapter aims at bridging technological development with bodily self-consciousness research by suggesting that it is possible to develop and use technologies to modify the characteristics of bodily self-consciousness with the specific goal of improving the person's level of well-being.

4.2 Bodily Self-Consciousness

As underlined by Olaf Blanke (2012) in his recent paper for Nature Reviews Neuroscience:

> "Human adults experience a 'real me' that 'resides' in 'my' body and is the subject (or 'I') of experience and thought. This aspect of self-consciousness, namely the feeling that conscious experiences are bound to the self and are experiences of a unitary entity ('I'), is often considered to be one of the most astonishing features of the human mind." (p. 556).

The increasing interest of cognitive science, social and clinical psychology in the study of the experience of the body is providing a better picture of the process (Blanke, 2012;

Gallagher, 2005; Slaughter & Brownell, 2012; Tsakiris, Longo, & Haggard, 2010). First, even though bodily self-consciousness is apparently experienced by the subject as a unitary experience, neuroimaging and neurological data suggest that it includes different experiential layers that are integrated in a coherent experience (Blanke, 2012; Crossley, 2001; Pfeiffer et al., 2013; Shilling, 2012; Vogeley & Fink, 2003). In general, we become aware of our bodies through exteroceptive signals arising on (i.e., touch), or outside the body (i.e., vision) and through interoceptive (i.e., heart rate) and proprioceptive (i.e. skeletal striated muscles and joints) signals arising from within the body (Durlik, Cardini, & Tsakiris, 2014; Garfinkel & Critchley, 2013).

Second, these studies support the idea that body representations play a central role in structuring cognition and the self. For this reason, the experience of the body is strictly connected to processes like cognitive development and autobiographical memory.

But what is the role of bodily self-consciousness? We use the "feelings" from the body to sense both our physical condition and emotional state. These feelings range from proprioceptive and exteroceptive bodily changes that may be visible also to an external observer (i.e., posture, touch, facial expressions) to proprioceptive and interoceptive changes that may be not visibile to an external observer (i.e., endocrine release, heart rate, muscle contractions) (Bechara & Damasio, 2005).

As suggested by Craig (2002, 2003), all feelings from the body are represented in a hierarchical homeostatic system that maintains the integrity of the body. More, a re-mapping of this representation can be used to judge and predict the effects of emotionally relevant stimuli on the body with the aim of making rational decisions that affect survival and quality of life (Craig, 2010; Damasio, 1994). According to Damasio (1994), this "*collective representation of the body constitutes the basis for a 'concept' of self*" (p. 239) *that exists as "momentary activations of topographically organized representations*"(p. 240). This view is shared by different authors. For example, for Craig (2003) "*the subjective image of the ' material me' is formed on the basis of the sense of the homeostatic condition of each individual' s body*" (p. 503).

4.2.1 Bodily Self-Consciousness: its Role and Development

From this brief analysis is clear that bodily self-consciousness it is not a simple phenomenon. First, it includes different processes and neural structures that work together integrating different sources of input (see Figure 4.2).

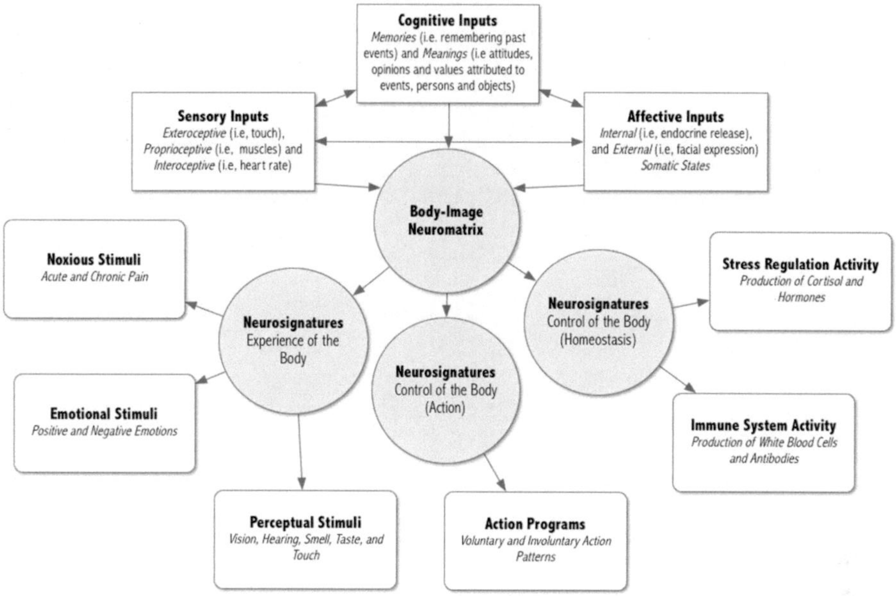

Figure 4.2: (Adapted from Melzack (2005)) Melzack, R. (2005). Evolution of the Neuromatrix Theory of Pain. The Prithvi Raj Lecture: Presented at the Third World Congress of World Institute of Pain, Barcelona 2004. Pain Practice, 5(2), 85–94.

Melzack (1999; 2013) defined this widely distributed neural network, including loops between the limbic system and cortex as well as between the thalamus and cortex, as the "body-self neuromatrix" (Melzack, 2005):

"The neuromatrix, distributed throughout many areas of the brain, comprises a widespread network of neurons which generates patterns, processes information that flows through it, and ultimately produces the pattern that is felt as a whole body. The stream of neurosignature output with constantly varying patterns riding on the main signature pattern produces the feelings of the whole body with constantly changing qualities". (p. 87).

More, the characteristics of bodily self-consciousness evolve over time following the ontogenetic development of the subject. Specifically, Riva (2014) suggested that we expand over time our bodily self-consciousness by progressively including new experiences – minimal selfhood, self location, agency, body ownership, third-person perspective, and body satisfaction – based on different and more sophisticated bodily representations (Figure 4.3).

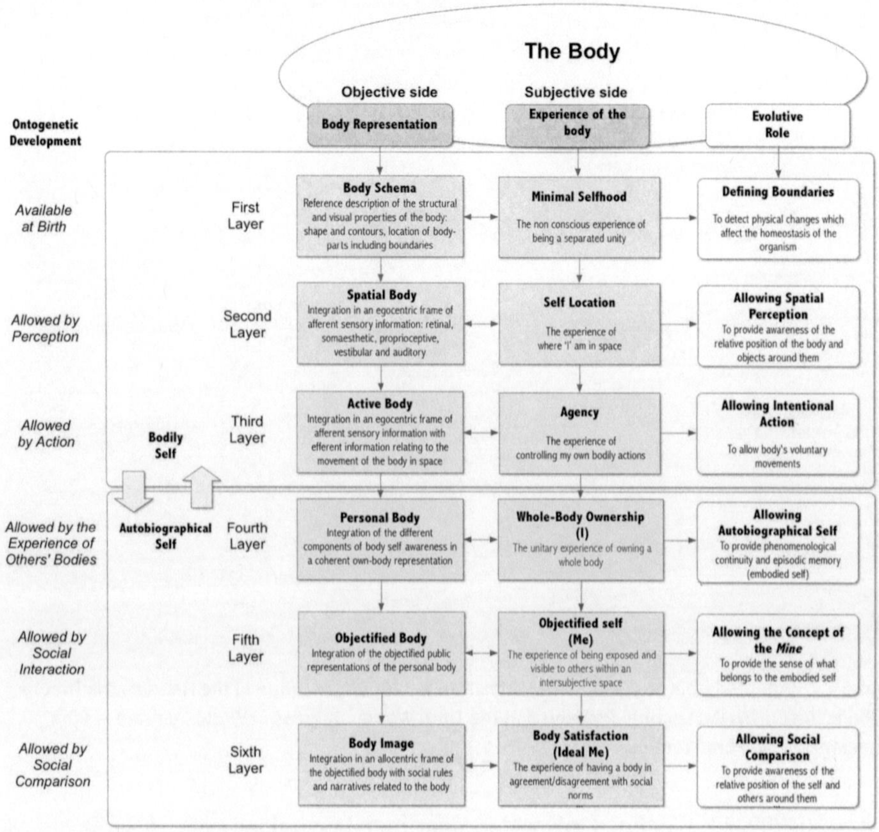

Figure 4.3: (Adapted from Riva (2014)) Riva, G. (2014). Out of my real body: cognitive neuroscience meets eating disorders. Front Hum Neurosci, 8, 236.

First, perception and action extend the minimal selhood (based on the body schema) existing at birth through two more online representations: "the spatial body," produced by the integration in an egocentric frame of afferent sensory information (retinal, somaesthetic, proprioceptive, vestibular, and auditory), and "the active body," produced by the integration of "the spatial body" with efferent information relating to the movement of the body in space. From an experiential viewpoint "the spatial body" allows the experience of where "I" am in space and that "I" perceive the world from there, while "the active body" provides to the self the sense of agency, the sense that we control our own bodily actions.

Then, through the maturation of the underlying neural networks and the progressive increase of mutual social exchanges, the embodied self is extended by further representations: "the personal body," integrating the different body locations in a whole body representation; "the objectified body," the integration of the objectified public representations of the personal body; the "body image," integrating the objectified representation of the personal body with the ideal societal body. From an experiential viewpoint these representations produce new bodily experiences: "the personal body" allows the "whole-body ownership", the unitary experience of owning a whole body (I); "the objectified body" allows the "objectified self", the experience of being exposed and visible to others within an intersubjective space (Me); the "body image" allows the "body satisfaction/dissatisfaction", the level of satisfaction the subject feels about the body in comparison to societal standards.

A first important characteristic (Galati, Pelle, Berthoz, & Committeri, 2010) of the different body representations described above is that they are both schematic (allocentric) and perceptual (egocentric). The role of the egocentric representations is "pragmatic" (Jeannerod & Jacob, 2005): the representation of an object using egocentric coordinates is required for reaching and grasping. Instead, the role of allocentric representations is "semantic" (Jeannerod & Jacob, 2005): the representation of an object using allocentric coordinates is required for the visual awareness of its size, shape, and orientation.

Another important characteristics of the different body representations involved is that each of them is characterized by a specific disorder (Riva, 2014) that significantly alters the experience of the body (Figure 4.4):

Phantom limb (body schema), the experience of a virtual limb, perceived to occupy body space and/or producing pain;

- *Unilateral hemi-neglect* (spatial body), the experience of not attending the contralesional side of the world/body;
- *Alien hand syndrome* (active body), the experience of having an alien hand acting autonomously;
- *Autoscopic phenomena* (personal body), the experience of seeing a second own body in extrapersonal space;
- *Xenomelia* (objectified body), the non-acceptance of one's own extremities and the resulting desire for elective limb amputation or paralysis;
- *Body dysmorphia* (body image), the experience of having a problem with a specific part of the body.

The features of these disorders suggest a third important characteristics of bodily representations (Melzack, 2005): they are usually produced and modulated by sensory inputs but they can act and produce qualitatively rich bodily experiences even in the absence of any input signal.

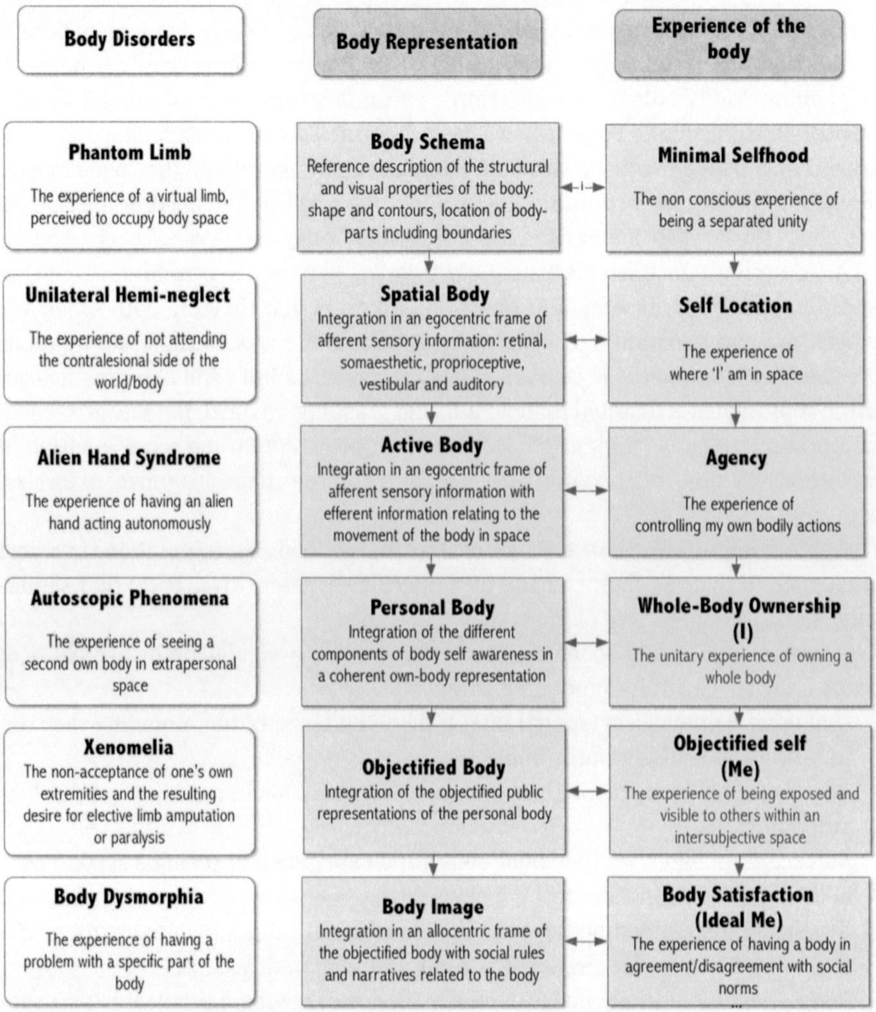
Body Disorders
Body Representation
Experience of the body
Phantom Limb
The experience of a virtual limb, perceived to occupy body space
Body Schema
Reference description of the structural and visual properties of the body: shape and contours, location of body-parts including boundaries
Minimal Selfhood
The non conscious experience of being a separated unity
Unilateral Hemi-neglect
The experience of not attending the contralesional side of the world/body
Spatial Body
Integration in an egocentric frame of afferent sensory information: retinal, somaesthetic, proprioceptive, vestibular and auditory
Self Location
The experience of where 'I' am in space
Alien Hand Syndrome
The experience of having an alien hand acting autonomously
Active Body
Integration in an egocentric frame of afferent sensory information with efferent information relating to the movement of the body in space
Agency
The experience of controlling my own bodily actions
Autoscopic Phenomena
The experience of seeing a second own body in extrapersonal space
Personal Body
Integration of the different components of body self awareness in a coherent own-body representation
Whole-Body Ownership (I)
The unitary experience of owning a whole body
Xenomelia
The non-acceptance of one's own extremities and the resulting desire for elective limb amputation or paralysis
Objectified Body
Integration of the objectified public representations of the personal body
Objectified self (Me)
The experience of being exposed and visible to others within an intersubjective space
Body Dysmorphia
The experience of having a problem with a specific part of the body
Body Image
Integration in an allocentric frame of the objectified body with social rules and narratives related to the body
Body Satisfaction (Ideal Me)
The experience of having a body in agreement/disagreement with social norms

Figure 4.4: The disturbances of bodily self-conciousness

Why? According to Melzack (2005; 2013), the different inputs received by the body-self neuromatrix are then converted in neurosignatures, patterns of brain cell activity (synaptic connections) and chemical releases that serve as the common repository of information about the different contents of our bodily experience in the brain. These neurosignatures, and not the original sensory inputs, are then projected in the "sentient neural hub" (brain areas in the central core of the brainstem) to be converted into a continually changing stream of awareness. In simple words, our experience of the body is not produced directly by sensory inputs, but it is mediated by neurosignatures that are influenced both by cognitive and affective inputs (see Figure 4.2). More, given their representational content – they are a memory of a specific bodily experience (Salt, 2002) – neurosignatures can produce an experience even without a specific sensory input or different time after it appeared (Melzack, 2005):

“When we reach for an apple, the visual input has clearly been synthesized by a neuromatrix so that it has three-dimensional shape, color, and meaning as an edible, desirable object, all of which are produced by the brain and are not in the object “out there.” (p. 88).

4.2.2 First-Person Spatial Images: the Common Code of Bodily Self-Consciousness

A key feature of the body-self neuromatrix is its ability of processing, integrating and generating a wide range of different inputs and patterns: sensory experiences, thoughts, feelings, attitudes, beliefs, memories and imagination. But how does it work? For a long time brain sciences considered action, perception, and interpretation as separate activities. However, recently brain sciences started to describe cognitive processes as *embodied* (J. Prinz, 2006). In this view, perception, execution, and imagination share a common spatial coding in the brain (Hommel, Müsseler, Aschersleben, & Prinz, 2001):

> “Cognitive representations of events (i.e., of any to-be-perceived or to-be-generated incident in the distal environment) subserve not only representational functions (e.g., for perception, imagery, memory, reasoning, etc.) but action-related functions as well (e.g., for action planning and initiation).” (p. 850).

Within this general view, the most important part for our discussion is the one related to the common coding (*Common Coding Theory*): *actions are coded in terms of the perceivable effects they should generate.* More in detail, when an effect is intended, the movement that produces this effect as perceptual input is automatically activated, because actions and their effects are stored in a common representational domain. As underlined by Prinz (1997):

> “Under conditions where stimuli share some features with planned actions, these stimuli tend, by virtue of similarity, either to induce those actions or interfere with them, depending on the structure of the task at hand. This implies that there are certain products of perception on the one hand and certain antecedents of action on the other that share a common representational domain.” (p. 152).

The *Common Coding Theory* may be considered a variation of the *Ideomotor Principle* introduced by William James (1890). According to James, imagining an action creates a tendency to its execution, if no antagonistic mental images are simultaneously present:

> "Every representation of a movement awakens in some degree the actual movement which is its object; and awakens it in a maximum degree whenever it is not kept from doing so by an antagonistic representation present simultaneously in the mind ." (p. 526).

Prinz (1997), suggests that the role of mental images is instead taken by the distal perceptual events that an action should generate. When the activation of a common code exceeds a certain threshold, the corresponding motor codes are automatically triggered.

Further, the *Common Coding Theory* extends this approach to the domain of event perception, action perception, and imitation. The underlying process is the following (Knoblich & Flach, 2003): first, common event representations become activated by the perceptual input; then, there is an automatic activation of the spatial codes attached to these event representations; finally, the activation of the spatial codes results in a prediction of the action results in terms of expected perceptual events on the common coding level.

Giudice and colleagues (2013) recently demonstrated that the processing of spatial representations in working memory is not influenced by its source. It is even possible to combine long-term memory data with perceptual images within an active spatial representation without influencing judgments of spatial relations.

A recent hypothesis is that these different representations can be integrated into an amodal spatial representational format, defined "spatial image" (see Figure 4.5), shared by both perceptual, memory and linguistic knowledge (Baddeley, 2012; Bryant, 1997; Kelly & Avraamides, 2011; Loomis, Klatzky, Avraamides, Lippa, & Golledge, 2007; Wolbers, Klatzky, Loomis, Wutte, & Giudice, 2011). Both Bryant and Loomis identified this representational format in a three-dimensional egocentric coordinate system (Bryant, 1997; Loomis et al., 2007; Loomis, Klatzky, & Giudice, 2013; Loomis, Lippa, Golledge, & Klatzky, 2002), available in the working memory, able to receive its contents both from multiple sensory input modalities (vision, tactile, etc.) and from multiple long-term memory contents (vision, language, etc.).

This vision fits well with the *Convergence Zone Theory* proposed by Damasio (1989). This theory has two main claims.

First, when a physical entity is experienced, it activates feature detectors in the relevant sensory-motor areas. During visual processing of an apple, for example, neurons fire for edges and planar surfaces, whereas others fire for color, configural properties, and movement. Similar patterns of activation in feature maps on other modalities represent how the entity might sound and feel, and also the actions performed on it. Second, when a pattern becomes active in a feature system, clusters of conjunctive neurons (*convergence zones*) in association areas capture the pattern for later cognitive use.

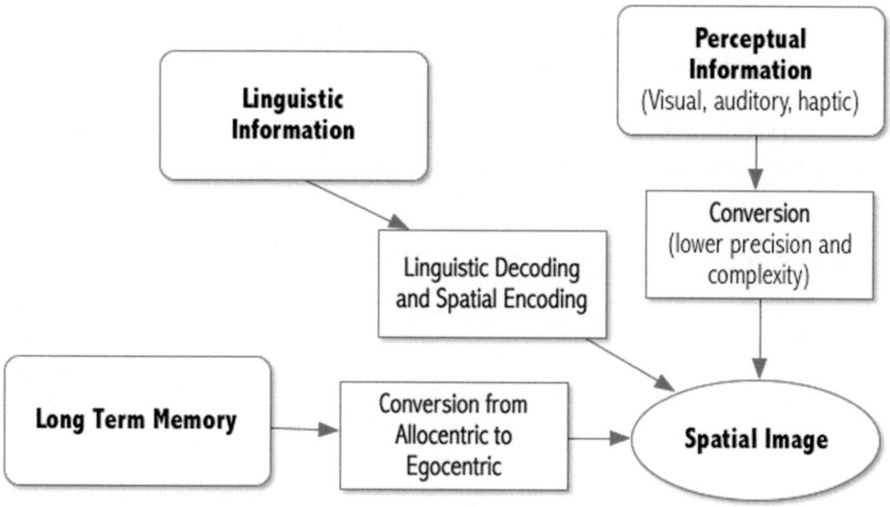

Figure 4.5: The "spatial image" amodal spatial representational format

Damasio assumes the existence of different convergence zones at multiple hierarchical levels, ranging from posterior to anterior in the brain. At a lower level, convergence zones near the visual system capture patterns there, whereas convergence zones near the auditory system capture patterns there. Further, downstream, higher-level association areas in more anterior areas, such as the temporal and frontal lobes conjoin patterns of activation *across* modalities.

In fact, a critical feature of convergence zones underlined by Simmons and Barsalou is *modality-specific re-enactments* (Barsalou, 2003; Simmons & Barsalou, 2003): once a convergence zone captures a feature pattern, the zone can later activate the pattern in the absence of bottom-up stimulation. In particular, the conjunctive neurons play the important role of reactivating patterns (*re-enactment*) in feature maps during imagery, conceptual processing, and other cognitive tasks. For instance, when retrieving the memory of an apple, conjunctive neurons partially reactivate the visual state active during its earlier perception. Similarly, when retrieving an action performed on the apple, conjunctive neurons partially reactivate the motor state that produced it.

According to this view, a fully functional conceptual system can be built on reenactment mechanisms: first, modality-specific sensorimotor areas become activated by the perceptual input (an apple) producing patterns of activation in feature maps; then, clusters of conjunctive neurons (convergence zones) identify and capture the patterns (the apple is red, has a catching size, etc.); later the convergence zone fire to partially reactivate the earlier sensory representation (I want to take a different apple); finally this representation reactivate a pattern of activation in feature maps similar, but not identical, to the original one (re-enactment) allowing the subject to predict the action results.

The final outcome of this vision is the idea of a spatial-temporal framework of virtual objects directly present to the subject: *an inner world simulation in the brain.* As described by Barsalou (2002):

> "In representing a concept, it is as people were being there with one of its instances. Rather than representing a concept in detached isolated manner, people construct a multimodal simulation of themselves interacting with an instance of the concept. To represent the concept they prepare for situated action with one of its instances." (p. 9).

In this view our body, too, can be considered the result of a multimodal simulation. Margaret Wilson clearly underlined (2006):

> "The human perceptual system incorporates an emulator... that is isomorphic to the human body. While it is possible that such an emulator is hard-wired into the perceptual system or learned in purely perceptual terms, an equally plausible hypothesis is that the emulator draws on body-schematic knowledge derived from the observer's representation of his own body." (p. 221).

Different clinical and experimental studies have shown that multimodal information about the body is coded in an egocentric spatial frame of reference (Fotopoulou et al., 2011; Loomis et al., 2013), suggesting that our bodily experience is build up using a first-person spatial code. However, differently from other physical objects, our body is experienced both as object (third-person) – we perceive our body as a physical object in the external world – and as subject (first-person) – we experience our body through different neural representations that are not related to its physical appearance (Legrand, 2010; Moseley & Brugger, 2009). Put differently, simulating the body is more complex than simulating an apple because it requires the integration/translation of both its first- (egocentric) and third-person (allocentric) characteristics (Riva, 2014) in a coherent representation. Knoblich and Flach clearly explained this point (2001):

> "First-person and third-person information cannot be distinguished on a common-coding level. This is because the activation of a common code can result either from one's own intention to produce a certain action effect (first person) or from observing somebody else producing the same effect (third person). Hence, there ought to be cognitive structures that, in addition, keep first- and third-person information apart." (p. 468).

But how do they interact? As suggested by Byrne and colleagues (Byrne, Becker, & Burgess, 2007):

> "Long-term spatial memory is modeled as attractor dynamics within medial temporal allocentric representations, and short-term memory is modeled as egocentric parietal representations driven by perception, retrieval, and imagery and modulated by directed attention. Both encoding

> and retrieval/imagery require translation between egocentric and allocentric representations, which are mediated by posterior parietal and retrosplenial areas and the use of head direction representations in Papez's circuit." (p.340).

Seidler and colleagues (2012) demonstrated the role played by working memory in two different types of motor skill learning – sensorimotor adaptation and motor sequence learning – confirming a critical involvement of this memory in the above interaction process. In general the interaction between egocentric perception and allocentric data happens through the episodic buffer of the working memory and involves all three of its components (Baddeley, 2012; Wen, Ishikawa, & Sato, 2013): verbal, spatial, and visuo-tactile.

4.3 The Impact of Altered Body Self-Consciousness on Health Care

The concept of neuromatrix was originally introduced by Melzack (2005) to explain the pain experience:

> "The neuromatrix theory of pain proposes that the neurosignature for pain experience is determined by the synaptic architecture of the neuromatrix, which is produced by genetic and sensory influences... In short, the neuromatrix, as a result of homeostasis-regulation patterns that have failed, may produce neural "distress" patterns that contribute to the total neuromatrix pattern... Each contribution to the neuromatrix output pattern may not by itself produce pain, but both outputs together may do so." (p. 90).

In his view, pain is a multidimensional experience produced by multiple influences. More, this experience is rooted in our bodily self-consciousness and mediated by a neurological representational system (neurosignatures produced by patterns of synaptic connections) that is the result of cognitive, affective and sensory inputs (see Figure 4.2). In particular, Melzack (2005) suggests that pain is the result of an abnormal representation of some bodily state:

> "Action-neuromodules attempt to move the body and send out abnormal patterns that are felt as shooting pain. The origins of these pains, then, lie in the brain... This suggests that an abnormal, partially genetically determined mechanism fails to turn off the stress response to viral, psychological, or other types of threat to the body-self.." (pp. 91–92).

The actual version of the "body-self neuromatrix" theory (Melzack, 2005) has a high explanatory power and it is able to account for a great deal of the variance found in the different pain related disorders. However, as this model has gained explanatory power, it has lost part of its predictive power: it is so general that it cannot be easily falsified. More, as we have seen previously, current advances in neuroscience suggest an important role played by the representational format of neurosignatures that is barely addressed by the theory.

The focus on the representational format is instead the main feature of the “dual representation theory of posttraumatic stress disorder (PTSD)” (Brewin, 2014; Brewin, Dalgleish, & Joseph, 1996) used to explain the visual intrusions (Brewin, Gregory, Lipton, & Burgess, 2010), sensory experiences of short duration, extremely vivid, detailed, and with highly distressing content, experienced by PTSD patients. According to this theory, patients during the traumatic event encode two different memory representations:

- *Sensory-bound representations* (S-rep): including sensory details and affective/emotional states;
- *Contextual representations* (C-rep): abstract structural descriptions, including the spatial and personal context of the person experiencing the event.

As explained by Brewin and Burgess (2014):

> “In healthy memory the S-rep and C-rep are tightly associated, such that an S-rep is generally retrieved via the associated C-rep. Access to C-reps is under voluntary control but may also occur involuntarily. According to the theory, direct involuntary activation and reexperiencing of S-reps occurs when the S-rep is very strongly encoded, due to the extreme affective salience of the traumatic event, and the C-rep is either encoded weakly or without the usual tight association to the S-rep. This might be due to stress-induced down-regulation of the hippocampal memory system and/or due to a dissociative response to the traumatic event.” (p. 217).

This description has many similarities with the one used by Melzack to explain pain. In both cases an abnormal process fails to turn off the stress response to a threat to the body-self. However, the added value of this theory is provided by the focus on the representational format: the problem is produced by the lack of coherence between two memories of the same event coded in different representational formats.

As we have seen before, the experience of the body is coded in two different formats – schematic (allocentric) and perceptual (egocentric) – that fit well with the descriptions provided by Brewin and colleagues (Brewin et al., 2010): one system encodes stimulus information from an egocentric viewpoint in a form similar to how it was originally experienced, allowing its storing and retrieval (involuntary only) into the episodic memory; the second system uses a set of abstract codes to translate the stimulus information in an allocentric format, allowing its storing and retrieval (both involuntary and voluntary) into the autobiographical memory.

A recent experiment using direct human neural activity recording from neurosurgical patients playing a virtual reality memory game provided a first, but important, evidence that in normal subjects these different representations are integrated in situated conceptualizations and retrieved using multimodal stimuli (from perception to language). In their study Miller and colleagues (2013) found that place-responsive cells (schematic) active during navigation were reactivated during the subsequent recall of navigation-related objects using language.

In the study, subjects were asked to find their way around a virtual world, delivering specific objects (e.g a zucchini) to certain addresses in that world (e.g. a bakery store). At the same time, the researchers recorded the activity in the hippocampus corresponding to specific groups of place cells selectively firing off when the subject was in certain parts of the game map. Using these brain recordings, the researchers were able to develop a neural map that corresponded to the city's layout in the hippocampus of the subject.

Next, the subjects were asked to recall, verbally, as many of the objects, in any order, they had delivered. Using the collected neural maps, the researchers were able to cross- reference each participant's spatial memories as he/she accessed his/her episodic memories of the delivered items (e.g. the zucchini). The researchers found that when the subject named an item that was delivered to a store in a specific region of the map the place cell neurons associated with it reactivated before and during vocalization.

This important experimental result suggests that schematic and perceptual representations are integrated in situated conceptualizations that allows us to represent and interpret the situation we are experiencing (Barsalou, 2013). Once these situated conceptualizations are assembled, they are stored in memory. When cued later, they reinstate themselves through simulation within the respective modalities producing pattern completion inferences (Barsalou, 2003).

In this way, a perceptual information stored in the episodic memory may be retrieved by corresponding emotional states or by sensory cues and modulated by activation of the associated schematic information (Brewin et al., 2010). Alternatively, schematic information may be retreived through language and activate associated perceptual information that provide additional sensory and emotional aspects to retrieval (Brewin et al., 2010).

Interestingly, the interaction between perceptual and schematic information happens both in memory and prospection (Zheng, Luo, & Yu, 2014). As explained by Brewin and colleagues (2010):

> "As part of the process of deliberately simulating possible future outcomes, some individuals will construct images (e.g., of worst possible scenarios) based on information in C-memory and generate images in the precuneus. These images may be influenced by related information held in C-memory or in addition the images may be altered by the involuntary retrieval of related material from S-memory. Novel images may also arise spontaneously in S-memory through processes of association... As a result, internallygenerated images may come to behave much like intrusive memories, being automatically triggered and accompanied by a strong sense of reliving." (p. 222).

In other words, as predicted by the neuromatrix theory, subjects to avoid stress may create new integrated conceptualizations producing simulation and pattern completion inferences that are indistinguishable from the ones closely reflecting actual experience. Considerable evidence suggests that the etiology of different disorders

– including PTSD, eating disorders, depression, chronic pain, phantom limb pain, autism, schizophrenia, Parkinson's and Alzheimer's – may be related to these processes. Specifically, these disorders may be produced by an abnormal interaction between perceptual and schematic contents in memory (both encoding and retrieval) and/or prospection (Brewin et al., 2010; Melzack, 2005; Riva, 2014; Riva, Gaudio, & Dakanalis, 2013; Serino & Riva, 2013, 2014; Zheng et al., 2014) that produces its effect on one or more layers of the bodily self-experience of the subjects.

4.4 The Use of Technology to Modify Our Bodily Self-Consciousness

Recently Riva and colleagues underlined that one of the fundamental objectives for human computer confluence in the coming decade will be to create technologies that contribute to enhancement of happiness and psychological well-being (Botella et al., 2012; Riva, Banos, Botella, Wiederhold, & Gaggioli, 2012; Wiederhold & Riva, 2012). In particular these authors suggested that it is possible to use technology to manipulate the quality of personal experience, with the goal of increasing wellness, and generating strengths and resilience in individuals, organizations and society (Positive Technology). But what is personal experience?

According to *Merriam Webster's Collegiate Dictionary* (http://www.merriam-webster.com/dictionary/experience), it is possible to define experience both as "a: direct observation of or participation in events as a basis of knowledge" (subjective experience) and "b: the fact or state of having been affected by or gained knowledge through direct observation or participation" (personal experience).

However, there is a critical difference between them (Riva, 2012). If subjective experience is the experience of being an intentional subject, personal experience is the experience affecting a particular subject. This difference suggests that, independently from the subjectivity/intentionality of any individual, it is possible to alter the features of our personal experience from outside.

Following the previous broad discussion that clearly identified in bodily self-consciousness the core of our personal experience, we can suggest that bodily self-consciousness may become the dependent variable that may be manipulated by external researchers using technologies to improve health and wellness. But why and how?

In the previous paragraph we suggested that many disorders may be produced by an abnormal interaction between perceptual and schematic contents in memory and/or prospection. A critical feature of the resulting abnormal representation is that in most situation they are not accessible to consciousness and cannot be directly altered. If this happens, the only working approach is to create or strengthen alternative ones (Brewin, 2006). This approach is commonly used by different cognitive-behavioral techniques. For example, the competitive memory training – COMET (Korrelboom, de Jong, Huijbrechts, & Daansen, 2009) has been used to improve low self esteem in individuals with eating disorders. This approach stimulate to retrieve and attend to positive autobiographical memories that are incompatible with low self-esteem by using self-esteem promoting imagery, self-verbalizations, facial and bodily expression, and music.

Another, potentially more powerful approach, is the use of technology for a direct modification of bodily self-consciousness. In general it is possible to modify our bodily self-consciousness in three different ways (Riva et al., 2012; Riva & Mantovani, 2014; Waterworth & Waterworth, 2014):

- *By structuring bodily self-consciousness* through the focus and reorganization of its contents (Mindful Embodiment).
- *By augmenting bodily self-consciousness* to achieve enhanced and extended experiences (Augmented Embodiment).
- *By replacing bodily self-consciousness* with a synthetic one (Synthetic Embodiment).
- The first approach – *mindful embodiment* – aims at helping the modification of our bodily experience by facilitating the availability of its content in the working memory. As we have seen previously, the availability of a spatial image in working memory from perception, language or long term memory, allows its updating (Loomis et al., 2013). Following this different techniques – from Vipassanā-meditation to Mindfulness – use focused attention to become aware of different bodily states (Pagnini, Di Credico, et al., 2014; Pagnini, Phillips, & Langer, 2014) to facilitate their reorganization and change by competing contents. Even if this approach does not necessarily requires technological support, technological tools can improve its effectiveness. For example, Chittaro and Vianello (2014) recently demonstrated that a mobile application could be beneficial in helping users practice mindfulness. The use of the App obtained better results in comparison to two traditional, well-known mindfulness techniques in terms of achieved decentering, level of difficulty and degree of pleasantness.

Another technologically enhanced approach to mindful embodiment is biofeedback: the use of visual or acoustic feedback for representing physiologic parameters like heart frequency or skin temperature to allow their voluntary control (Repetto et al., 2009; Repetto & Riva, 2011).

The second approach – *augmented embodiment* – aims at enhancing bodily self-consciousness by altering/extending its boundaries. As noted by Waterworth and Waterworth (2014), it is possible to achieve this goal through two different methods. The first, that the authors define “altered embodiment”, is achieved by mapping the contents of a sensory channel to a different one. An example of this approach is the “vOICe system” (http://www.seeingwithsound.com) that convert video camera images into sound to enable the blind to navigate the world (and other information) by hearing instead of seeing. The second, that the authors define “extended embodiment", is achieved through the active use of tools. Riva and Mantovani identified two different types of tool-mediated actions (Riva & Mantovani, 2012, 2014): *first-order* or *second-order*:

- *First-order mediated action:* the body is used to control a proximal tool (an artifact present and manipulable in the peripersonal space) to exert an action upon an external object. An example is the videogame player using a joystick (proximal tool) to move an avatar (distal tool) to pick up a sword (external object).
- *Second-order mediated action*: the body is used to control a proximal tool that controls a different distal one (a tool present and visible in the extrapersonal space, either real or virtual) to exert an action upon an external object. An example is the cranemen using a lever (proximal tool) to move a mechanical boom (distal tool) to lift materials (external objects).

In their view, which is in agreement with and supported by different scientific and research data (Balakrishnan & Shyam Sundar, 2011; Blanke, 2012; Clark, 2008; Herkenhoff Carijó, de Almeida, & Kastrup, in press; Jacobs, Bussel, Combeaud, & Roby-Brami, 2009; Slater, Spanlang, Sanchez-Vives, & Blanke, 2010), these two mediated actions have different effects on our spatial and bodily experience (see Figure 4.1):

- *Incorporation:* the proximal tool extends the peripersonal space of the subject;
- *Telepresence*: the user experiences a second peripersonal space centered on the distal tool.

A successfully learned first-order mediated action produces incorporation – the proximal tool extends the peripersonal space of the acting subject. In other words, the acquisition of a motor skill related to the use of a proximal tool extends the body model we use to define the near and far space. From a neuropsychological view point the tool is incorporated in the near space, prolonging it till the end point of the tool. From a phenomenological view point, instead, we are now present in the tool and we can use it intuitively as we use our hands and our fingers.

A successfully learned second-order mediated action, produces incarnation, too – a second body representation centered on the distal tool. In fact, second-order mediated actions are based on the simultaneous handling of two different body models – one centered on the real body (based on proprioceptive data) and a second centered on the distal tool (visual data) – that are weighted in a way that minimizes the uncertainty during the mediated action. In other words, this second peripersonal space centered on the distal tool competes with the one centered on the body to drive action and experience. Specifically, when the distal-centered peripersonal space becomes the prevalent one, it also shifts the extrapersonal space to the one surrounding the distal tool. From an experiential viewpoint the outcome is simple (Riva, Waterworth, Waterworth, & Mantovani, 2011; Waterworth, Waterworth, Mantovani, & Riva, 2010, 2012): the subject experiences presence in the distal environment (telepresence).

A final approach – *synthetic embodiment* – aims at replacing bodily self-consciousness with a synthetic one (incarnation). As also discussed in the chapter by Herbelin and colleagues in this volume, it is possible to use a specific technology – virtual reality (VR) – to reach this goal. But what is VR?

The basis for the VR idea is that a computer can synthesize a three-dimensional (3D) graphical environment from numerical data. Using visual, aural or haptic devices, the human operator can experience the environment as if it were a part of the world. This computer generated world may be either a model of a real-world object, such as a house; or an abstract world that does not exist in a real sense but is understood by humans, such as a chemical molecule or a representation of a set of data; or it might be in a completely imaginary science fiction world.

Usually VR is described as a particular collection of technological hardware. However, given the properties of distal tools described before, we can describe VR as an "embodied technology" for its ability of modifying the feeling of presence (Riva, 2009; Riva et al., 2014): the human operator can experience the synthetic environment as if it were "his/her surrounding world" (*telepresence*) or can experience the synthetic avatar (user's virtual representation) as if it were "his/her own body" (*synthetic embodiment*).

Different authors showed that is possible to use VR both to induce an illusory perception of a fake limb (Slater, Perez-Marcos, Ehrsson, & Sanchez-Vives, 2009) or a fake hand (Perez-Marcos, Slater, & Sanchez-Vives, 2009) as part of our own body, and to produce an out-of-body experience (Lenggenhager et al., 2007), by altering the normal association between touch and its visual correlate. It is even possible to generate a body transfer illusion (Slater et al., 2009): Slater and colleagues substituted the experience of male subjects' own bodies with a life-sized virtual human female body. To achieve synthetic embodiment – the user experiences a synthetic new body – a spatio-temporal correspondence between the multisensory signals and sensory feedback experienced by the user and the visual data related to the distal tool is required. For example, users are embodied in an avatar if the movements of the avatar are temporally synchronized with their own movements and there is a synchronous visuotactile stimulation of their own and avatar's body.

4.5 Conclusions

In this chapter we claimed that the structuration, augmentation and replacement of bodily self-consciousness is at the heart of the research in Human Computer Confluence, requiring knowledge from both cognitive/social sciences and advanced technologies. More, the chapter suggested that this research has a huge societal potential: it is possible to use different technological tools to modify the characteristics of bodily self-consciousness with the specific goal of improving the person's level of well-being.

In the first part of the chapter we explored the characteristics of bodily self-consciousness.

- *Even though bodily self-consciousness is apparently experienced by the subject as a unitary experience, neuroimaging and neurological data suggest that it includes different experiential layers that are integrated in a coherent experience.* First, in the chapter we suggested the existence of six different experiential layers – minimal selfhood, self location, agency, whole-body ownership, objectified self, and body satisfaction – evoving over time by integrating six different representations of the body characterized by specific pathologies – body schema (phantom limb), spatial body (unilateral hemi-neglect), active body (alien hand syndrome), personal body (autoscopic phenomena), objectified body (xenomelia) and body image (body dysmorphia); second, we do not experience these layers separately except in some neurological disorders; third, there is a natural, intermodal communication between them; and fourth, changes in one component can educate and inform other ones (Gallagher, 2005).
- *The different pathologies involving the different bodily representations suggest a critical role of the brain in the experience of the body*: our experience of the body in not direct, but mediated by neurosignatures that are influenced both by cognitive and affective inputs and can produce an experience even without a specific sensory input or different time after it appeared (Melzack, 2005):
- *Neurosignatures share spatial images as a common representational format.* To interact between them, neurosignatures share a common representational code (Loomis et al., 2013): spatial images. Main features of spatial images are: a) they are relatively short-lived and, as such, resides within working memory; b) they are experienced as entities external to the head and body; c) they can be based on inputs from the three spatial senses, from language, and from long term memory; d) they represents space in egocentric coordinates. This suggests that dysfunctions in bodily self-consciousness may arise from two possible sources: a failure in the conversion/update between these representations or errors in perception of spatial relations by a given perceptual/cognitive system (Bryant, 1997).

In the second part of the chapter we discussed how different mental health disorders may be produced by an abnormal interaction between perceptual and schematic contents in memory (both encoding and retrieval) and/or prospection. A critical feature of the resulting abnormal representation is that not always they are accessible to consciousness So, it is possible to counter them only by creating or strengthening alternative ones (Brewin, 2006).

A possible strategy to achieve this goal is using technology. As discussed in the chapter it is possible to modify our bodily self-consciousness in three different ways (Riva et al., 2012; Riva & Mantovani, 2014; Waterworth & Waterworth, 2014):

- *By structuring bodily self-consciousness* through the focus and reorganization of its contents (*Mindful Embodiment*). In this approach individual use focused attention to become aware of different bodily states. Particulary relevant is biofeedback, a technology that use visual or acoustic feedback for representing physiologic parameters like heart frequency or skin temperature.

- *By augmenting bodily self-consciousness* to achieve enhanced and extended experiences (*Augmented Embodiment*). In this approach it is possible to use technology either to map the contents of a sensory channel to a different one, or to extend the boundaries of the body through the incorporation of the tool of the incarnation of the subject in a virtual space (telepresence).
- *By replacing bodily self-consciousness* with a synthetic one (*Synthetic Embodiment*). In this approach it is possible to use virtual reality for creating synthetic avatar (user's virtual representation) experienced by the user as if it were "his/her own body". To achieve synthetic embodiment a spatio-temporal correspondence between the multisensory signals and sensory feedback experienced by the user, and the visual data related to the avatar, is required.

In conclusion, the contents of this chapter constitute a sound foundation and rationale for future researches aimed at the definition and development of technologies and procedures aimed at the structuration, augmentation and replacement of bodily self-consciousness. In particular, the chapter provides the preliminary evidence required to justify future research to identify the most effective technological interventions and the optimal amount of technological support needed for improving our level of well-being.

References

Baddeley, A. (2012). Working memory: theories, models, and controversies. *Annu Rev Psychol, 63*, 1–29.

Balakrishnan, B., & Shyam Sundar, S. (2011). Where Am I? How Can I Get There? Impact of Navigability and Narrative Transportation on Spatial Presence. *Human – Computer Interaction, 26*(3), 161–204.

Barsalou, L.W. (2002). Being there conceptually: Simulating categories in preparation for situated action. In N.L. Stein, P.J. Bauer & M. Rabinowitz (Eds.), *Representation, memory and development: Essays in honor of Jean Mandler* (pp. 1–15). Mahwah, NJ: Erlbaum.

Barsalou, L.W. (2003). Situated simulation in the human conceptual system. *Language and Cognitive Processes, 18*, 513–562.

Barsalou, L.W. (2013). Mirroring as Pattern Completion Inferences within Situated Conceptualizations. *Cortex, 49*(10), 2951–2953.

Bechara, A., & Damasio, A. (2005). The somatic marker hypothesis: A neural theory of economic decision. *Games and Economic Behavior, 52*, 336–372.

Bermúdez, J., Marcel, A.J., & Eilan, N. (1995). *The Body and the Self.* Cambridge, MA: MIT Press.

Blanke, O. (2012). Multisensory brain mechanisms of bodily self-consciousness. [Research Support, Non-U.S. Gov't Review]. Nature reviews. Neuroscience, 13(8), 556–571.

Review]. *Nature reviews. Neuroscience, 13*(8), 556–571.

Botella, C., Riva, G., Gaggioli, A., Wiederhold, B. K., Alcaniz, M., & Banos, R. M. (2012). The present and future of positive technologies. *Cyberpsychology, behavior and social networking, 15*(2), 78–84.

Brewin, C. R. (2006). Understanding cognitive behaviour therapy: A retrieval competition account. *Behav Res Ther, 44*(6), 765–784.

Brewin, C. R. (2014). Episodic memory, perceptual memory, and their interaction: Foundations for a theory of posttraumatic stress disorder. *Psychol Bull, 140*(1), 69–97.

Brewin, C. R., & Burgess, N. (2014). Contextualisation in the revised dual representation theory of PTSD: a response to Pearson and colleagues. *J Behav Ther Exp Psychiatry, 45*(1), 217–219.

Brewin, C. R., Dalgleish, T., & Joseph, S. (1996). A dual representation theory of posttraumatic stress disorder. *Psychol Rev, 103*(4), 670–686.

Brewin, C. R., Gregory, J. D., Lipton, M., & Burgess, N. (2010). Intrusive images in psychological disorders: characteristics, neural mechanisms, and treatment implications. [Research Support, Non-U.S. Gov't

Review]. *Psychological review, 117*(1), 210–232.

Brugger, P., Lenggenhager, B., & Giummarra, M. J. (2013). Xenomelia: a social neuroscience view of altered bodily self-consciousness. *Frontiers in psychology, 4*, 204.

Bryant, D.J. (1997). Representing Space in Language and Perception. *Mind & Language, 12*(3/4), 239–264.

Byrne, P., Becker, S., & Burgess, N. (2007). Remembering the Past and Imagining the Future: A Neural Model of Spatial Memory and Imagery. *Psychological Review, 114*(2), 340–375.

Chittaro, L., & Vianello, A. (2014). Computer-supported mindfulness: Evaluation of a mobile thought distancing application on naive meditators. *International Journal of Human-Computer Studies, 72*(3), 337–348.

Clark, A. (2008). *Supersizing the mind: embodiment, action and cognitive extension*. Oxford, UK: Oxford University Press.

Craig, A. D. (2002). How do you feel? Interoception: the sense of the physiological condition of the body. *Nature Reviews Neuroscience, 3*(8), 655–666.

Craig, A. D. (2003). Interoception: the sense of the physiological condition of the body. *Current Opinion in Neurobiology, 13*(4), 500–505.

Craig, A. D. (2010). The sentient self. *Brain Structure & Function, 214*(5–6), 563–577.

Crossley, N. (2001). *The Social Body: Habit, Identity and Desire*. London: SAGE.

Damasio, A. (1989). Time-locked multiregional retroactivation: a systems-level proposal for the neural substrates of recall and recognition. *Cognition, 33*, 25–62.

Damasio, A. (1994). *Decartes' error: Emotion, reason, and the brain*. New York: Grosset/Putnam.

Damasio, A. (1996). The somatic marker hypothesis and the possible functions of the prefrontal cortex. *Philosophical Transactions of the Royal Society B-Biological Sciences, 351*(1346), 1413–1420.

Damasio, A. (1999). *The Feeling of What Happens: Body, Emotion and the Making of Consciousness*. San Diego, CA: Harcourt Brace and Co, Inc.

Durlik, C., Cardini, F., & Tsakiris, M. (2014). Being watched: The effect of social self-focus on interoceptive and exteroceptive somatosensory perception. *Consciousness and Cognition, 25*, 42–50.

Ferscha, A. (Ed.). (2013). *Human Computer Confluence – The Next Generation Humans and Computers Research Agenda*. Linz: Johannes Kepler University.

Fotopoulou, A., Jenkinson, P. M., Tsakiris, M., Haggard, P., Rudd, A., & Kopelman, M. D. (2011). Mirror-view reverses somatoparaphrenia: Dissociation between first- and third-person perspectives on body ownership. *Neuropsychologia, 49*(14), 3946–3955.

Galati, G., Pelle, G., Berthoz, A., & Committeri, G. (2010). Multiple reference frames used by the human brain for spatial perception and memory. *Exp Brain Res, 206*(2), 109–120.

Gallagher, S. (2005). *How the Body Shapes the Mind*. Oxford.

Garfinkel, S. N., & Critchley, H. D. (2013). Interoception, emotion and brain: new insights link internal physiology to social behaviour. Commentary on: "Anterior insular cortex mediates bodily sensibility and social anxiety" by Terasawa et al. (2012). *Social Cognitive and Affective Neuroscience, 8*(3), 231–234.

Giudice, N.A., Klatzky, R.L., Bennett, C.R., & Loomis, J.M. (2013). Combining Locations from Working Memory and Long-Term Memory into a Common Spatial Image. *Spatial Cognition & Computation: An Interdisciplinary Journal, 13*(2), 103–128.

Herkenhoff Carijó, F., de Almeida, M.C., & Kastrup, V. (in press). On haptic and motor incorporation of tools and other objects. *Phenomenology and the Cognitive Sciences, doi: 10.1007/s11097-012-9269-8.*

Hommel, B., Müsseler, J., Aschersleben, G., & Prinz, W. (2001). The Theory of Event Coding (TEC): A framework for perception and action planning. *Behavioral and Brain Sciences, 24*(5), 849–937.

Jacobs, S., Bussel, B., Combeaud, M., & Roby-Brami, A. (2009). The use of a tool requires its incorporation into the movement: Evidence from stick-pointing in apraxia. *Cortex, 45*(4), 444–455.

James, W. (1890). *The principles of psychology*. New York: Holt.

Jeannerod, M., & Jacob, P. (2005). Visual cognition: a new look at the two-visual systems model. [Review]. *Neuropsychologia, 43*(2), 301–312.

Kelly, J. W., & Avraamides, M. N. (2011). Cross-sensory transfer of reference frames in spatial memory. *Cognition, 118*(3), 444–450.

Knoblich, G., & Flach, R. (2001). Predicting the effects of actions: Interactions of perception and action. *Psychological Science, 12*(6), 467–472.

Knoblich, G., & Flach, R. (2003). Action identity: Evidence from self-recognition, prediction, and coordination. *Consciousness and Cognition, 12*, 620–632.

Korrelboom, K., de Jong, M., Huijbrechts, I., & Daansen, P. (2009). Competitive memory training (COMET) for treating low self-esteem in patients with eating disorders: A randomized clinical trial. *J Consult Clin Psychol, 77*(5), 974–980.

Legrand, D. (2010). Subjective and physical dimensions of bodily self-consciousness, and their dis-integration in anorexia nervosa. [Research Support, Non-U.S. Gov't]. *Neuropsychologia, 48*(3), 726–737.

Lenggenhager, B., Tadi, T., Metzinger, T., & Blanke, O. (2007). Video ergo sum: manipulating bodily self-consciousness. *Science, 317*(5841), 1096–1099.

Loomis, J.M., Klatzky, R.L., Avraamides, M.N., Lippa, Y., & Golledge, R.G. (2007). Functional equivalence of spatial images produced by perception and spatial language. In F. Mast & L. Jancke (Eds.), *Spatial processing in navigation, imagery, and perception* (pp. 29–48). New York: Springer.

Loomis, J.M., Klatzky, R.L., & Giudice, N.A. (2013). Representing 3D space in working memory: Spatial images from vision, hearing, touch, and language. In S. Lacey & R. Lawson (Eds.), *Multisensory Imagery* (pp. 131–155). New York: Springer.

Loomis, J.M., Lippa, Y., Golledge, R.G., & Klatzky, R.L. (2002). Spatial updating of locations specified by 3-d sound and spatial language. *J Exp Psychol Learn Mem Cogn, 28*(2), 335–345.

Melzack, R. (1999). From the gate to the neuromatrix. *Pain*, S121–S126.

Melzack, R. (2005). Evolution of the Neuromatrix Theory of Pain. The Prithvi Raj Lecture: Presented at the Third World Congress of World Institute of Pain, Barcelona 2004. *Pain Practice, 5*(2), 85–94.

Melzack, R., & Katz, J. (2013). Pain. *Wiley Interdisciplinary Reviews-Cognitive Science, 4*(1), 1–15.

Miller, J. F., Neufang, M., Solway, A., Brandt, A., Trippel, M., Mader, I., et al. (2013). Neural activity in human hippocampal formation reveals the spatial context of retrieved memories. *Science, 342*(6162), 1111–1114.

Moseley, G. L., & Brugger, P. (2009). Interdependence of movement and anatomy persists when amputees learn a physiologically impossible movement of their phantom limb. *Proc Natl Acad Sci U S A, 106*(44), 18798–18802.

Pagnini, F., Di Credico, C., Gatto, R., Fabiani, V., Rossi, G., Lunetta, C., et al. (2014). Meditation training for people with amyotrophic lateral sclerosis and their caregivers. *J Altern Complement Med, 20*(4), 272–275.

Pagnini, F., Phillips, D., & Langer, E. (2014). A mindful approach with end-of-life thoughts. *Front Psychol, 5*, 138.

Perez-Marcos, D., Slater, M., & Sanchez-Vives, M. V. (2009). Inducing a virtual hand ownership illusion through a brain-computer interface. *Neuroreport, 20*(6), 589–594.

Pfeiffer, C., Lopez, C., Schmutz, V., Duenas, J. A., Martuzzi, R., & Blanke, O. (2013). Multisensory origin of the subjective first-person perspective: visual, tactile, and vestibular mechanisms. *PLoS One, 8*(4), e61751.

Prinz, J. (2006). Putting the brakes on Enactive Perception. *PSYCHE, 12*(1), 1–12; online: http://psyche.cs.monash.edu.au.

Prinz, W. (1997). Perception and action planning. *European Journal of Cognitive Psychology, 9*(2), 129–154.

Repetto, C., Gorini, A., Vigna, C., Algeri, D., Pallavicini, F., & Riva, G. (2009). The use of biofeedback in clinical virtual reality: the INTREPID project. *J Vis Exp*(33).

Repetto, C., & Riva, G. (2011). From virtual reality to interreality in the treatment of anxiety disorders. *Neuropsychiatry, 1*(1), 31–43.

Riva, G. (2009). Is presence a technology issue? Some insights from cognitive sciences *Virtual Reality, 13*(3), 59–69.

Riva, G. (2012). Personal experience in positive psychology may offer a new focus for a growing discipline. *American Psychologist, 67*(7), 574–575.

Riva, G. (2014). Out of my real body: cognitive neuroscience meets eating disorders. *Front Hum Neurosci, 8*, 236.

Riva, G., Banos, R. M., Botella, C., Wiederhold, B. K., & Gaggioli, A. (2012). Positive technology: using interactive technologies to promote positive functioning. *Cyberpsychology, behavior and social networking, 15*(2), 69–77.

Riva, G., Gaudio, S., & Dakanalis, A. (2013). I'm in a virtual body: a locked allocentric memory may impair the experience of the body in both obesity and anorexia nervosa. *Eating and weight disorders: EWD*.

Riva, G., & Mantovani, F. (2012). From the body to the tools and back: a general framework for presence in mediated interactions. *Interacting with Computers, 24*(4), 203–210.

Riva, G., & Mantovani, F. (2014). Extending the Self through the Tools and the Others: a General Framework for Presence and Social Presence in Mediated Interactions. In G. Riva, J. A. Waterworth & D. Murray (Eds.), *Interacting with Presence: HCI and the sense of presence in computer-mediated environments* (pp. 12–34). Berlin: De Gruyter Open – Online: http://www.presence-research.com.

Riva, G., & Waterworth, J. A. (2014). Being present in a virtual world. In M. Grimshaw (Ed.), *The Oxford Handbook of Virtuality* (pp. 205–221). New York: Oxford University Press.

Riva, G., Waterworth, J. A., & Murray, D. (2014). *Interacting with Presence: HCI and the sense of presence in computer-mediated environments*. Berlin: De Gruyter Open – Online: http://www.presence-research.com.

Riva, G., Waterworth, J.A., Waterworth, E.L., & Mantovani, F. (2011). From intention to action: The role of presence. *New Ideas in Psychology, 29*(1), 24–37.

Salt, W. (2002). *Irritable Bowel Syndrome and The Mind Body Connection*. Columbus, OH: Parkview Publishing.

Seidler, R. D., Bo, J., & Anguera, J. A. (2012). Neurocognitive contributions to motor skill learning: the role of working memory. *J Mot Behav, 44*(6), 445–453.
Serino, S., & Riva, G. (2013). Getting lost in Alzheimer's disease: a break in the mental frame syncing. *Medical Hypotheses, 80*(4), 416–421.
Serino, S., & Riva, G. (2014). What is the role of spatial processing in the decline of episodic memory in Alzheimer's disease? The "mental frame syncing" hypothesis. [Perspective]. *Frontiers in Aging Neuroscience, 6*(33), 1–7.
Shilling, C. (2012). *The Body & Social Theory*. London: SAGE.
Simmons, K.W., & Barsalou, L.W. (2003). The similarity-in-topography principle: reconciling theories of conceptual deficits. *Cognitive Neuropsychology, 20*, 451–486.
Slater, M., Perez-Marcos, D., Ehrsson, H. H., & Sanchez-Vives, M. V. (2009). Inducing illusory ownership of a virtual body. *Front Neurosci, 3*(2), 214–220.
Slater, M., Spanlang, B., Sanchez-Vives, M. V., & Blanke, O. (2010). First person experience of body transfer in virtual reality. *PLoS One, 5*(5), e10564.
Slaughter, V., & Brownell, C. (Eds.). (2012). *Early development of body representations*. Cambridge, UK: Cambridge University Press.
Tsakiris, M., Hesse, M. D., Boy, C., Haggard, P., & Fink, G. R. (2007). Neural signatures of body ownership: a sensory network for bodily self-consciousness. *Cereb Cortex, 17*(10), 2235–2244.
Tsakiris, M., Longo, M. R., & Haggard, P. (2010). Having a body versus moving your body: neural signatures of agency and body-ownership. [Research Support, Non-U.S. Gov't]. *Neuropsychologia, 48*(9), 2740–2749.
Vogeley, K., & Fink, G. R. (2003). Neural correlates of the first-person-perspective. *Trends Cogn Sci, 7*(1), 38–42.
Waterworth, J.A., & Waterworth, E.L. (2014). Altered, expanded and distributed embodiment: the three stages of interactive presence. In G. Riva, J. A. Waterworth & D. Murray (Eds.), *Interacting with Presence: HCI and the sense of presence in computer-mediated environments* (pp. 36–50). Berlin: De Gruyter Open–Online: http://www.presence-research.com.
Waterworth, J.A., Waterworth, E.L., Mantovani, F., & Riva, G. (2010). On Feeling (the) Present: An evolutionary account of the sense of presence in physical and electronically-mediated environments. *Journal of Consciousness Studies, 17*(1–2), 167–178.
Waterworth, J.A., Waterworth, E.L., Mantovani, F., & Riva, G. (2012). Special Issue: Presence and Interaction. *Interacting with Computers, 24*(4), 190–192.
Wen, W., Ishikawa, T., & Sato, T. (2013). Individual Differences in the Encoding Processes of Egocentric and Allocentric Survey Knowledge. *Cognitive Science, 37*(1), 176–192.
Wiederhold, B.K., & Riva, G. (2012). Positive technology supports shift to preventive, integrative health. *Cyberpsychology, behavior and social networking, 15*(2), 67–68.
Wilson, M. (2006). Covert Imitation. In G. Knoblich, I.M. Thornton, M. Grosjean & M. Shiffrar (Eds.), *Human body perception from the inside out* (pp. 211–228). New York: Oxford University Press.
Wolbers, T., Klatzky, R.L., Loomis, J.M., Wutte, M.G., & Giudice, N.A. (2011). Modality-independent coding of spatial layout in the human brain. *Curr Biol, 21*(11), 984–989.
Zheng, H., Luo, J., & Yu, R. (2014). From memory to prospection: The overlapping and the distinct components between remembering and imagining. *Frontiers in psychology, 5*(856).

Bruno Herbelin, Roy Salomon, Andrea Serino and Olaf Blanke

5 Neural Mechanisms of Bodily Self-Consciousness and the Experience of Presence in Virtual Reality

Abstract: Recent neuroscience research emphasizes the embodied origins of the experience of the self. This chapter shows that further advances in the understanding of the phenomenon of VR-induced presence might be achieved in connection with advances in the understanding of the brain mechanisms of bodily self-consciousness. By reviewing the neural mechanisms that make the virtual reality experience possible and the neurocognitive models of bodily self-consciousness, we highlight how the development of applied human computer confluence technologies and the fundamental scientific investigation of bodily self-consciousness benefit from each other in a symbiotic manner.

Keywords: Bodily Self-consciousness, Presence, Virtual Reality, Out-of-body Experience, Agency, Body Ownership, Self-location.

5.1 Introduction

The ultimate goal of virtual reality (VR) is to produce the authentic experience of being 'present' in an artificial environment. To achieve this, VR technologies have been classically conceived within a cybernetic approach, placing the human subject at the core of a feedback control loop where multi-media technologies substitute all interaction with the external world. Pioneers of VR began to describe this 'presence' as the "illusion of non-mediation" (Lombard & Ditton, 1997) or the "suspension of disbelief" (Slater & Usoh, 1993), which occurs when the subject reports a transfer of presence from reality to the immersive virtual environment. This is directly linked to the mechanisms by which our experience of being a self in the world, termed bodily self-consciousness, is constructed using multisensory information.

The study of bodily self-consciousness has been based on the findings from altered experiences of the self, such as out of body experiences (OBE). During an OBE, a subject (or self) experiences states in which he/she feels as though he/she occupies a spatial location separated from that of his/her own physical body and perceives the world from a disembodied perspective. Alterations in bodily self-consciousness, whether of neurological origin or induced experimentally, shed light on the components and mechanisms that structure our natural and typical sense of presence. We suggest here that the presence in VR relies on these mechanisms, and as such, one should consider scientific insights about bodily self-consciousness and its neural origins in order to understand how presence in a virtual environment can be achieved.

This chapter aims to bridge the VR development and the neuroscience of self-consciousness by showing that VR profits from concepts and knowledge developed in cognitive neuroscience, which help us understand and perfect the technology that gives rise to presence in VR environments. Additionally, it highlights that cognitive neuroscience benefits from the unique opportunities offered by VR technologies to manipulate perception and consciousness and study the brain mechanisms underlying self-consciousness.

We first illustrate the close association of the origins of tele presence technologies with altered forms of self-consciousness. We then discuss attempts to establish models of presence in virtual reality and neurocognitive models of bodily self-consciousness. Finally, we conclude by examining the reciprocal relationship between these fields and consider the direction of future interactions.

5.2 Tele-Presence, Cybernetics, and Out-of-Body Experience

The possibility to experience tele-presence in a distant or even an artificial reality was first realized when the technologies of video transmission and computer graphics allowed individuals to wear displays mounted on the head and see pictures of a world captured at another location – or through fully generated by a mathematical computer model. Howard Rheingold experimented with this idea in Dr. Tashi's Laboratory (Tsukuba, Japan, in 1990) with a remotely controlled robotic head and head mounted displays (HMD). At one point, turning his head as he was looking through the robot's eyes, the cameras installed inside the robot caused the robot to turn toward his physical body. Speaking of the body he saw, Rheingold said; "He looked like me and abstractly I could understand that he was me, but I know who me is, and me is here. He, on the other hand, was there. It doesn't take a high degree of verisimilitude to create a sense of remote presence" (Rheingold, 1991). Rheingold concluded, "What you don't realize until you do it is that tele-presence is a form of out-of-the-body experience."

It may not come as a surprise that we owe the invention of the head-mounted graphical displays in 1963 to a brilliant engineer and scientist Marvin Minsky who had an out of body experience. He indeed revealed, "One day, at age 17, I was walking alone at night during a snowstorm in a singularly quiet place. I noticed that the ground looked further away than usual, and then it seems that I was looking down from a height of perhaps 10 meters, watching myself crossing the field" (reported in Grossinger, 2006). Minsky, a pioneer in cybernetics and artificial intelligence, was a highly influential thinker since the invention of tele-presence and immersion systems. Following the cybernetic principles in which a person can be considered an 'entity' reacting to 'inputs' through 'output' channels, it was hypothesized that an ultimate and total mediation of all the input-output channels would lead to a replacement of what a person perceives as being their environment. In other words, a person could be fooled into believing that the experienced situation is real if his/her mind cannot detect any discrepancy between the expected and the mediated outcome of their actions (e.g., the head-camera feedback-loop that Rheingold experienced). Using VR systems, which consider the human "senses as channels to the mind" and the "body as a communication device" (Biocca, 1997), it became possible to explore cyberspace and to contemplate a generalization of Minsky's idea of tele-presence in a distant location (Minsky, 1980) to the broader concept of presence in an immersive virtual environment. Pioneers in VR soon observed that users of virtual reality systems "are in a world other than where their real bodies are located" (Slater & Usoh, 1992) and that they experience the troubling "sense of being" in a non-existing environment (Heeter, 1992). Interestingly, these accounts resemble Rheingold's reference to an artificial form of "out-of-the-body experience" (Rheingold, 1991).

What exactly are out-of-body experiences (OBE) of neurological origin? An OBE is an autoscopic phenomenon during which people have the impression of having left their body, of floating above it, and of observing it from outside. During an OBE, one is subjected to a displacement of their point of view out of the boundaries of the physical body. OBEs may occur during epileptic seizures, but they have also been observed in other neurological or psychiatric conditions. They may also occur in neurologically healthy individuals. OBEs have even been directly evoked by administering electrical stimulation to the brain during the treatment of an epileptic patient, specifically at the right angular gyrus (Blanke, Landis, Spinelli, & Seek, 2002). Blanke and colleagues proposed that an OBE involves an alteration in bodily self-consciousness (BSC) caused by selective deficits in integrating multisensory body-related information into a coherent neural representation of one's body and of its position in extrapersonal space (Blanke, Landis, Spinelli, & Seek, 2004; Blanke, 2012). In the normally functioning brain, self-consciousness arises at different levels, ranging from the "the very simple (the automatic sense that I exist separately from other entities) to the very complex (my identity, complete with a variety of biographical details)" (Damasio, 2003). Blanke and Metzinger (2009) described a low-level account of the bodily self and termed it minimal phenomenal selfhood. Focusing on the experience of the bodily self, minimal phenomenal selfhood comprises three main components, (i) self-identification with the body as a whole (rather than ownership of body parts), (ii) self-location, and (iii) the first person perspective (1PP). Using this concept, an OBE can be described as an incoherence in the integration of 1PP, self-identification, and self-location. Interestingly, the alteration of the three components of BSC also applies to the description of tele-presence phenomenon reported by Rheingold. A similar parallel can also be drawn between autoscopic hallucinations (the experience of viewing one's own body in extracorporeal space) and multimedia setups (an example of which is "Video Place", an interactive installation created by Krueger in 1985 where people play with interactive video silhouettes of themselves).

Apart from pathological cases of altered bodily self-consciousness, such as OBE and autoscopic hallucinations that may strike us as rather strange phenomena (see also heautoscopy and feeling-of-a-presence; Lopez et al., 2008; Heydrich, Blanke, & Brain, 2013), it might seem quite astonishing that in most instances, we experience a presence inside a body and rarely question how this is achieved. Similarly, the experience of being in the world that is perceived from the perspective of the body (1PP) is rarely challenged in reality. It is only under the artificial mediation of perception induced by VR technologies that a subject questions the limits of the natural and usual experience of self-consciousness. What makes the condition of tele-presence induced by VR interesting as a phenomenon is the intangibility of those limits, with an experience of presence (almost) as authentic as that experienced in reality on the one hand and an unusual experience closer to an actual OBE on the other hand. As such, trying to understand the presence in virtual reality is similar to investigating the ability of the brain to integrate artificial perceptions into a coherent representation. As such, presence might better be described "as an immediate feeling produced by some fundamental evaluation by the brain of one's current circumstances" (Slater, 2009) or as the "neuropsychological phenomenon evolved from the interplay of our biological and cultural inheritance" (Riva, Waterworth, & Waterworth, 2004).

5.3 Immersion, Presence, Sensorimotor Contingencies, and Self-Consciousness

In the previous section, we highlighted similarities between the experience of tele-presence in VR and the neurological phenomenon of OBEs, suggesting a stronger link between VR research on presence and neuroscientific research on self-consciousness. In the next section, we first consider more recent developments regarding the experience of presence in the context of VR and then focus on neuroscience research elucidating its neural mechanisms.

As mentioned in Lombard and Jones (2007), various terms have been used to discuss the concept of presence in the 1800 articles, which the authors reviewed over more than twenty years. Today, the terminology benefits from these decades of refinement based on which several terms have been distinctively identified. In particular, Slater defined 'immersion' as the ability of a VR system to induce an experiential displacement of a person inside what is called an immersive virtual environment (Slater, 2003). Presence should be distinguished from immersion and considered more correctly as "a 'response' to a system of a certain level of immersion" (Slater, 2003). Compared to Lombard and Ditton's (1997) original conception of presence as the "perceptual illusion of non-mediation" or to the previous definition "suspension of disbelief" proposed by Slater and Usoh (1993), this distinction between immersion and presence disuntangle the concept of presence as an experience from the technological and artificial substrates that are used to generate it.

Later, Slater introduced two concepts with an aim to establish two levels of presence (Slater, 2009), the place illusion (PI) and the plausibility illusion (Psi). The PI phenomenon is arising directly from the integration of multiple cues from the virtual environment, whereas the Psi is the result of higher-level cognitive processes accepting a virtual scenario as plausible and therefore potentially real. The PI may therefore be more closely related to different bottom-up levels of sensorimotor immersion generated by VR, whereas the Psi acts on specific cognitive mechanisms. These distinctions are fundamental for engineers to evaluate the immersive power of their systems and for researchers to target how to generate a more substantial experience of presence. Importantly, it is generally accepted that the key mechanism for generating the PI is the implementation of a set of sensorimotor contingencies (SCs) supported by the virtual environment. Thus, the corresponding set of valid actions available to the user corresponds to a given sensory feedback, and it is implemented as action-effect feedback loops. It is useful for programmers of VR simulation systems to understand that the feedback loop is not simply a design pattern but a necessary condition for SCs, as the richness and extent of the SCs contribute to the experience by augmenting the PI level in response to the subject's exploration of the virtual environment.

To explain with greater concision its separate experiential states, Riva and Waterworth described the presence in VR as a three-level hierarchical process (Riva, Waterworth & Waterworth, 2004); (i) the proto-presence, i.e., an embodied presence related to the level of perception-action coupling, (ii) the core presence emerging from conscious and selective activity in order to integrate sensory occurrences into coherent percepts, and (iii) the extended presence linking the current core-presence to the past experience in a way that challenges the significance of the lived experience. Riva and Waterworth's different levels of presence in VR closely correspond to the 'layers of the self' proposed by Damasio (1999), i.e., the proto-self (to which the proto-presence corresponds), the core-self (the core-presence in VR), and the autobiographical self (the extended presence in VR). To situate these levels of presence within the general picture of VR, Riva and Waterworth introduced additional dimensions of focus, locus, and sensus (Riva, Waterworth & Waterworth, 2004; see also Waterworth & Waterworth, 2001). "Focus can be seen as the degree to which the three layers of presence are integrated toward a particular situation" and is maximal "when the three levels are working in concert", i.e., proto, core, and extended presence are coherent. The locus dimension or "the extent to which the observer is attending to the real world or to a world conveyed through the media" is more about contrasting the virtual to the physical world. Finally, sensus (defined as "the level of consciousness or attentional arousal of the observer") denotes one's awareness of 'feeling present' during immersion, and it is also referred to as the sense of presence (SoP). Estimations of SoP through questionnaire have been proposed as a mean to quantify presence (see review Herbelin, 2005). However, in the same way in which "participants know that nothing is 'really' happening, and they can consciously decide to modify their automatic behavior accordingly" (Slater, 2009), participants are made aware of the artificial nature of their feeling of presence in VR and evaluate it in comparison with what they think it should be in reality. To avoid this bias, a direct approach based on low-level bodily experience, as studied in cognitive science of self-consciousness, seems preferable.

This refinement of the concept of presence highlights its experiential nature and thus its link to aspects of consciousness, particularly bodily self-consciousness. To address this link further, we review selected findings on bodily self-consciousness and its neural underpinnings.

5.4 Presence and Bodily Self-Consciousness

A system based purely on sensory-motor contingencies cannot account for the experiential nature of presence. The experience of 'being here' (in a physical reality or in VR) implies that a *subject* is having this experience. According to Damasio (1999), the minimal level of experience, also defined as the "core consciousness", arises at the interplay between two components, "the organism" and "the object". Thus, a pre-reflexive, non-verbal representation of the "organism" as the subject of experience, which Damasio conceptualized as the Self (i.e., the "core Self"), precedes any experience. Recent research in neuroscience has suggested a systematic relationship between the subject of experience and the specific representations of the body in the brain. We experience the world from the physical location and with an egocentric perspective of the body, which we feel as our own. The concept of minimal phenomenal selfhood corresponds to such a proposal of the embodied self (Blanke and Metzinger, 2009) and of bodily self-consciousness (Blanke, 2012).

According to a prominent view in neuroscience, the embodied self is characterized by two major aspects of bodily experience, i) the sense of agency, i.e., the subjective experience of being the author of one's own actions, and ii) the sense of ownership, the feeling that this body is mine (Gallagher, 2000; van den Bos & Jeannerod, 2002). Both may be selectively impaired by neurological and psychiatric disorders. For example, in somatoparaphrenia (typically occurs following right parietal brain damage), patients feel that their contralesional hand is not their own (Vallar & Ronchi, 2009). In the 'Anarchic Hand' syndrome, patients feel a loss of volitional control over their hand while maintaining ownership (Della Sala, 1998). The double dissociations observed in these disorders support the notion that agency and ownership rely on separate brain mechanisms. On the one hand, the brain seeks correspondence between internally generated motor commands and the re-afferent sensory feedback caused by their consequences. Some neuroscientists believe that this correspondence is crucial for generating the experience of being the agent of the movement. On the other hand, our brain also constantly receives and integrates multisensory information from different parts of our body, and the integration of these different multisensory body-related signals is assumed an important mechanism for generating body ownership.

Recent developments in VR have captured these basic mechanisms of bodily self-consciousness and used them to introduce a new and potentially more powerful account of VR experience, the sense of embodiment. Kilteni, Groten, and Slater (2012) defined it as "the ensemble of sensations that arise in conjunction with being inside, having, and controlling a body". Accordingly, the sense of embodiment is generated in conjunction with the sense of agency, the sense of body ownership, and the sense of self-location. The latter is defined as a position in space where the self is experienced to be, according to the model of bodily self-consciousness by Blanke and Metzinger (2009). Kilteni and colleagues suggested that, "self-location refers to one's spatial experience of being inside a body, and it does not refer to the spatial experience of being inside a world"; thus, it may be that self-location does not entirely correspond to the place illusion. Although different, sense of presence and sense of embodiment certainly share most mechanisms described above. It has even been proposed that the sense of embodiment "potentially includes the presence subcomponent" (Kilteni, Groten, & Slater, 2012).

Research on cognitive neuroscience has shown that critical concepts in the VR field, such as presence and sense of embodiment, are better understood in terms of neural mechanisms of bodily self-consciousness. Critical components of bodily self-consciousness are associated with integrated sensorimotor and multisensory body-related signals, generating agency, body ownership, self-location, and the first person perspective (see Blanke & Metzinger, 2009; Blanke, 2012). In the next sections, we will review major achievements in neuroscience that support this view, starting with studies on agency and following with research on body ownership and self-location.

5.4.1 Agency

The predominant model that reflects our sense of agency is often referred to as the "forward model". Following the original idea of Von Helmholtz (1866), it posits that when we make a movement, our sensorimotor systems generate an "efferent copy" of that movement, i.e., an internal representation of the sensory consequences of the planned movement (Wolpert, Ghahramani & Jordan, 1995). This internal representation is compared to the actual re-afferent sensory inputs related to the action (e.g., visual, proprioceptive). Under normal conditions, the sensory feedback matches signals predicted by the efferent copy, and such a match generates the attribution of the action to oneself, i.e., the sense of agency (Blakemore & Frith, 2003; Jeannerod, 2006). To experimentally test the sense of agency, neuroscientists have introduced systematic perturbations of the sensory (mostly visual) feedback for movements (Georgieff & Jeannerod, 1998). Early experiments on agency used ingenious manipulations, employing mirrors to achieve visuo-motor discrepancies, such as in the classical paradigm proposed by Nielsen (1963), which indicated, for the first time, the dissociation between the unconscious monitoring of our hand motor actions and our sense of agency for them.

While mirror based paradigms contributed to our initial understanding of the sensorimotor mechanisms underlying the sense of agency, the advent of computer and video technology gave rise to novel possibilities to test sensorimotor mismatch. As the control of digitally represented outcomes (such as cursor movements) entered many research laboratories, several paradigms utilizing these new sensorimotor contingencies appeared. The use of computers allowed the introduction of precise and well controlled deviations between motor actions and their visual outcomes and made it possible to precisely test the effect on the attribution of those actions to the self (David et al., 2007; Salomon, Szpiro-Grinberg & Lamy, 2011). For example, Farrer and colleagues (2007) joined such conflicts with functional magnetic resonance imaging (fMRI) to study brain activity in participants while controlling the movement of a circle along a T shaped path. In some trials, the participants had full control over the movement of the circle while in other trials, the computer controlled the shown trajectory. The results showed that when the participants felt in control over the reproduced movement, this was associated with the activation of the insular cortex, an area that processes and integrates several bodily-related signals (Craig, 2009; Tsakiris et al., 2007). When the participants felt no control over the movement, a different region was activated, specifically, the right inferior parietal cortex. This region has been related to many spatial functions, particularly to self-attribution of actions (Salomon, Malach, & Lamy, 2009; Tsakiris, Longo & Haggard, 2010) and awareness of one's own actions (Lau et al., 2004; Sirigu et al., 2004). Moreover, lesions to this region may lead to loss of agency, as in the anarchic hand syndrome (Bundick & Spinella, 2000). These and other findings are consistent with the observation that the inferoparietal cortex is responsible (together with areas not reviewed here, such as the supplementary motor area and the cerebellum) for capturing discrepancies between the efferent copy and the actual sensory consequence of actions, thus for monitoring action attribution (Chaminade & Decety, 2002; David, Newen, & Vogeley, 2008; Farrer et al., 2003; Farrer et al., 2007).

Other paradigms based on live and recorded video images of movements have also been employed to study the mechanisms underlying self-attribution of actions (Farrer et al., 2008; Sirigu et al. 1999; Tsakiris et al., 2005). In a classic experiment, Van de Bos and Jeannerod asked participants to make one of several possible hand gestures and showed them, by means of a video setup, their own hand or that of an experimenter making the same or a different gesture. Additionally, the presented hands were also rotated, such that the participants or experimenter's hand could appear to be facing down, up, left or right (van den Bos & Jeannerod, 2002; see also Kannape et al., 2010, 2012). Their results indicated that when the participant and experimenter made different actions, almost no self-attribution errors occurred. However, when the actions were identical, the spatial orientation of the hand served as a strong cue for self-attribution of that action to the self or the other – that is when the hand of the experimenter was shown in the same posture and from the same perspective as one's own hand, participants more frequently misattributed that hand to themselves. Thus, although action-based self-attribution related to the forward model, proprioceptive and spatial cues strongly affected self-judgments of the depicted actions when dynamic cues were non-informative.

Technological advances allowing more controlled manipulation of sensorimotor contingencies, such as computer-based control of the visual consequences of actions and real time video presentations, have increased our understanding of the sense of agency. The advantages inherent in these methods have now been combined with those of VR. Modern VR, including full body motion tracking and realistic avatar modeling, offer an optimal environment to study the sense of agency and body ownership as well as their effect on presence. For instance, Salomon and colleagues (2013) used a visual search task with multiple full body avatars animated in real time, with one avatar mimicking the participants' movements precisely while the others movements are spatially or temporally deviated. The participants had to find the avatar moving in accordance with their own movements among the distractor avatars when their movements were self-initiated or when being moved passively by the experimenter. The results showed that during self-initiated trials, the participants detected the self-avatar more rapidly, even when more distractor avatars were present.

Finally, VR has allowed studies to be extended beyond specific limb representations into full body representations of action in space. In a full body version of Nielsen's and Jeannerod's agency experiments, Kanappe and colleagues used full body tracking and avatar animation to test agency of locomotion. The results showed that we have limited conscious monitoring of our locomotive actions, indicating the limits of agency for full body motion (Kannape et al., 2010; see also Mentzer et al., 2010 for a related paradigm using auditory-motor conflicts). Once again, the relationship between technological advances in video and VR and the study of the sense of agency highlights the symbiosis between the study of the self and the emulation of self-related processes in virtual environments.

5.4.2 Body Ownership and Self-Location

The findings of the sense of agency over one's own movements, however, does not sufficiently account for the experience of the embodied self, in particular of body ownership. Simply consider the example that another person is lifting your arm. You perceive no sense of agency, but a preserved sense of body ownership. Research has shown that the subjective feeling that this hand and body is mine originates from the integration of different sensory cues. This is difficult to test experimentally because of the complexity of manipulating the experience of one's own body. In research on the awareness for external events, researchers can manipulate the sensory features of external stimuli and then measure the effects of such manipulations on perceptual and neural mechanisms. In the case of body ownership, however, such a classical experimental approach is much more difficult for the simple reason, which is that the body is always present to the subject, as William James noticed. Some of the first insights on bodily self-consciousness arose from Ambroise Paré's description in 1551 of the illusory presence of a missing limb, i.e., the 'phantom limb' experience frequently reported by amputee patients. Phantom limb phenomenon shows that the brain can generate the experience of a limb and body ownership (because phantom limbs generally are experienced as own limbs) even if the respective body part is absent. Neuroscientists, more than 400 years later, were able to experimentally reproduce an analogous phenomenon, i.e., extending the sense of bodily ownership to an artificial object. In the so-called "rubber hand illusion", synchronous stroking of a seen fake hand and of one's own unseen (real) hand cause the fake hand to be attributed to the subject's body ("I feel like it is my hand"; Botvinick & Cohen, 1998; Ehrsson et al., 2007; Tsakiris & Haggard, 2005). The rubber hand illusion is also associated with a misperception of the position of the participant's own hand relative to the fake hand and even with changes in the physiology of one's own hand. For instance, if a harmful stimulus suddenly approaches the rubber hand while the illusion occurs, subject's skin conductance response increases (neurophysiological marker of increased arousal to a threat, see Armel & Ramachandran, 2003; Ehrsson et al., 2007). Others have reported a reduction in temperature of the real limb 'perceptually' substituted by the rubber hand (Moseley, Olthof et al., 2008). Sanchez-Vives and colleagues demonstrated the rubber hand illusion in VR by showing that illusory ownership of an artificial hand could be obtained when a virtual hand, instead of a rubber hand, is presented in a virtual environment (Sanchez-Vives et al., 2010). VR provided Evans and Blanke (2012) with the ability to induce illusory hand ownership in a systematic and computer-controlled manner, thus allowing for the simultaneous recording of high-density EEG, revealing that illusory ownership and motor imagery share the same neural substrates in fronto-parietal areas of the brain. Neuroimaging techniques, such as fMRI (Ehrsson et al., 2007; Tsakiris et al., 2007), transcranial magnetic stimulation (TMS; Kammers et al., 2009; Tsakiris et al., 2008), and electroencephalography (EEG, Kanayama et al., 2007), have been applied to study the neural correlates of the rubber hand illusion, pointing to a fronto-parietal network of brain areas involving the premotor cortex and the posterior parietal cortex, which normally integrate multisensory stimuli (somatosensory, visual, auditory) occurring on or close to the body. The experience of ownership of the rubber hand is also associated with activity in the (predominantly right) insular cortex, an area receiving multiple sensory inputs from 'exteroceptive' senses as well as from 'interoceptive' channels monitoring internal body states (Craig, 2009). These neuroimaging results are important in showing that body ownership is obtained though activation of brain regions that integrate multisensory body-related signals to construct multiple representations of one's own body.

The paradigm generating the rubber hand illusion has also been extended to face perception. In the so-called 'enfacement' illusion, viewing another person's face being touched while feeling touch on one's own face results in perceiving the other person's face as similar to one's own (see Apps & Tsakiris, 2013 for a review; Sforza et al., 2008; Tsakiris et al., 2008). Showing a change in the perception of one' own face following such short sensory stimulation is particularly interesting, as one's own face is the part of the body that most strongly defines one's own visual identity and is shown to others during social interactions (Rochat & Zahavi, 2011). Self-face recognition is considered an important component of self-consciousness, such that self-face recognition in the mirror-test is considered a hallmark of self-consciousness in non-human species and in human infants (see, e.g., Gallup, 1970; Povinelli, 2001). A recent fMRI study investigating the neural correlates of the enfacement illusion has shown that it is generated by modulation of activity in the right temporo-parietal junction and intraparietal sulcus, areas that normally integrate multisensory body-related information (Apps et al., 2013).

Thus, an abundance of evidence from both the rubber hand illusion and enfacement illusion has contributed to the establishment of some of the mechanisms which allow manipulating BSC. Specifically, synchronous multisensory inputs related to a part of the real body and to an artificial replacement of that body part activate brain areas, which normally integrate multisensory information related to one's own body. Such stimulations induce an extension of the limits of BSC from the physical body to its artificial or virtual replacement. However, although these studies have important contributions to the understanding of BSC, they focus on separate (body part centered) representations of the body. On the contrary, a fundamental feature of self-consciousness is that it is characterized by the experience of a single and coherent whole body rather than of multiple separated body parts. For this reason, Blanke (2012) proposed the concept of self-identification in order to reflect full-body ownership, as opposed to the feeling of ownership of single body parts. Lenggenhager and colleagues (2007) used VR technology to study this global aspect of BSC experimentally. In what it is referred to as the full body illusion, subjects see a virtual body (avatar) placed 2 meters in front of them while being stroked on their back (Lenggenhager et al., 2007). When the viewed and felt stroking is synchronous, participants report perceiving the virtual body as their own (change in self-identification) and feel displacement toward the virtual body (change in self-location). Other variants of the full-body illusion have been reported. For instance, in the so-called body swap illusion, participants observe, via head-mounted display and the first-person perspective, a mannequin being stroked on its chest, which is congruent with a stroking of their own chest (Ehrsson, 2007; Petkova & Ehrsson, 2008). When interviewed about such experience, participants scored high on questions such as, "I had the impression that the fake body was my own body", and they physiologically reacted strongly to harmful stimuli approaching the fake body (Petkova & Ehrsson, 2008).

Ionta, Heydrich, and colleagues (2011) used fMRI to study the neural mechanism of the full body illusion. They showed that self-location induced by synchronous stroking of the virtual body and of one's own body activated the temporo-parietal junctions (TPJ). Interestingly, the focus of TPJ activity found in fMRI was close to the area of brain damage in nine patients suffering OBEs of neurological origin. Further, functional connectivity analyses of the fMRI data showed that right and left TPJ are bilaterally connected to the supplementary motor area, ventral premotor cortex, insula, intraparietal sulcus, and occipito-temporal cortex and that changes in self-location modulated brain activity among right TPJ, right insula, and right supplementary motor area and between left TPJ and right insula (Ionta, Martuzzi et al., 2014). These recent data, together with the previously reviewed neuroimaging studies (see also Serino et al., 2013), point to an extended network of multisensory areas underlying BSC, which involve premotor and posterior parietal cortices as well as the temporal parietal junction and the insula, predominantly in the right hemisphere.

5.5 Conclusion

The early VR developments were based on the concepts from cybernetics, that is, an artificial system which would be capable of emulating sensory inputs, thus removing the person from his/her true environment and placing him/her into an artificial one. This view initiated the quest for fully immersive systems, which would surround entirely the human body and its senses, transporting people into 'cyberspace'. These technological developments in sensing, display, and immersion technologies have since evolved symbiotically with research on the cognitive mechanisms of presence.

The present selective review of recent literature in neurology and neuroscience of bodily self-consciousness crucially highlights how new technologies have enabled experimental manipulations that contribute to the understanding of bodily self-consciousness and therefore of presence itself. In particular, these technologies offer novel methodological approaches, and they have provided researchers in neuroscience with unprecedented experimental opportunities for approaching high level and complex mechanisms of self-consciousness, such as agency, body ownership, and self-location. Research on these aspects of embodiment and bodily self-consciousness, and the neural underpinnings of both, have been investigated in the last 15 years, and are beginning to contribute to our understanding of the mechanisms of presence in VR. For instance, although the VR community has highlighted sensorimotor contingency as the prominent factor for presence, neuroscience research shows that multisensory integration of bodily signals is also critical for the presence, embodiment, and related aspects of bodily self-consciousness.

As illustrated throughout this chapter, research on the cognitive neuroscience of bodily self-consciousness is gradually merging with the investigation of presence in VR. Neurological observations of altered bodily self-consciousness (employing VR technologies) might eventually lead to a better understanding of self-consciousness in its most basic form, arising when the "I" of the conscious self declares to be present at a given place. While a definitive model of presence is yet to be achieved, cognitive neuroscience has enriched the field with novel paradigms, allowing qualification and quantification of the multisensory integrative mechanisms with which bodily self-consciousness is constructed. This model of how the mind gives rise to our presence in the world promises to introduce original perspectives for approaching immersive embodiment systems.

When observing the increasing complex nature of human-computer confluence technologies, it appears that the evolution of research on the presence in VR can be seen as a precursor of how interactions within the digital world should be considered using a neurological perspective and how they may eventually shape our bodily self.

Acknowledgements: The VERE project (FP7-ICT-2009-5, Project 257695) and the industrial grant EPFL-WInvestments 'RealiSM' provided support for this work.

References

Apps, M. A., & Tsakiris, M. (2013). The free-energy self: A predictive coding account of self-recognition. *Neuroscience & Biobehavioral Reviews* . 85–97. doi: 10.1016/j.neubiorev.2013.01.029.

Apps, M. A., Tajadura-Jiménez, A., Sereno, M., Blanke, O., & Tsakiris, M. (2013). Plasticity in unimodal and multimodal brain areas reflects multisensory changes in self-face identification. *Cerebral Cortex*, 25, 46–55.

Armel, K. C., & Ramachandran, V. S. (2003). Projecting sensations to external objects: evidence from skin conductance response. *Proceedings. Biological Sciences, The Royal Society*, 270(1523), 1499–1506.

Barnsley, N., McAuley, J. H., Mohan, R., Dey, A., Thomas, P., & Moseley, G. L. (2011). The rubber hand illusion increases histamine reactivity in the real arm. Current Biology, 21(23), 945–946.

Blakemore, S. J., & Frith, C. (2003). Self-awareness and action. *Current Opinion in Neurobiology*, 13(2), 219–224.

Blanke, O. (2012). Multisensory brain mechanisms of bodily self-consciousness. *Nature Review Neuroscience*, 13(556–571).

Blanke, O., Ortigue, S., Landis, T., & Seeck, M. (2002). Stimulating illusory own-body perceptions. *Nature*, 419(6904), 269–270.

Blanke, O., Landis, T., Spinelli, L., & Seeck, M. (2004). Out-of-body experience and autoscopy of neurological origin. *Brain: A Journal of Neurology*, 127(Pt 2), 243–258.

Blanke, O., & Metzinger, T. (2009). Full-body illusions and minimal phenomenal selfhood. *Trends in Cognitive Sciences*, 13(1), 7–13.

Botvinick, M., & Cohen, J. (1998). Rubber hands "feel" touch that eyes see. *Nature*, 391(6669).

Bremmer, F., Schlack, A., Shah, N. J., Zafiris, O., Kubischik, M., Hoffmann, K.-P., et al. (2001b). Polymodal Motion Processing in Posterior Parietal and Premotor Cortex: A Human fMRI Study Strongly Implies Equivalencies between Humans and Monkeys. *Neuron*, 29(1), 287–296.

Bundick, T., & Spinella, M. (2000). Subjective experience, involuntary movement, and posterior alien hand syndrome. *Journal of Neurology, Neurosurgery & Psychiatry*, 68(1), 83–85.

Chaminade, T., & Decety, J. (2002). Leader or follower? Involvement of the inferior parietal lobule in agency. *NeuroReport*, 13(15), 1975.

Craig, A. D. B. (2009). How do you feel – now? The anterior insula and human awareness. *Nature Reviews Neuroscience*, 10(1) 59-70.

Damasio, A. (1999). The feeling of what happens: body, emotion and the making of consciousness. San Diego: Harcourt Brace.

Damasio, A. (2000). The feeling of what happens: Body and emotion in the making of consciousness: Harvest Books.

Damasio, A. (2003). Mental self: The person within. *Nature*, 423(6937), 227.

David, N., Bewernick, B., Cohen, M., Newen, A., Lux, S., Fink, G., . . . Vogeley, K. (2006). Neural representations of self versus other: visual-spatial perspective taking and agency in a virtual ball-tossing game. *Journal of cognitive neuroscience*, 18(6), 898–910.

David, N., Cohen, M., Newen, A., Bewernick, B., Shah, N., Fink, G., & Vogeley, K. (2007). The extrastriate cortex distinguishes between the consequences of one's own and others' behavior. *Neuroimage*, 36(3), 1004–1014.

David, N., Newen, A., & Vogeley, K. (2008). The "sense of agency" and its underlying cognitive and neural mechanisms. *Consciousness and Cognition*.

Della Sala, C. M. (1998). Disentangling the alien and anarchic hand. *Cognitive Neuropsychiatry*, 3(3), 191–207.

di Pellegrino, G., Ladavas, E., & Farne, A. (1997). Seeing where your hands are. *Nature*, 388(6644), 730.

Ehrsson, H. H. (2007). The experimental induction of out-of-body experiences. *Science* 317, 1048–1048.

Evans, N. and Blanke, O. (2012). Shared electrophysiology mechanisms of body ownership and motor imagery. *NeuroImage* 204, 2016–228.

Farne, A., & Ladavas, E. (2000). Dynamic size-change of hand peripersonal space following tool use. *Neuroreport*, 11(8), 1645–1649.

Farrer, C., Franck, N., Georgieff, N., Frith, C., Decety, J., & Jeannerod, M. (2003). Modulating the experience of agency: a positron emission tomography study. *Neuroimage*, 18(2), 324–333.

Farrer, C., Frey, S. H., Van Horn, J. D., Tunik, E., Turk, D., Inati, S., & Grafton, S. T. (2008). The Angular Gyrus Computes Action Awareness Representations. *Cerebral Cortex*, 18(2), 254–261.

Fink, G., Marshall, J., Halligan, P., Frith, C., Driver, J., Frackowiak, R., & Dolan, R. (1999). The neural consequences of conflict between intention and the senses. *Brain*, 122(3), 497.

Fogassi, L., Gallese, V., Fadiga, L., Luppino, G., Matelli, M., & Rizzolatti, G. (1996). Coding of peripersonal space in inferior premotor cortex (area F4). *Journal of Neurophysiology*, 76(1), 141–157.

Gallagher, S. (2000). Philosophical conceptions of the self: Implications for cognitive science. *Trends in Cognitive Sciences*, 4(1), 14–21.

Gallup, G.G. (1970). Chimpanzees: self-recognition. *Science* 167(3914), 86-87

Gentile, G., Petkova, V. I., & Ehrsson, H. H. (2011). Integration of visual and tactile signals from the hand in the human brain: an FMRI study. *Journal of Neurophysiology*, 105(2), 910–922.

Georgieff, N., & Jeannerod, M. (1998). Beyond consciousness of external reality: a "who" system for consciousness of action and self-consciousness. *Consciousness and Cognition*, 7(3), 465–477.

Grossinger, R. (2006). Migraine Auras: When the Visual World Fails. North Atlantic Books.

Heeter, C. (1992). Being there: the subjective experience of presence. *Presence: Teleoperators and Virtual Environments*, 1(2), 262–271.

Herbelin, B. (2005). Virtual Reality Exposure Therapy of Social Phobia. Ph.D. thesis No 3351, Virtual Reality Laboratory, School of Computer and Communication Sciences, École Polytechnique Fédérale de Lausanne, Lausanne.

Heydrich, L., & Blanke, O. (2013). Distinct illusory own-body perceptions caused by damage to posterior insula and extrastriate cortex. *Brain : A Journal of Neurology*, 136(Pt 3), 790-803.

Ionta, S., Heydrich, L., Lenggenhager, B., Mouthon, M., Fornari, E., Chapuis, D., Gassert, R and Blanke, O. (2011). Multisensory mechanisms in temporo-parietal cortex support self-location and first-person perspective. *Neuron*, 70(2), 363–74.

Ionta, S., Martuzzi, R., Salomon, R., & Blanke, O. (2014). The brain network reflecting bodily self-consciousness: a functional connectivity study. *Social Cognitive and Affective Neuroscience* 9, 1904-1913.

Jeannerod M. Motor cognition: What actions tell the Self. (2006). Oxford University Press.

Kammers, M. P. M., Verhagen, L., Dijkerman, H. C., Hogendoorn, H., De Vignemont, F., & Schutter, D. J. L. G. (2009). Is this hand for real? Attenuation of the rubber hand illusion by transcranial magnetic stimulation over the inferior parietal lobule. *Journal of Cognitive Neuroscience*, 21(7), 1311–1320.

Kanayama, N., Sato, A., & Ohira, H. (2007). Crossmodal effect with rubber hand illusion and gamma-band activity. *Psychophysiology*, 44(3), 392-402.

Kannape, O., Schwabe, L., Tadi, T., & Blanke, O. (2010). The limits of agency in walking humans. *Neuropsychologia*, 48(6), 1628–1636.

Kilteni, K., Groten, R., & Slater, M. (2012). The Sense of Embodiment in Virtual Reality. *Presence: Teleoperators and Virtual Environments*, 21(4), 373–387.

Krueger, M. W., Gionfriddo, T., & Hinrichsen, K. (1985). VIDEOPLACE – an artificial reality. *ACM SIGCHI Bulletin* 16(4), 35–40

Ladavas, E., di Pellegrino, G., Farne, A., & Zeloni, G. (1998). Neuropsychological evidence of an integrated visuotactile representation of peripersonal space in humans. *J Cogn Neurosci*, 10(5), 581–589.

Ladavas, E., & Serino, A. (2008). Action-dependent plasticity in peripersonal space representations. *Cognitive Neuropsychology*, 25(7–8), 1099–1113.

Lau, H. C., Rogers, R. D., Haggard, P., & Passingham, R. E. (2004). Attention to intention. *Science* 303(5661), 1208–1210. doi:10.1126/science.1090973

Lenggenhager, B., Tadi, T., Metzinger, T., Blanke, O. (2007). Video ergo sum: manipulating bodily self-consciousness. *Science* 317, 1096–1099.

Lenggenhager, B., Tadi, R. T. S., Metzinger, T. and Blanke, O. (2007b). Response to: “Virtual reality and telepresence”. *Science* 318 (5854), 1241–1242.

Lombard, M., & Ditton, T. (1997). At the Heart of It All: The Concept of Presence. *Journal of Computer-Mediated Communication*, 3(2).

Lombard, M., & Jones, M. T. (2007). Identifying the (Tele) Presence Literature. *PsychNology Journal*, 5(2), 197–206.

Lopez, C., Halje, P., & Blanke, O. (2008). Body ownership and embodiment: Vestibular and multisensory mechanisms. *Neurophysiologie Clinique*, 38(3), 149–161.

Minsky, M. (1980). Telepresence. *Omni*, 2(9), 45–51.

Moseley, G. L., Olthof, N., Venema, A., Don, S., Wijers, M., Gallace, A., & Spence, C. (2008). Psychologically induced cooling of a specific body part caused by the illusory ownership of an artificial counterpart. *Proceedings of the National Academy of Sciences of the United States of America*, 105(35), 13169–13173.

Nielsen, T. I. (1963). Volition: A new experimental approach. *Scandinavian journal of psychology*, 4(1), 225–230.

Petkova, V. I., Ehrsson, H. H. (2008). If I were You: perceptual illusion of body swapping. *PLoS ONE* 3, e3832.10.1371/journal.pone.0003832.

Povinelli D.J. (2991). The Self: Elevated in consciousness and extended in time. In Moore C, Lemmon K (Eds.). The self in time: Developmental perspectives. Pp. 73–94. Cambridge University Press.

Ramachandran, V. S., & Rogers-Ramachandran, D. (1996). Synaesthesia in phantom limbs induced with mirrors. *Proceedings of the Royal Society of London. Series B: Biological Sciences*, 263(1369), 377–386.

Rheingold, H. (1991). Virtual Reality: Exploring the Brave New Technologies. Simon & Schuster Adult Publishing Group.

Riva, G., Waterworth, J. A., & Waterworth, E. L. (2004). The layers of presence: a bio-cultural approach to understanding presence in natural and mediated environments. *Cyberpsychology & Behavior*: The Impact of the Internet, Multimedia and Virtual Reality on Behavior and Society, 7(4), 402–416.

Riva, G. (2008). Presence and Social Presence: From Agency to Self and Others. Proc. 11th International Workshop on Presence, Padova (IT), 16–18 Oct. 2008, pp. 66–72.

Rochat P, Zahavi D. (2011). The uncanny mirror: a re-framing of mirror self-experience. *Conscious Cogn*. 20(2):204–13.

Salomon, R., Lim, M., Kannape, O., Llobera, J., & Blanke, O. (2013). "Self pop-out": agency enhances self-recognition in visual search. *Experimental brain research*, 1–9.

Salomon, R., Malach, R., & Lamy, D. (2009). Involvement of the Intrinsic/Default System in Movement-Related Self Recognition. *PLoS ONE*, 4(10), e7527.

Salomon, R., Szpiro-Grinberg, S., & Lamy, D. (2011). Self-Motion Holds a Special Status in Visual Processing. *PLoS ONE*, 6(10), e24347. doi: 10.1371/journal.pone.0024347

Sanchez-Vives, M. V., & Slater, M. (2005). From presence to consciousness through virtual reality. *Nature Reviews Neuroscience*, 6(4), 332–339.

Serino, A., Alsmith, A,, Costantini, M., Mandrigin, A., Tajadura-Jimenez, A., Lopez, C. (2013). Bodily ownership and self-location: components of bodily self-consciousness, *Consciousness and Cognition*, 22(4):1239–1252.

Sirigu, A., Daprati, E., Pradat-Diehl, P., Franck, N., & Jeannerod, M. (1999). Perception of self-generated movement following left parietal lesion. *Brain*, 122(10), 1867–1874.

Sirigu, A., Daprati, E., Ciancia, S., Giraux, P., Nighoghossian, N., Posada, A., & Haggard, P. (2004). Altered awareness of voluntary action after damage to the parietal cortex. *Nature Neuroscience*, 7(1), 80–84.

Sforza A, Bufalari I, Haggard P, Aglioti SM. (2010). My face in yours: Visuo-tactile facial stimulation influences sense of identity. *Soc Neurosci*. 2010;5(2):148–162.

Slater, M. (2003). A note on Presence terminology. *Presence-Connect*, 3(1). Jan. 2003. On-line: http://presence.cs.ucl.ac.uk/presenceconnect/.

Slater, M. (2009). Place illusion and plausibility can lead to realistic behaviour in immersive virtual environments. *Philosophical Transactions of the Royal Society of London. Series B, Biological Sciences*, 364(1535), 3549–3557.

Slater, M., & Usoh, M. 1993. Representations systems, perceptual position, and presence in immersive virtual environments. *Presence: Teleoperators and Virtual Environments,* 2(3), 221–233.

Tsakiris M. (2008). Looking for myself: current multisensory input alters self-face recognition. *PLoS One*. 3(12):e4040.

Tsakiris, M., & Haggard, P. (2005). The rubber hand illusion revisited: visuotactile integration and self-attribution. *Journal of Experimental Psychology. Human Perception and Performance*, 31(1).

Tsakiris, M., Haggard, P., Franck, N., Mainy, N., & Sirigu, A. (2005). A specific role for efferent information in self-recognition. *Cognition*, 96(3), 215–231.

Tsakiris, M., Hesse, M. D., Boy, C., Haggard, P., & Fink, G. R. (2007). Neural signatures of body ownership: A sensory network for bodily self-consciousness. *Cerebral Cortex*, 17(10), 2235–2244.

Tsakiris, M., Longo, M. R., & Haggard, P. (2010). Having a body versus moving your body: Neural signatures of agency and body-ownership. [doi: DOI: 10.1016/j.neuropsychologia.2010.05.021]. *Neuropsychologia*, 48(9), 2740–2749.

Vallar, G., & Ronchi, R. (2009). Somatoparaphrenia: a body delusion. A review of the neuropsychological literature. *Experimental brain research*, 192(3), 533–551.

van den Bos, E., & Jeannerod, M. (2002). Sense of body and sense of action both contribute to self-recognition. *Cognition*, 85(2), 177–187.

von Helmholtz, H. (1866). Handbuch der Physiologischen Optik, Leipzig: Leopold Voss.

Waterworth, J. A., & Waterworth, E. L. (2001). Focus, Locus, and Sensus: The three dimensions of virtual experience. *Cyberpsychology and Behavior*, 4(2), 203–213.

Waterworth J.A. & Waterworth E.L. (2008). Presence in the Future. Proc. 11th International Workshop on Presence, Padova (IT), 16–18 Oct. 2008, pp. 61–65.

Waterworth, J. A., & Waterworth, E. L. (2006). Presence as a Dimension of Communication: Context of Use and the Person. Chapter 4 in G. Riva, M.T. Anguera, B.K. Wiederhold and F. Mantovani (Eds.) From Communication to Presence: Cognition, Emotions and Culture towards the Ultimate Communicative Experience. IOS Press, Amsterdam, 2006, http://www.emergingcommunication.com.

Wolpert, D. M., Ghahramani, Z., & Jordan, M. I. (1995). An internal model for sensorimotor integration. *Science*, 269(5232), 1880.

Andrea Gaggioli

6 Transformative Experience Design

Abstract: Until now, information and communication technologies have been mostly conceived as a mean to support human activities – communication, productivity, leisure. However, as the sophistication of digital tools increases, researchers are starting to consider their potential role in supporting the fullfilment of higher human needs, such as self-actualization and self-transcendence. In this chapter, I introduce Transformative Experience Design (TED), a conceptual framework for exploring how next-generation interactive technologies might be used to support long-lasting changes in the self-world. At the center of this framework is the elicitation of transformative experiences, which are experiences designed to facilitate an epistemic expansion through the (controlled) alteration of sensorial, perceptual, cognitive and affective processes.

Keywords: Transformative Experience, Complex Systems, Virtual Reality, Neuroscience, Art

6.1 Introduction

I have experienced several transformative moments in my life. The first that comes to my mind occurred when I was as young adolescent, as I watched the movie "Dead Poets Society". Another transformative moment occurred when I was in my twenties, as I first surfed the web using the then-popular Netscape Navigator browser. In both circumstances, I felt that I was discovering new truths about myself and new purpose in life. These experiences deeply affected my perspective on the world, changing my values and beliefs. Simply put, after these experiences I was not the same person I had been before. Retrospectively, I can say that without these milestone experiences, I would probably not be the person I am today.

How do transformative experiences occur? Do they play a role in our personal development? And if they do, can we design technologies that support them?

Throughout time and across cultures, human beings have developed a number of transformative practices to support personal growth. These include, for example, meditation, hypnosis, and several techniques to induce altered states of consciousness (Tart, 1972). However, other media such as plays, storytelling, imagery, music, films and paintings can also be regarded as possibile means to elicit transformative experiences (Gaylinn, 2005).

In the rest of this chapter, I will introduce Transformative Experience Design (TED) as a new conceptual framework for the design of self-actualization experiences. In the theoretical introduction, I draw on the existing literature to argue three key theses that are central to the development of TED. First, a transformative experience is a sudden and profound change in the self-world, which has peculiar phenomenological features that distinguish it from linear and gradual psychological change. Second, a transformative experience has an epistemic dimension and a personal dimension: not only it changes what you know, it also changes how you experience being yourself. Third, a transformative experience can be modelled as an emergent phenomenon that results from complex self-organization dynamics. In the methodological section that follows, I build up on these conceptual pillars to explore possible principles and ways in which transformative experiences may be invited or elicited combining interactive technologies, cognitive neuroscience and art.

6.2 Transformation is Different From Gradual Change

Most experiences of everyday life are mundane and tend to be repeated over time. However, in addition to these ordinary moments, there exists a special category of experiences – transformative experiences – which can result in profound and longlasting restructuration of our worldview (Miller & C'de Baca, 2001). The characteristics of these experiences, which can take the form of an epiphany or a sudden insight, are reported to be remarkably consistent across cultures. Their phenomenological profile often encompasses a perception of truth, a synthesis of conflicting ideas and emotions, and a new sense of order and beauty. A further distinguishing feature of a transformative experience is a perception of discontinuity between the present and the past self, in terms of beliefs, character, identity, and interpersonal relationships. By virtue of this radical transformation of the self-world, the individual can find new meaning in life, turning his view in a totally new direction. Despite the abundance of historical, anthropological and psychological evidence of the occurrence of transformative experiences across cultures, these moments represent one of the least understood mechanism of human change (C'De Baca & Wilbourne, 2004).

William James pioneered the exploration of transformative experience while examining the phenomenon of religious conversions. In his work *The Varieties of Religious Experience* (James, 1902), he distinguished two types of conversions: a volitional type, in which "the regenerative change is usually gradual, and consists in the building up, piece by piece, of a new set of moral and spiritual habits" (p. 189), and a self-surrender type, unconscious and involuntary, in which "the subconscious effects are more abundant and often startling" (p. 191). According to James, the self-surrender type is characterized by an intense struggle toward an aspiration that is perceived as true and right, as well as a resistance to its actualization; this struggle is eventually resolved when the person "surrenders" (i.e., stop resisting).

Abraham Maslow introduced the term "peak experience" to describe a moment of elevated inspiration and enhanced well-being (Maslow, 1954). According to Maslow, a peak experience can permanently affect one's attitude toward life, even if it never happens again. However, differently from James, Maslow noted that peak experiences are not necessarily mystical or religious in the supernaturalistic sense. To investigate the characteristics of peak experiences, Maslow examined personal interviews, personal reports and surveys of mystical, religious and artistic literature (Maslow, 1964). This analysis generated a list of characterizing features of peak experiences, including disorientation in space and time; ego transcendence and self-forgetfulness; a perception that the world is good, beautiful, and desirable; feeling passive, receptive, and humble; a sense that polarities and dichotomies have been transcended or resolved; and feelings of being lucky, fortunate, or graced. After a peak experience, the individual may have enjoy several beneficial effects, including a more positive view of the self, other people, and the world, as well as renewed meaning in life. Maslow contended that peak experiences are perceived as a state of great value and significance for the life of the individual and play a chief role in the self-actualization process. According to Maslow, self-actualization refers to "the desire for self-fulfillment" or "the desire to become more and more what one is, to become everything that one is capable of becoming" (1954, pp. 92–93). Maslow considered self-actualization to be the universal need for personal growth and discovery that is present throughout a person's life (Maslow, 1962b). He argued that self-actualization is the apex of the motivation hierarchy, and it can be achieved only after the lower needs – physiological, safety, love and belongingness, and esteem needs – have been reasonably satisfied (Maslow, 1962a). As he noted: "When we are well and healthy and adequately fulfilling the concept 'Human Being' then experiences of transcendence should in principle be commonplace" (p. 32). Maslow (1954) identified the following key characteristics of self-actualized individuals: accurate, unbiased perception of reality; greater acceptance of the self and the others; nonhostile sense of humor; spontaneity; task centering; autonomy; need for privacy; sympathy for humankind; intimate relationships with a few, specially loved people; democratic character structure; discrimination between means and ends; creativeness; resistance to enculturation; and peak experience. He argued that peak experiences can help people to change and grow, overcome emotional blocks, and achieve a stronger sense of identity and fulfillment. According to Maslow, peak experiences can be triggered by specific settings and activities, such as listening to music, being in nature (particularly in association with water, wild animals, sunsets, and mountains), meditation, prayer, deep relaxation, and physical accomplishment (Maslow, 1964).

A common characteristic of peak experiences is that they often involve a heightened sense of *awe*, a multifaceted emotion in which fear is blended with astonishment, admiration and wonder. Despite the fact that awe is not included as one of Eckman's basic emotions (Coghlan, Buckley, & Weaver, 2012; Ekman, 1992), this feeling has been regarded as a "foundational human experience that defines the human existence" (Schneider, 2011). In a seminal article, Keltner and Haidt (Keltner & Haidt, 2003) identified two prototypical elicitors of awe: *perceived vastness* (something that is experienced as being much larger than the self's ordinary frame of reference) and a *need for accommodation*, defined as an "inability to assimilate an experience into current mental structures" (p. 304). Accommodation refers to the Piagetian process of adjusting cognitive schemas that cannot assimilate a new experience (Piaget & Inhelder, 1969). According to Keltner and Haidt, accomodation can be either successful, leading to an enlightening experience (associated with an expansion of one's frame of reference); or unsuccessful (when one fails to understand), leading to terrifying and upsetting feelings. Keltner and Haidt suggest that nature, supernatural experiences, and being in the presence of powerful or celebrated individuals are frequent elicitors of awe; however, human arts and artifact – such as songs, symphonies, movies, plays, paintings and architectural buildings (skyscrapers, cathedrals, etc.) are also able to induce this feeling. According to Keltner and Haidt, awe is more likely to occur in response to highly unusual or even magical or impossible objects, scenes or events, or in response to products that provide the spectator with novel ways of viewing things. Shiota, Keltner, and Mossman (Shiota, Keltner, & Mossman, 2007) found that awe is elicited by different kinds of experiences, the most common of which are experiences of natural and artistic beauty, and of exemplary or exceptional human actions or abilities. Keltner and Haidt believe that the study of awe has important scientific and societal implications, since its transformative potential can reorient individuals' lives, goals, and values. Furthermore, these authors hold that a better comprehension of how awe is induced could be of help in definining new methods of personal change and growth (Keltner & Haidt, 2003).

The feeling of awe has often been found to be associated with sudden personal transformation, which William Miller and C' de Baca have defined as "quantum psychological change" (Miller & C'de Baca, 2001). These authors have described two types of quantum changes: insightful and mystical (Miller & C'De Baca, 1994; Miller & C'de Baca, 2001). Insightful changes are described as breakthrough of internal awareness, such as those occurring in psychotherapy. These are "a-ha" experiences in which the person comes to a new realization, a new way of thinking or understanding. Insightful transformations grow out of life experiences, in that they tend to follow personal development. In contrast, mystical quantum changes – or epiphanies – have no continuity with "ordinary" reality and are characterized by a sense of being acting upon by an outside force. The person knows immediately that something major has happened, and that life will never be the same again. According to Miller and C' de Baca, although insightful and mystical transformations are qualitatively different experiences, they both usually involve a significant alteration in how the person perceives him- or herself, others and the world.

As recent research has suggested, not only positive events but also psychological trauma and suffering may bring about genuine transformations of the individual. In particular, Tedeschi and Calhoun (Tedeschi & Calhoun, 2004) introduced the concept of Posttraumatic Growth, to refer to positive changes experienced as a result of the struggle with major life crises; such changes include the development of new perspectives and personal growth, the perception of new opportunities or possibilities in life, changes in relationships with others, and a richer existential and spiritual life.

6.2.1 Transformative Experiences Have an Epistemic Dimension and a Personal Dimension

As we have seen, transformative experiences differ from mere psychological change; specifically, all transformations involve change, but not all changes result in transformations. A transformative experience can completely alter one's relationship with the self-world: the individual builds up a new worldview, and this new perspective supports lasting change.

In psychological terms, a worldview (also world-view) has been defined by Koltko-Rivera (Koltko-Rivera, 2004) as "a way of describing the universe and life within it, both in terms of what is and what ought to be" (p. 4). A worldview is at the heart of one's knowledge: it encompasses a collection of beliefs about the fundamental aspects of reality, which allow us to understand and interact with the physical and social world. According to Koltko-Rivera (2004, p. 5) a worldview includes three different types of beliefs: existential, evaluative, and prescriptive/proscriptive. Existential beliefs describe either entities thought to exist in the world (e.g., "There exists a God or Goddess who cares for me personally") or statements concerning the nature of what can be known or done in the world (e.g., "There is such a thing as free will"). Evaluative beliefs are judgments of human beings or actions (e.g., "Those who fight against my nation are evil"). Finally, prescriptive/proscriptive beliefs are values, intended as descriptions of preferred means or ends (e.g., "The right thing to do in life is to live in the moment"). According to Mezirow's Transformative Learning Theory, a learning experience is transformative when it causes the learner to restructure his or her perspective towards more functional frames of reference (Mezirow, 1991). As he notes: "Perspective transformation is the process of becoming critically aware of how and why our assumptions have come to constrain the way we perceive, understand, and feel about our world; changing these structures of habitual expectation to make possible a more inclusive, discriminating, and integrating perspective; and finally, making choices or otherwise acting upon these new understandings" (p. 167). In Mezirow's theory, a disorienting dilemma can help this process by inducing the learners to examine, challenge and revise his assumptions and beliefs. For Mezirow, a disorienting dilemma is ususally triggered by a life crisis or major life transition (e.g. death, ilness, separation or divorce), but it can also result from "an eyeopening discussion, book, poem, or painting or from efforts to understand a different culture with customs that contradict our own previously accepted presuppositions" (p. 168). Mezirow identified three types of reflection that can occur when we face a dilemma: content reflection, process reflection, and premise reflection. The first two are involved when we reflect on the content of an actual issue (i.e., "what are the key issues to examine?") or on the process by which we solved a specific problem (i.e. "how did I get here?"). These areas of reflection result in the transformation of meaning schemes, which is a common, everyday occurrence. In contrast, premise reflection concerns the relevance of the problem itself (i.e. "why did this happen?") and involves a critique of the presuppositions on which our beliefs have been built. According to Mezirow, premise reflection can bring about the most significant learning, as it results in the transformation of one's meaning structure.

The philosopher Paul (Paul, 2014) argues that transformative experiences have an epistemic dimension and a personal dimension. Epistemically-transformative experiences are those that allow an individual to grasp new knowledge, which would be inaccessible to the knower until he or she has such an experience. For example, if you have never seen color, you cannot know "what it is like" to see red; similarly, if you have never heard music, you cannot know "what is like" to hear music. However, Paul points out that not all epistemic experiences hold the same transformative potential, as not all of them are able to change our self-defining preferences or worldview. In Paul's example, tasting a durian for the first time is epistemically transformative, as the taste experience of the durian is revealed to the individual and allows him or her to gain new subjective knowledge. On the other hand, it is unlikely that this new taste will radically change the individual's perspective on life. According to Paul, there is another type of experience that can really change who a person is; these are called personally transformative experiences. For example, Paul notes, the experience of having a child is not only epistemically transformative, it is also personally transformative. This experience not only provides new knowledge about what is like to have a baby but can also change a person's values, priorities, and self-conception in ways that are deep and unpredictable. For Paul, personally transformative experiences can be of various natures, such as "(experiencing) a horrific physical attack, gaining a new sensory ability, having a traumatic accident, undergoing major surgery, winning an Olympic gold medal, participating in a revolution, having a religious conversion, having a child, experiencing the death of a parent, making a major scientific discovery, or experiencing the death of a child" (p. 16). In particular, Paul notes that "If an experience changes you enough to substantially change your point of view, thus substantially revising your core preferences or revising how you experience being yourself, it is a personally transformative experience" (p. 16). Thus, according to Paul personally transformative experiences can change our worldview; that is, they can change not only *what* we know but also *how* we experience being who we are. In this sense, transformative experiences are potential sources of epistemic expansion, because they teach us something that we could not have known before having the experience, while at the same time changing us as a person. As Paul notes: "Such experiences are very important from a personal perspective, for transformative experiences can play a significant role in your life, involving options that, speaking metaphorically, function as crossroads in your path towards self-realization" (p. 17). Paul argues that transformative experiences are also philosophically important, as they challenge our ordinary conception of major life-changing decisions as rational decisions. Rational decision-making models assume that when we choose a course of action, we try to maximize the expected value of our phenomenological preferences. However, Paul contends that, since we don't know what it will be like to have the experience until we have it, then it follows that some life-changing decisions – like whether or not to have a child – cannot be made rationally (Paul, 2015): "The trouble comes from the fact that, because having one's first child is epistemically transformative, one cannot determine the value of what it's like to have one's own child before actually having her" (p. 11). Thus, in reality, the kind of epistemic discoveries related to what it is like to be a parent (in terms of emotions, beliefs, desires, and dispositions) are made only upon entering parenthood. Paul's claim regarding the irreducible subjective dimension of transformative experiences is analogous to Nagel's (Nagel, 1974) famous thought experiment regarding whether it is possible to know what it is like to be a bat. According to Nagel, regardless of all objective scientific information that we can obtain by investigating a bat's brain, it is not possible to know how it *feels* to be a bat, since we will never be able to take the exact perspective of a bat. In Nagel's own terms: "I want to know what it is like for a bat to be a bat. Yet if I try to imagine this, I am restricted to the resources of my own mind, and those resources are inadequate to the task. I cannot perform it either by imagining additions to my present experience, or by imagining segments gradually subtracted from it, or by imagining some combination of additions, subtractions, and modifications" (p. 220).

Although Paul's argument is philosophically controversial (Dougherty, Horowitz, & Sliwa, 2015), it nevertheless supports the idea that transformative experiences have the potential to extend our (subjective) epistemic horizon, which is hedged-in by our unactualized possible selves. Of course, one might disagree that having a transformative experience is the only means to know how that experience feels. For example, it could be argued that it is possible to rely on imagination and assess the way that we would react to the transformative event. However, the bulk of empirical evidence shows that people are not good at predicting their own future feelings, an ability known as "affective forecasting" (for a review, see (Dunn & Laham, 2006)). For example, young adults overestimate how happy they will feel in the event of having a date on Valentine's Day, and overestimate how unhappy they will feel if they do not have a date (Hoerger & Quirk, 2010; Hoerger, Quirk, Chapman, & Duberstein, 2012). A possible explanation that has been raised to explain this biased affective prediction is that people tend to overlook coping strategies that attenuate emotional reactions to events – a phenomenon known as "immune neglect" (Gilbert, Pinel, Wilson, Blumberg, & Wheatley, 1998). According to Epstein's (Epstein, 1994, 2003) Cognitive-Experiential Self Theory, humans operate through the use of two fundamental information-processing systems, a rational system (driven by reason) and an experiential system (driven by emotions), which operate in an interactive and parallel fashion. The rational system, which has a short evolutionary history, is based on logical inference and operates in an analytically, relatively slow and affect-free fashion. Encoding of reality in this system involves abstract symbols, words and numbers, linked together by logical relations. In contrast, the experiential system has a much longer evolutionary history and is present in both humans and non-human animals. It processes information automatically, rapidly and holistically, creating associative connections that are closely linked to emotions such as pleasure and pain. In the experiential system, encoding of reality occurs in metaphors, images and narratives. Drawing on Epstein's theory, it has been proposed that when people engage in affective forecasting, immune neglect emerges because the rational system fails to appreciate the important role that the experiential system plays in shaping emotional experience (Dunn, Forrin, & Ashton-James, 2009). Because of the fundamental difference by which these two systems operate, as Kushlev and Dunn (Kushlev & Dunn, 2012) efficiently summarize, "trying to use the rational system to predict the outputs of the experiential system is a little like asking a robot to analyze a poem, and a diverse array of affective forecasting errors arise from this fundamental mismatch" (p. 279).

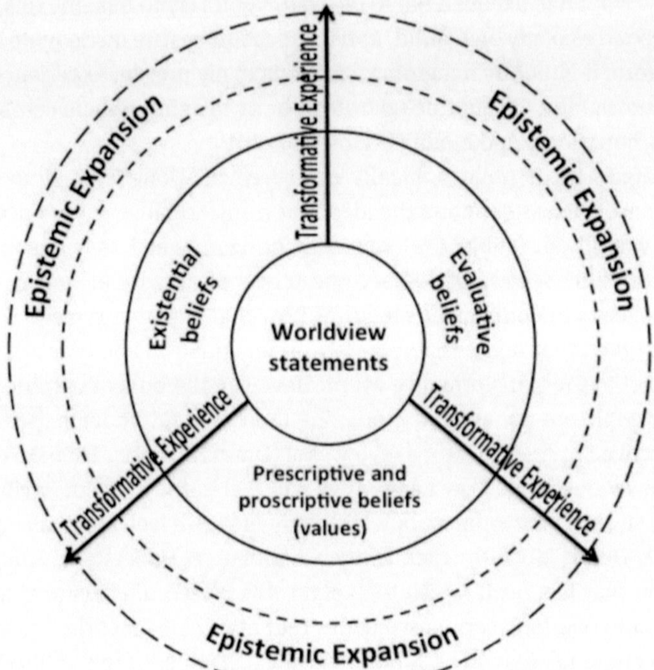

Figure 6.1: A conceptual representation of the process of epistemic expansion driven by transformative experience (adapted from Koltko-Rivera, 2004)

6.2.2 Transformative Experience as Emergent Phenomenon

The review of previous research on personally transforming experiences suggests that, in spite of commonly held assumptions, psychological change is not always the result of a gradual and linear process that occurs under conscious control (C'De Baca & Wilbourne, 2004; Miller & C'De Baca, 1994). Rather, under certain circumstances, enduring transformations can be the result of epiphanies and sudden insights. But how do these transformations occur? The theory of complex dynamical systems (Haken, 2002, 2004; Prigogine, 1984; Scott Kelso, 1995), which has been applied across disciplines as diverse as physics, biology, ecology, chemistry, political science , may offer an useful framework to address this question. From the perspective of complexity theory, humans, like all living organisms, are open, self-organizing systems that attain increasing levels of complexity and adaptation through the continuous exchange of energy and information with the environment. Dynamic systems evolve in complexity through the generation of *emergent properties*, which can be defined as properties that are possessed by a system as a whole but not by its constituent parts (Haken, 2002, 2004; Prigogine, 1984; Scott Kelso, 1995). These emergent phenomena are the result of feedback loop mechanisms that affect the system's equilibrium state, either amplifying an initial change in a system (positive feedback) or dampening an effect (negative feedback). Perturbation studies in dynamic systems research have revealed that an important predictor of transition is a type of discontinuity called critical fluctuations (Bak, Chen, & Creutz, 1989; Hayes, Laurenceau, Feldman, Strauss, & Cardaciotto, 2007). When the system has a stable or equilibrium structure, the fluctuation is usually very slight and can be offset by the negative feedback effect of the structure. However, even a single fluctuation, by acting synergistically with other fluctuations, may become powerful enough (i.e., a giant fluctuation) to reorganize the whole system into a new pattern. The critical points at which this happens are called "bifurcation points," at which the system experiences a phase transition towards a new structure of higher order (Tsonis, 1992). When seen through the lens of complexity theory, a quantum psychological change may occur when the person perceives an inability to assimilate an experience into current mental structures following an event that is experienced as being much larger than the self's ordinary frame of reference (as in Keltner and Haidt's model of awe). During this critical fluctuation, the system is destabilized but also open to new information and to the exploration of potentially more adaptive associations and configurations (Hayes et al., 2007). Interestingly, psychotherapists are starting to consider dynamic systems principles to conceptualize their interventions (Hayes & Strauss, 1998; Hayes et al., 2007; Heinzel, Tominschek, & Schiepek, 2014). According to Hayes and Yasins (Hayes & Yasinski, 2015), effective therapy involves exposure to corrective information and new experiences that challenge patients to develop new cognitive-affective-behavioral-somatic patterns, rather than to assimilate new information into old patterns. In the view of these authors, destabilization of pathological patterns can facilitate new learning, a shift in meaning and affective response, and an integration of cognitive and affective experiences.

6.2.3 Principles of Transformative Experience Design

The theoretical framework introduced in the previous paragraphs has allowed us to identify key features of transformative experiences. As I move forward to explore how these concepts might be turned into design principles, it is important to stress a central tenet of TED: *transformative experiences cannot be constructed but can only be invited*. Although the term "design" is commonly used to denote a set of explicit rules for achieving a product (in this case, a transformative experience) a key assumption of TED is that no subjective transformation can be imposed or constructed using technology the way marble is modelled by a sculptor. Authentic transformation requires the active involvement of the individual in the generation of new meanings as well as the perception that the experience being lived is self-relevant. Furthermore, since any personal transformation has an inherent subjective dimension, it is not possible to know in advance how the experience will feel for the individual, before it is actually lived through. Rather, TED argues that it is possible to define some specific *transformative affordances*, which are theoretically-based design guidelines for inviting, eliciting or facilitating a transformative experience. To illustrate the framework, I will focus on four different but interrelated aspects of TED: (i) medium; (ii) content; (iii) form; (iv) purpose.

6.2.3.1 The Transformative Medium

In principle, a transformative experience could be elicited by various media – including plays, storytelling, imagery, music, films and paintings. However, I argue that a specific technology – immersive virtual reality (VR) – holds the highest potential to foster a transformative process, since it is able to meet most of the key conceptual requirements of quantum psychological change. As previously argued, transformative experiences are sources of epistemic expansion, however we cannot benefit from this epistemic expansion until these transformations have been actualized. In addition, mental simulation of our "possible selves" cannot offer much help, as the rational system (which we use to run the simulation) is essentially different from what we are trying to predict (the experiential outcome): that's why simulations and actual perceptions systematically diverge (Kushlev & Dunn, 2012). As Gilbert and Wilson (Gilbert & Wilson, 2007) argue, "Compared to sensory perceptions, mental simulations are mere cardboard cut-outs of reality" (p. 1354). What if we had a technology that could fill this "epistemic gap", enabling one to experience a possible self, from a subjective perspective? Could such a technology be used as a medium to support, foster, or invite personally-transformative experiences?

A VR system is the combination of stereoscopic displays, real-time motion-tracking, stereo headphones and other possible sensory replications (i.e., tactile, olfactory, and gustatory senses), which provide the users a sense of presence – that is, the perception of "being there" (Barfield & Weghorst, 1993; Riva, Waterworth, & Waterworth, 2004; Riva, Waterworth, Waterworth, & Mantovani, 2011). Thanks to these unique characteristics, VR can be used to generate an infinite number of "possible selves", by providing a person a "subjective window of presence" into unactualized but possible worlds. From this perspective, virtual reality may be referred to as an *epistemically transformative technology*, since it allows individuals to encounter totally new experiences from a first-person, embodied perspective. The ability of VR to allow an individual to enact a possible self from a first-person perspective has been effectively exploited in psychotherapy (Riva, 2005). For example, virtual reality worlds are currently used to expose phobic patients to 3D simulations of the feared object or situation, in order to help them to handle the unsettling emotional reactions (Meyerbroker & Emmelkamp, 2010).

However, I contend that beyond clinical uses, the potential of VR for eliciting epistemically transformative experiences is still largely unexplored. The possible uses of VR range from the simulation of "plausible" possible worlds and possible selves to the simulation of realities that break the laws of nature and even of logic. These manipulations could be used as cognitive perturbations, since, as previously noted, appraisal of uncanny events (such as seeing an object levitate for no reason), causes a massive need for accommodation. Hence, the experience of such VR paradoxes may offer new opportunities for epistemic expansions, providing the participant with new potential sources of insight and inspiration. Researchers are already looking at ways in which VR can be used to hack our ordinary perception of self and reality in order to observe what happens to specific brain or psychological processes when a person is exposed to alterations of the bodily self using multisensory conflicts. By virtue of this manipulation researchers hope to cast light on the neurobiological process underlying self-consciousness. However, the experimental paradigms used in these studies may offer new, powerful tools to provide people with sources of awe and therefore trigger the active process of assimilation/accommodation. For the present discussion, I will consider three kinds of transformative potentials that are unique to VR: (i) manipulating bodily self-consciousness; (ii) embodying another person's subjective experience; and (iii) altering the laws of logic and nature.

6.2.3.1.1 I Am a Different Me: Altering Bodily Self-Consciousness

VR is able to generate an artificial sense of embodiment, or the subjective experience of using and having a body (Blanke & Metzinger, 2009) by acting on three multisensory brain processes: the sense of self-location (the feeling of being an entity localized at a position in space and perceiving the world from this position and perspective), the sense of agency (the sense that I am causing the action) and the sense of body ownership (the sense of one's self-attribution of a body, or self-identification) (Kilteni, Groten, & Slater, 2012).

Thanks to this feature, by using VR it is possible to alter body self-consciousness to give people the illusion that they have a different body. This type of manipulation uses video, virtual reality and/or robotic devices to induce changes in self-location, self-identification and first-person perspective in healthy subjects. By altering the neurophysiological basis of self experiences (*self as an object*), VR allows for experimenting with a different "ontological self" (*self as a subject*). For example, Lenggenhager et al. (Lenggenhager, Tadi, Metzinger, & Blanke, 2007) applied VR to induce an out-of-body experience by using conflicting visual-somatosensory input to disrupt the spatial unity between the self and the body. Riva (in this volume) has three possible strategies that can be used to alter bodily self-consciousness using virtual reality and brain-based technologies: (i) mindful embodiment, which consists in the modification of the bodily experience by facilitating the availability of its content in the working memory; augmented embodiment, which is based on the enhancement of bodily self-consciousness by altering/extending its boundaries; and (iii) synthetic embodiment, which aims at replacing bodily with synthetic self-consciousness (incarnation). Interestingly, VR is a technology that allows for not only simulating a plausible possible self, but even simulating the self-experience of another living organism, thus providing access to what Nagel considered impossible to access – that is, "what is like to be a bat". This potential of VR was already recognized by Charles Tart, one of the leading researchers in the field of altered states of consciousness and transpersonal psychology, at the very beginning of VR technology. In a 1990 article, Tart wrote (Tart, 1990): "Suppose everything that has been learned to date about ground squirrels, rattlesnakes, their interactions, and their environment could be put into a simulation world, a computer-generated virtual reality. To a much greater extent than is now possible, you (and your colleagues) could see and hear the world from the point of view of a ground squirrel, walk through the tunnels a ground squirrel lives in, know what it is perceptually like to be in a world where the grass is as tall as you, and what it is like when a rattlesnake comes slithering down your tunnel! What kind of insights would that give you into what it is like to live in that kind of world?" (p. 226).

6.2.3.1.2 I Am Another You: Embodying The Other

In the movie *Being John Malkovich* the main character Craig, a failed puppeteer, enters a portal into the mind of actor John Malkovich. After this discovery, Craig goes into business with a coworker with whom he is secretly in love, selling fifteen-minute "rides" in Malkovich's head. Suppose that you were able to enter someone's else body in this way: how would this experience change you? A potential of immersive VR as a transformative tool lies in its capability to render an experience from the perspective of another individual, by seeing what another saw, hearing what another heard, touching what another touched, saying what another said, moving as another moved, and – through narrative and drama – feeling the emotions another felt (Raij, Kotranza, Lind, Pugh, & Lok, 2009). Thanks to the ability of VR of enabling social-perspective taking, different experiments have been carried out to test the potential of this technology for enhancing empathy, prosocial behavior and moral development. In one such study, Yee and Bailenson (Yee & Bailenson, 2007) observed that participants spending several minutes in a virtual world embodying a tall virtual self-representation were found to be prone to choose more aggressive strategies in a negotiation task compared to participants who were given short avatars. These authors called this phenomenon the "Proteus Effect", a reference to the Greek sea-god Proteus, who was noted for being capable of assuming many different forms. More recently, Ahn, Tran Le and Bailenson (Ahn, Le, & Bailenson, 2013) carried out three experiments to explore whether embodied experiences via VR would elicit greater self-other merging, favorable attitudes, and helping efforts toward persons with a visual disability (colorblindness) compared to imagination alone. Findings showed that participants in the embodied experience condition experienced greater self-other merging compared to those in the imagination condition, and this effect generalized to the physical world, leading participants to voluntarily spend twice as much effort to help persons with colorblindness compared to participants who had only imagined being colorblind. Peck et al. (2013) demonstrated that embodiment of light-skinned participants in a dark-skinned virtual body significantly reduced implicit racial bias against dark-skinned people, in contrast to embodiment in light-skinned, purple-skinned or no virtual body.

It should be noted that, although VR is one of the most advanced technologies to embody another person's visual perspective, this experience could be further enhanced by integrating VR with other kinds of first-person simulation technologies. For example, age simulation suits have been designed to enable younger persons to experience common age-related limitations such as sensory impairment, joint stiffness or loss of strength. Schmidt and Jekel (Schmidt & Jekel, 2013) carried out experimental study that evaluated the potential of a realistic simulation of physical decline to stimulate empathy for older people in society. The simulated impairments were rated as realistic, and a majority of participants reported a higher mental strain during the tasks. After the session, understanding for typical everyday problems of older people increased. In part, the simulation evoked fear and negative attitudes towards aging. I argue that the potential of these age simulators could be even further enhanced having participants wear these suits in immersive VR scenarios, in which the older person might interact in realistic ageing-related contexts and situations.

6.2.3.1.3 I Am in a Paradoxical Reality: Altering the Laws of Logic

A further opportunity offered by VR as a transformative medium is the possibility of simulating impossibile worlds – that is, worlds that do not conform to the fundamental laws of logic and nature (Orbons & Ruttkay, 2008). The simulated violation of real-world constraints has been used to explore cognitive and metacognitive processes, yet this impossible-world paradigm could be also used to trigger the active process of assimilation/accommodation, which fosters epistemic expansion. Moreover, the manipulation of fundamental physical parameters, such as space and time, could be used to help people to grasp complex metaphysical questions in order to stimulate reflection on philosophical and metaphysical issues that are critical to understanding the self-world relationship. As Tart suggested, "A virtual reality could readily be programmed to accentuate change in virtual objects, virtual people and virtual events. Would the experience of such a world, even though artificial, sensitize a person so that they could learn the lesson of recognizing change and becoming less attached to the illusion of permanence more readily in subsequent meditation practice?" (p. 229).

Suzuki et al. (Suzuki, Wakisaka, & Fujii, 2012) developed a novel experimental platform, referred to as a "substitutional reality" (SR) system, for studying the conviction of the perception of live reality and related metacognitive functions. The SR system was designed to allow for manipulating participants' perception of reality by allowing participants to experience live scenes (in which they were physically present) and recorded scenes (which were recorded and edited in advance) in an alternating manner. Specifically, the authors' goal was to examine whether participants were able to identify a reality gap. Findings showed that most of the participants were induced to believe that they had experienced live scenes when recorded scenes were presented. However, according to Suzuki et al., the SR system offers several other ways to manipulate participants' reality. Authors suggest that for example, the SR can be used to cause participants to experience inconsistent or contradictory episodes, such as encountering themselves, or to experience déjà vu-like situations (e.g., repetitions of same event such as conversations or one-time-only events, such as breaking a unique piece of art). Furthermore, SR allows for the implementation of a visual experience of worlds with different natural laws (e.g., weaker gravity or faster time).

Time alterations and time paradoxes (i.e., the possibility of changing history) represent another kind of impossible manipulation of physical reality that might be feasible in virtual reality. For example, Friedman et al. (Friedman et al., 2014) described a method based on immersive virtual reality for generating an illusion of having traveled backward through time to relive a sequence of events in which the individual can intervene and change history. The authors consider this question: what if someone could travel back through time to experience a sequence of events and be able to intervene in order to change history? To answer this question, Friedman et al. simulated a sequence of events with a tragic outcome (deaths of strangers) in which the participant can virtually travel back to the past and undo actions that originally led to the unfortunate outcome. The participant is caught in a moral dilemma: if the subject does nothing, then five people will die for certain; if he acts then five people might be saved but another would die. Since the participant operates in a synthetic reality that does not obey the laws of physics (or logic), he is able to affect past events (therefore changing history), but in doing so he intervenes as a "ghost" that cannot be perceived by his past Doppelgänger. One of the goals of the experiment was to examine the extent to which the experience of illusory time travel might influence attitudes toward morality, moral dilemmas and "bad decisions" in personal history. The epistemic value of the experience, if successful, is that the subject would implicitly learn that the past is mutable. In particular, the authors speculated that the illusion of traveling in time might influence present-day attitudes – in particular possibly lessening negative feelings associated with past decisions and giving a different perspective on past actions, including those associated with the experienced scenario. Findings showed that the virtual experience of time travel produced an increase in guilt feelings about the events that had occurred and an increase in support of utilitarian behavior as the solution to the moral dilemma. The experience of time travel also produced an increase in implicit morality as judged by an implicit association test. Interestingly for the present discussion, the time travel illusion was associated with a reduction of regret associated with bad decisions in the participants' own lives. The authors also argue that this kind of epistemic expansion (the illusion that the past can be changed) might have important consequences for present-day attitudes and beliefs, including implications for self-improvement and psychotherapy; for example, giving people an implicit sense that the past is mutable may be useful in releasing the grip of past traumatic memories in people suffering from post-traumatic stress disorder.

6.2.3.2 Transformative Content

Transformative content refers to the content and structure of the designed experience. To understand the nature of transformative content, it is important to emphasize that from the perspective of complexity theory, a transformative experience is conceptualized as a "perturbation experiment", which attempts to facilitate a restructuration of meaning and beliefs by exposing the participant to experiences that induce destabilization within stable boundary conditions. As I will argue, this goal can be achieved by presenting the participant with high emotional and cognitive challenges, which may lead the individual to enter a mindset that is more flexible and open to the exploration of new epistemic configurations.

In the TED framework, such transformative content is delivered through a set of *experiential affordances*, which are stimuli designed to elicit emotional and cognitive involvement in the designed experience. Here, I will introduce two types of experiential affordances: (i) emotional affordances; (ii) epistemic affordances.

6.2.3.2.1 Emotional Affordances

Emotional affordances are perceptual cues or stimuli that are aimed to elicit a deep emotional involvement in the user, i.e. by evoking feelings of interest, inspiration, curiosity, wonder and awe. Previous research has shown that emotions of awe can be elicited by presenting participants with multimedia stimuli (e.g. images) which depict vast, mentally overwhelming, and realistic scenarios (Rudd, Vohs, & Aaker, 2012). To further elucidate the concept of *emotional affordance*, consider a recent study by Gallagher et al. (Gallagher, Reinerman, Sollins, & Janz, 2014), who used mixed-reality simulations in an attempt to elicit the experiences of awe and wonder reported by astronauts in their journals during space flight and in interviews after returning to the earth. Based on these reports, the authors created a virtual simulation (the "Virtual Space Lab") resembling an International Space Station workstation, which was designed to expose subjects to simulated stimuli of the earth and deep space (including physical structure plus simulated visuals). During and after exposure, researchers collected and integrated first-person subjective information (i.e. psychological testing, textual analysis, and phenomenological interviews) with third-person objective measures (i.e. physiological variables), following the "neurophenomenology method" (Gallagher & Brøsted Sørensen, 2006; Varela, 1996). Findings indicated that, despite some limitations, the Virtual Space Lab was able to induce awe experiences similar to those reported in the astronauts' reports. Thus, as noted by the authors, findings show promise for using a simulative technology in a laboratory when eliciting and assessing deeply involving experiences such as awe and wonder, otherwise very difficult to investigate (because unfeasible or too expensive) in real-world contexts.

6.2.3.2.2 Epistemic Affordances

In TED, emotional affordances have the goal of providing novel and awe-eliciting information, which can trigger the complementary processes of assimilation and accommodation, and by the virtue of the complex interplay of these processes, drive the system to a new order of complexity. However, in order to provide the participant with the opportunity to integrate new knowledge structures, it is necessary to present the participant with *epistemic affordances*, which are cues/information/narratives designed to trigger reflection and elicit insight. Epistemic affordances might be either represented by *explicit* dilemmatic situations – e.g., a provocative or paradoxical question, like a Zen *kōan* – but they could also be conveyed through *implicit* or evocative contents, that is, symbolic-metaphoric situations (i.e. one bright and one dark path leading from a crossroads). For example, going back to the Virtual Space Lab' study, Gallagher and his team demonstrated the feasibility of inducing awe within a simulated environment, which individuals previously had only in extraterrestrial space. In TED terms, this may be regarded as an instance of emotional affordance. Now assume that a designer would like to add to the Virtual Space Lab experience an epistemic affordance. To do that, the designer should create a dilemmatic situation to allow the participant not just to experience the same feeling of awe of an astronaut, but also to an opportunity to develop new insight. For example, such epistemic affordance could be resembled by the "floating dilemma" faced by *Gravity*'s main character Stone (played by Sandra Bullock), which represents a metaphor for a life that's in permanent suspension. From this perspective, an epistemic affordance could be also the simulated situation itself, to the extent it is able to provide a (virtual) space for self-reflection and self-experimentation.

6.2.3.3 The Transformative Form

The form dimension of the TED framework is different from the transformative content, in that it is less concerned with the *subject* of the experience that is represented, and more concerned with the *style* through which the transformative content is conveyed/delivered. Thus far, I have identified two components of form: (i) cinematic codes; (ii) narratives.

6.2.3.3.1 Cinematic Codes

In cinema, it is possible to enhance the emotional and cognitive involvement of the spectator in the storyline using audiovisual effects, such as lighting, camera angles, and music. For example, it is well known that the inclusion of a music "soundtrack" plays a key role in heightening not only the dramatic effects but also the faces, voices and the personalities of the players. As noted by Fischoff (Fischoff, 2005), "Music adds something we might call heightened realism or supra-reality. It is a form of theatrical, filmic reality, different from our normal reality." (p. 3). Thus, a key challenge related to the form dimension of TED is to examine the possibility of adapting/reinventing the cinematic codes with the specific objective of inducing more compelling VR-based transformative experiences. The potential of translating the cinematic audiovisual language to the context of interactive media has already been extensively explored in the video game domain (Girina, 2013). This attempt has led to the development of specific games, such as adventure and role-playing games, which make massive use of the expressive potential of cinematic techniques.

6.2.3.3.2 Narratives

In addition to the possibility of taking advantage of cinematic audiovisual codes, a further component of the form dimension is the creation of a dramatic and engaging *narrative* or story. In his lecture "Formal Design Tools" at the 2000 Game Developers' Conference, Marc LeBlanc introduced a distinction between *embedded* and *emergent* narrative (LeBlanc, 2000). Embedded narrative is the story implemented by the game designer; it includes a set of fixed narrative units (i.e. texts or non-interactive cut scenes) that exist prior to the player's interaction with the game and are used to provide the player with a fictional background, motivation for actions in the game and development of the story arc. In contrast, emergent narrative is the story that unfolds in the process of playing – that is, the storytelling generated by player actions within the rule structure governing interaction with the game system. In TED, both embedded and emergent narratives may play a key role in facilitating a transformative experience. Embedded narrative can be used to provide a context for enhancing the participant's sense of presence in the simulated environment. As previous research has shown, a meaningful narrative context can have a significant influence on the user's sense of presence, providing a more compelling experience compared to non-contextualized virtual environments (Gorini, Capideville, De Leo, Mantovani, & Riva, 2011). Emergent narrative, on the other hand, can be employed to influence the way the transformative content/story is created, making the story experience potentially more engaging (i.e., both attentionally and emotionally involving) for the participant. Further, since emergent narratives allow the participant to interactively create the narrative of the experience, they generate feedback loop mechanisms, which in turn can trigger the complex self-organization dynamics that facilitate transformations.

An example of how cinematic codes and emergent narratives have been used in combination with immersive virtual reality to support positive psychological change is provided by EMMA's World (Banos, Botella, Quero, Garcia-Palacios, & Alcaniz, 2011), a therapeutical virtual world designed to assist patients in confronting situations in which they have suffered or are suffering a stressful experience. EMMA's World includes five different evocative scenarios or "landscapes": a desert, an island, a threatening forest, a snow-covered town and a meadow. These virtual worlds have been designed to reflect/induce different emotions (e.g., relaxation, elation, sadness). However, the type of scenario that is selected is not pre-defined according to a fixed narrative; rather, it depends on the context of the therapeutic session and can be chosen by the therapist in real time. The goal of this strategy is to reflect and enhance the emotion that the user is experiencing or to induce certain emotions. The control tools of EMMA's World provide also the possibility to modify the scenarios and graduate their intensity in order to reflect the changes in the participants' mood states.

Another important component of EMMA's World is the Book of Life, a virtual book in which patients can reflect upon feelings and experiences. The goal of the Book of Life is to represent the most important moments, people and situations in the person's life (related to the traumatic or negative experience). Anything that is meaningful for the patient can be incorporated into the system: photos, drawings, phrases, videos. This last feature of EMMA's World allows it to exemplify a further design principle of TED: *personalization*. This concerns the possibility of including personal details of the participant in the immersive experience, with particular reference to autobiographically-relevant elements (e.g., videos, photos, music, song lyrics) that have an important personal meaning and therefore are able to elicit emotions (e.g., nostalgia) related to the intimate sphere of the participant.

6.2.3.4 The Transformative Purpose

The central tenet of TED is that it is possible to design technologically-mediated transformative experiences that support epistemic expansions and personal development. However, since the outcome of a personally transformative experience is inherently subjective and therefore not predictable, the idea of transformative design might seem contradictory in itself. Nevertheless, there is another, more open-ended way in which one might define the purpose of a (designed) transformative experience, which places more focus on the transformative process than on the transformative outcome: that is, considering an interactive experience as a space for transformative possibilities.

6.2.3.4.1 Transformation as Liminality

Winnicot (Winnicott, 1971) described a "potential space" as a metaphorical space that is intermediate between fantasy and reality, an area of experiencing which opens up new possibilities for imagination, symbolization and creativity. According to Winnicot, potential space is inhabited by play, which has a central importance in developmental processes. Winnicot believed that engaging in play is important not only during childhood, but also during adulthood: "It is in playing and only in playing that the individual child or adult is able to be creative and to use the whole personality, and it is only in being creative that the individual discovers the self" (p. 54). A closely related concept is "liminality", intended as a space of transformation wherein the human being is between past and future identities. The notion of liminality (from the latin term *limen*: threshold, boundary) was first introduced by the ethnologist Arnold van Gennep (Van Gennep, 1908/1960) to describe the initiation rites of young members of a tribe, which fall into three structural phases: separation, transition, and incorporation. Van Gennep defined the middle stage in a rite of passage (transition) as a "liminal period". Elaborating on van Gennep's work, anthropologist Victor Turner (V. Turner, 1974) argued that, in postindustrial societies, traditional rites of passage had lost much of their importance and have been progressively replaced by "liminoid" spaces. There are defined by Turner as "out-of-the-ordinary" experiences set aside from productive labor, which are found in leisure, arts, and sports (e.g., extreme sports). These liminoid spaces have similar functions and characteristics to as liminal spaces, disorienting the individual from everyday routines and habits and situating him in unfamiliar circumstances that deconstruct the "meaningfulness of ordinary life" (V. Turner, 1985).

The metaphors of potential space and liminality/liminoid space provide a platform for further elaborating the purpose of transformative design as the realization of interactive systems that allow participants to experience generative moments of change, which situate them in creative learning spaces where they can challenge taken-for-granted ways of knowing and being. From this perspective, interactive transformative experiences may function both as potential spaces and liminal spaces, offering participants novel opportunities for promoting creativity and personal growth. However, as open-ended "experiments of the self", such interactive, transformative experience may also situate the participants in situations of discomfort, disorientation and puzzlement, which are also turning points out of which new possibilities arise.

6.2.3.4.2 The Journey Matters, Not the Destination

To reach this goal, TED can take advantage of the ability to integrate the language of arts. Indeed, art provides a vocabulary that is rich, multisensory, and at the same time able to elicit experiences of dislocation, evocativeness, ambiguity, and openness that can be effectively combined to generate powerful liminal spaces. As noted by Preminger (Preminger, 2012), art can contribute in several ways to the design of transformative experiences. First of all, the immersive and holistic nature of the experience of art is supportive of cognitive and emotional involvement, which in turn can enhance learning. Second, art can be a vehicle for more efficient access to and modification of brain representations. Third, the evocative nature of some artworks requires the experiencer to use internally generated cognitive processes (i.e. imagery, introspection, self-representation, autobiographic and prospective memory, and volition), which allows for enhanced immersion and identification. In addition to these characteristics, which are common to art domains where the induced experience involves mainly perceptual and cognitive processes, interactive arts (including games) can also involve motor functions and behavioral control in dynamically changing environments, which can further enhance the transformative potential of the designed experience.

An interesting example of how arts can be combined with interactive design to create emotionally-rich, memorable and transformative experiences is provided by the games developed by computer scientist Jenova Chen. Chen believes that for video games to become a mature medium like film, it is important to create contents that are able to induce different emotional responses in the player than only excitement or fear (Chen, 2009). This design philosophy is best exemplified in the critically-acclaimed video game *Journey* (Chen, 2012), a mysterious desert adventure in which the player takes the role of a red-robed figure in a desert populated by supernatural ruins. On the far horizon is a big mountain with a light beam shooting straight up into the sky, which becomes the natural destination of the adventurer. While walking towards the mountain, the avatar can encounter other players, one at a time, if they are online; they cannot speak but can help each other in their journey if they wish. The goal of the game is to take the player on an emotional and artistic journey that evokes feelings of spirituality and a sense of smallness, wonder and awe, as well as to foster an emotional connection with the anonymous players encountered along the way (Pantazis, 2010). To achieve this, the game uses a very sophisticated visual aesthetics, in combination with music that dynamically responds to the player's actions, building a single theme to represent the game's emotional arc throughout the story. A further

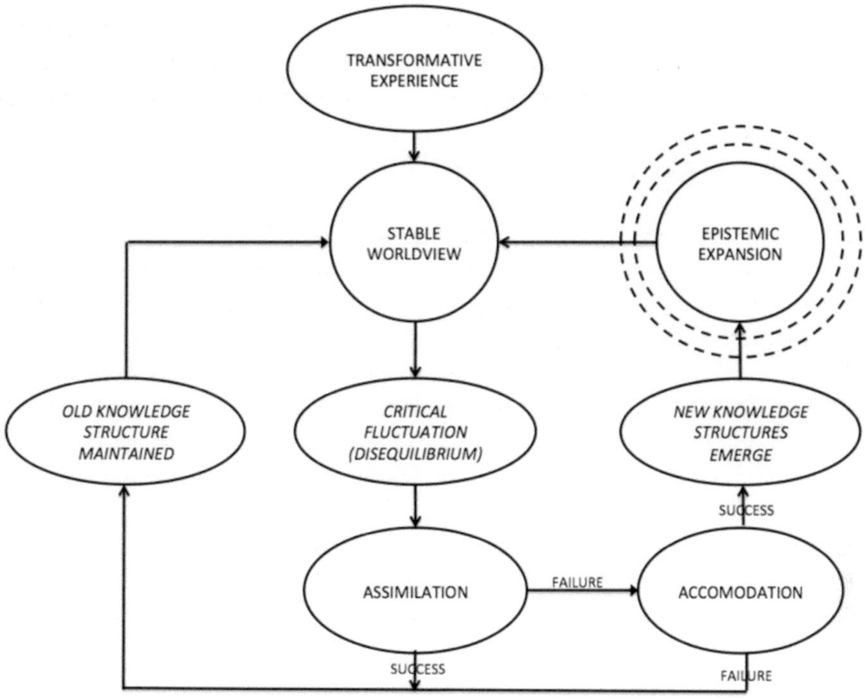

Figure 6.2: A possible schematization of the transformative process. The exposure to novel information (i.e. awe-inducing stimuli) triggers the process of assimilation. If integration fails, the person experiences a critical fluctuation that can either lead to rejection of novelty or to an attempt to accommodate existing schema, eventually generating new knowledge structures and therefore producing an epistemic expansion

relevant feature of *Journey* for the TED framework is that, unlike conventional games, its goal is not clearly set, as it places greater emphasis on enjoying the experience as it unfolds during play.

6.3 Conclusion: the Hallmarks of Transformative Experience Design

This chapter aimed at providing a first framework for Transformative Experience Design, which refers to the use of interactive systems to support long-lasting changes in the self-world. In particular, the goal of this chapter was two-fold: (i) to provide background knowledge on the concepts of transformative experience, as well as its implications for individual growth and psychological wellbeing; and (ii) to translate such knowledge into a tentative set of design principles for developing transformative applications of technology.

The central assumption of TED is that the next generation of interactive systems and brain-based technologies will offer the unprecedented opportunity to develop synthetic, controlled transformative experiences to foster epistemic expansion and personal development. For the first time in its history, the human being has the possibility of developing technologies that allow for experimenting the "Other-than-Self" and, by doing so, exploring new means of epistemic expansion. This Other-than-Self encompasses a broad spectrum of transformative possibilities, which include "what it is like" to be another self, another life form, or a possible future or past self. These designed experiences can be used to facilitate self-knowledge and self-understanding, foster creative expression, develop new skills, and recognize and learn the value of others.

Although the present discussion is largely exploratory and speculative, I believe this initial analysis of TED has some significant potential. First, the analysis of transformative experience can inspire new applications of VR that go beyond gaming and therapy to address issues related to personal development and self-actualization. Furthermore, the analysis of the characteristics of transformative experience has intrinsic scientific value, since it can promote a deeper understanding of this complex psychological phenomenon at multiple levels of analysis – neuropsychological, phenomenological, and technological. Finally, the further development of TED may also contribute to redefinining our conceptualization of information technologies, from tools of mass consumption to potential means to satisfy the highest psychological needs for growth and fulfillment.

However, a caveat is necessary before this research moves forward. I believe that the study of how to use technology to support positive transformations of the self should not be considered a deterministic, technologically-centered perspective on human personal development. The final aim of transformative design, as I see it, should not be confused with the idea of "engineering self-realization". Rather, I hold that the objective of this endeavour should be to explore new possible technological means of supporting human beings' natural tendency towards self-actualization and self-transcendence. As Haney (Haney, 2006) beautifully puts it: "each person must choose for him or herself between the technological extension of physical experience through mind, body and world on the one hand, and the natural powers of human consciousness on the other as a means to realize their ultimate vision" (ix, Preface).

References

Ahn, S. J., Le, A. M. T., & Bailenson, J. N. (2013). The effect of embodied experiences on self-other merging, attitude, and helping behavior. *Media Psychology, 16*(1), 7–38.

Bak, P., Chen, K., & Creutz, M. (1989). Self-organized criticality and the 'Game of Life'. *Nature, 342*, 780–782.

Banos, R., Botella, C., Quero, S., Garcia-Palacios, A., & Alcaniz, M. (2011). Engaging Media for Mental Health Applications: the EMMA project. *Stud Health Technol Inform, 163*, 44–50.

Barfield, W., & Weghorst, S. (1993). The Sense of Presence within Virtual Environments – a Conceptual-Framework. *Human-Computer Interaction, Vol 2, 19*, 699–704.

Blanke, O., & Metzinger, T. (2009). Full-body illusions and minimal phenomenal selfhood. *Trends Cogn Sci, 13*(1), 7–13. doi: 10.1016/j.tics.2008.10.003.

C'De Baca, J., & Wilbourne, P. (2004). Quantum change: ten years later. *J Clin Psychol, 60*(5), 531–541. doi: 10.1002/jclp.20006.

(2009, January 28, 2009). *Full Interview: Jenova Chen* [MP3/Audio Podcast]. Retrieved from http://web.archive.org/web/20090213221451/http://www.cbc.ca/spark/2009/01/full-interview-jenova-chen/.

Chen, J. (2012). Journey: Thatgamecompany, Sony Computer Entertainment.

Coghlan, A., Buckley, R., & Weaver, D. (2012). A framework for analysing awe in tourism experiences. *Annals of Tourism Research, 39*(3), 1710–1714.

Dougherty, T., Horowitz, S., & Sliwa, P. (2015). Expecting the Unexpected. *Res Philosophica*.

Dunn, E. W., Forrin, N., & Ashton-James, C. E. (2009). On the excessive rationality of the emotional imagination: A two-systems account of affective forecasts and experiences. In K. D. Markman, W. M. P. Klein & J. A. Suhr (Eds.), *The Handbook of Imagination and Mental Simulation*. New York: Psychology Press.

Dunn, E. W., & Laham, S. A. (2006). A user's guide to emotional time travel: Progress on key issues in affective forecasting. In J. Forgas (Ed.), *Hearts and minds: Affective influences on social cognition and behavior*. New York: Psychology Press.

Ekman, P. (1992). Are there basic emotions? *Psychological Review, 99*(550–553).

Epstein, S. (1994). An integration of the cognitive and psychodynamic unconscious. *American Psychologist, 49*, 709–724.

Epstein, S. (2003). *Cognitive-experiential self-theory of personality* (Vol. 5: Personality and Social Psychology). Hoboken, NJ: Wiley & Sons.

Fischoff, S. (2005). *The Evolution of Music in Film and its Psychological Impact on Audiences*. Retrieved from http://web.calstatela.edu/faculty/abloom/tvf454/5filmmusic.pdf.

Friedman, D., Pizarro, R., Or-Berkers, K., Neyret, S., Pan, X., & Slater, M. (2014). A method for generating an illusion of backwards time travel using immersive virtual reality-an exploratory study. *Front Psychol, 5*, 943. doi: 10.3389/fpsyg.2014.00943.

Gallagher, S., & Brøsted Sørensen, J. (2006). Experimenting with phenomenology. *Conscious Cogn, 15*(1), 119–134.

Gallagher, S., Reinerman, L., Sollins, B., & Janz, B. (2014). Using a simulated environment to investigate experiences reported during space travel. *Theoretical Issues in Ergonomic Sciences, 15* (4), 376–394.

Gaylinn, D. L. (2005). Reflections on Transpersonal Media: An Emerging Movement. *The Journal of Transpersonal Psychology, 37*(1), 1–8.

Gilbert, D. T., Pinel, E. C., Wilson, T. D., Blumberg, S. J., & Wheatley, T. P. (1998). Immune neglect: a source of durability bias in affective forecasting. *J Pers Soc Psychol, 75*(3), 617–638.

Gilbert, D. T., & Wilson, T. D. (2007). Prospection: experiencing the future. *Science, 317*(5843), 1351–1354. doi: 10.1126/science.1144161.

Girina, I. (2013). Video game Mise-En-Scene remediation of cinematic codes in video games. In H. Koenitz , I. S. Tonguc , D. Sezen, M. Haahr, G. Ferri & G. ̧Catak (Eds.), *Interactive Storytelling* (Vol. 8230, pp. 45–54). Berlin Heidelberg: Springer.

Gorini, A., Capideville, C. S., De Leo, G., Mantovani, F., & Riva, G. (2011). The role of immersion and narrative in mediated presence: the virtual hospital experience. *Cyberpsychol Behav Soc Netw, 14*(3), 99–105. doi: 10.1089/cyber.2010.0100.

Haken, H. (2002). *Haken, H. (2002). Brain Dynamics*. Berlin: Springer.

Haken, H. (2004). *Synergetics. Introduction and Advanced Topics*. Berlin: Springer.

Haney, W. S. (2006). *Cyberculture, cyborgs and science fiction: consciousness and the posthuman*. Amsterdam: Rodopi.

Hayes, A., & Strauss, J. (1998). Dynamic systems theory as a paradigm for the study of change in psychotherapy: An application to cognitive therapy for depression. *Journal of Consulting and Clinical Psychology, 66*, 939–947.

Hayes, A. M., Laurenceau, J. P., Feldman, G., Strauss, J. L., & Cardaciotto, L. (2007). Change is not always linear: the study of nonlinear and discontinuous patterns of change in psychotherapy. *Clin Psychol Rev, 27*(6), 715–723. doi: 10.1016/j.cpr.2007.01.008

Hayes, A. M., & Yasinski, C. (2015). Pattern destabilization and emotional processing in cognitive therapy for personality disorders. *Frontiers in Psychology, 6*(107).

Heinzel, S., Tominschek, I., & Schiepek, G. (2014). Dynamic patterns in psychotherapy – discontinuous changes and critical instabilities during the treatment of obsessive compulsive disorder. *Nonlinear Dynamics Psychol Life Sci, 18*(2), 155–176.

Hoerger, M., & Quirk, S. W. (2010). Affective forecasting and the Big Five. *Pers Individ Dif, 49*(8), 972–976. doi: 10.1016/j.paid.2010.08.007

Hoerger, M., Quirk, S. W., Chapman, B. P., & Duberstein, P. R. (2012). Affective forecasting and self-rated symptoms of depression, anxiety, and hypomania: evidence for a dysphoric forecasting bias. *Cogn Emot, 26*(6), 1098–1106. doi: 10.1080/02699931.2011.631985.

James, W. (1902). *The Varieties of Religious Experience: A Study in Human Nature* J. Manis (Ed.) (pp. 469).

Keltner, D., & Haidt, J. (2003). Approaching awe, a moral, spiritual, and aesthetic emotion. *Cognition and Emotion, 17*, 297–314.

Kilteni, K., Groten, R., & Slater, M. (2012). The Sense of Embodiment in Virtual Reality *Presence: Teleoperators and Virtual Environments, 21* (4), 373–387.

Koltko-Rivera, M. E. (2004). The psychology of worldviews. *Review of General Psychology, 8*(1), 3–58.

Kushlev, K., & Dunn, E. W. (2012). Affective forecasting: Knowing how we will feel in the future. In S. Vazire & T. Wilson (Eds.), *Handbook of self-knowledge* (pp. 277–292). New York: Guilford Press.

LeBlanc, M. (2000). *Formal Design Tools: Feedback Systems and the Dramatic Structure of Competition*. Paper presented at the Game Developers Conference, San Jose, California. http://algorithmancy.8kindsoffun.com/.

Lenggenhager, B., Tadi, T., Metzinger, T., & Blanke, O. (2007). Video ergo sum: manipulating bodily self-consciousness. *Science, 317*(5841), 1096–1099. doi: 10.1126/science.1143439.

Maslow, A. (1962a). Lessons from the peak-experiences. *Journal of Humanistic Psychology, 2*, 9–18.

Maslow, A. (1962b). *Towards a psychology of being*. Princeton: D. Van Nostrand Company.

Maslow, A. (1954). *Motivation and personality*. New York: Harper and Row.

Maslow, A. (1964). *Religions, Values and Peak Experiences*. Columbus, Ohio: Ohio State University Press.

Meyerbroker, K., & Emmelkamp, P. M. G. (2010). Virtual Reality Exposure Therapy in Anxiety Disorders: A Systematic Review of Process-and-Outcome Studies. *Depression and Anxiety, 27*(10), 933–944. doi: Doi 10.1002/Da.20734.

Mezirow, J. (1991). *Transformative Dimensions of Adult Learning*. San Francisco, CA: Jossey-Bass.

Miller, W. R., & C'De Baca, J. (1994). Can personality change? In T. F. Heatherton & J. L. Weinberger (Eds.), *Quantum change: Toward a psychology of transformation* (pp. 253–280). Washington D.C.: American Psychological Association.

Miller, W. R., & C'de Baca, J. (2001). *Quantum Change: When Epiphanies and Sudden Insights Transform Ordinary Lives, New York: Guilford Press.* New York: Guilford Press.

Nagel, T. (1974). What is it like to be a bat? *Philosophical Review, 83*, 435–450.

Orbons, E., & Ruttkay, Z. (2008). *Interactive 3D Simulation of Escher-like Impossible Worlds.* Paper presented at the Bridges Leeuwarden Mathematics, Music, Art, Architecture, Culture, Leeuwarden. The Netherlands.

Pantazis, N. (2010). E3 Preview: Journey – Preview. Retrieved 18 October, 2014, from http://www.gamrreview.com/preview/80568/e3-pjourney/.

Paul, L. A. (2014). *Transformative Experience*. Oxford: Oxford University Press.

Paul, L. A. (2015). What You Can't Expect When You're Expecting. *Res Philosophica, 92*(2).

Piaget, J., & Inhelder, B. (1969). *The psychology of the child* (H. Weaver, Trans.). New York: Basic Books, Inc.

Preminger, S. (2012). Transformative art: art as means for long-term neurocognitive change. *Frontiers in Human Neuroscience, 6*, 96. doi: 10.3389/fnhum.2012.00096.

Prigogine, I. (1984). *Order out of Chaos : Man's New Dialogue with Nature*. New York: Bentam.

Raij, A., Kotranza, A., Lind, D. S., Pugh, C. M., & Lok, B. (2009, Mar. 14–18). *Virtual Experiences for Social Perspective Taking*. Paper presented at the IEEE Virtual Reality 2009, Lafayette, LA.

Riva, G. (2005). Virtual reality in psychotherapy: Review. *Cyberpsychology & Behavior, 8*(3), 220–230. doi: Doi 10.1089/Cpb.2005.8.220

Riva, G., Waterworth, J. A., & Waterworth, E. (2004). The layers of presence: A bio-cultural approach to understanding presence in natural and mediated environments. *Cyberpsychology & Behavior, 7*(4), 402–416. doi: Doi 10.1089/Cpb.2004.7.402.

Riva, G., Waterworth, J. A., Waterworth, E. L., & Mantovani, F. (2011). From intention to action: The role of presence. *New Ideas in Psychology, 29*(1), 24–37. doi: Doi 10.1016/J. Newideapsych.2009.11.002.

Rudd, M., Vohs, K. D., & Aaker, J. (2012). Awe expands people's perception of time, alters decision making, and enhances well-being. *Psychol Sci, 23*(10), 1130–1136. doi: 10.1177/0956797612438731.

Schmidt, L. I., & Jekel, K. (2013). "Take a Look through My Glasses": An Experimental Study on the Effects of Age Simulation Suits and their Ability to Enhance Understanding and Empathy. *The Gerontologist,, 53*(624). doi: doi:10.1093/geront/gnt151.

Schneider, K. J. (2011). Awakening to an Awe-Based Psychology. *The Humanist Psychologist, 39*, 247–252.

Scott Kelso, J. A. (1995). *Dynamic Patterns: The Self-organization of Brain and Behavior*. Cambridge, MA: The MIT Press.

Shiota, M. N., Keltner, D., & Mossman, A. (2007). The nature of awe: Elicitors, appraisals, and effects on self-concept. *Cognition & Emotion, 21*, 944–963.

Suzuki, K., Wakisaka, S., & Fujii, N. (2012). Substitutional reality system: a novel experimental platform for experiencing alternative reality. *Sci Rep, 2*, 459. doi: 10.1038/srep00459

Tart, C. T. (1972). States of consciousness and state-specific sciences. *Science, 176*(4040), 1203–1210. doi: 10.1126/science.176.4040.1203.

Tart, C. T. (1990). Multiple personality, altered states, and virtual reality: The world simulation approach. *Dissociation, 4* (3), 222–223.

Tedeschi, R. G., & Calhoun, L. G. (2004). Posttraumatic growth: Conceptual foundations and empirical evidence. *Psychological Inquiry, 15*(1), 1–18.

Tsonis, A. A. (1992). *Chaos: from theory to applications*. New York: Plenum.

Turner, V. (1974). Liminal to Liminoid in Play, Flow, and Ritual. *Rice University Studies, 60*(3), 53–92.

Turner, V. (1985). Process, System, and Symbol: A New Anthropological Synthesis. In E. Turner (Ed.), *On the Edge of the Bush: Anthropology as Experience* (pp. 151–173). Tucson: University of Arizona Press.

Van Gennep, A. (1908/1960). *The Rites of Passage*. Chicago: University of Chicago Press.

Varela, F. (1996). Neurophenomenology: A Methodological Remedy for the Hard Problem. *Journal of Consciousness Studies, 3*, 330–349.

Winnicott, D. W. (1971). *Playing and reality* London: Routledge.

Yee, N., & Bailenson, J. N. (2007). The Proteus Effect: The Effect of Transformed Self-Representation on Behavior. *Human Communication Research, 33*, 271–290.

Section II: **Emerging Interaction Paradigms**

Frédéric Bevilacqua and Norbert Schnell

7 From Musical Interfaces to Musical Interactions

Abstract: In this chapter, we review research that was conducted at Ircam in the Real-Time Musical Interactions team on motion-based musical interactions. First, we developed various tangible motion-sensing interfaces and interactive sound synthesis systems. Second, we explored different approaches to design motion-sound relationships, which can be derived from object affordances, metaphors or from embodied listening explorations. Certain scenarios utilize machine-learning techniques we shortly describe. Finally, some examples of collaborative musical interactions are presented, which represents an important area of development with the rapidly increased capabilities of embedded and mobile computing. We argue that the research we report relates to challenges posed by the Human Computer Confluence research agenda.

Keywords: Gesture, Sound, Music, Sensorimotor, Interactive Systems, Sound Synthesis, Sensors

7.1 Introduction

Musical instruments have always made use of the "novel technology" of their time, and the appearance of electronics in the 20th century has stimulated numerous new musical instruments, more than generally acknowledged. Several of them were groundbreaking by introducing novel types of interfaces for music performance, significantly ahead of their time. To cite a few: non-contact sound control by Leon Theremin in the 1920' (the Thereminvox), sonification of electroencephalography by Avin Lucier in 1965 (Music for Solo Performer), active force feedback interfaces by Claude Cadoz and colleagues starting in the 1970', bi-manual tangible and motion-based interfaces in the 1984 by Michel Waisviz (The Hands), full body video capture by David Rokeby starting in the 1980' (VeryNervousSystem), use of electromyography by Atau Tanaka starting the 1990'. Interestingly, these musical systems can be seen as precursors of several computer interfaces nowadays popularized by the gaming industry (Wiimote, Kinect, Leapmotion, MyndBrain etc...).

Most of these original musical instrument prototypes were played principally by their inventors, who developed simultaneously technology (interfaces, sound processing), artistic works and often idiosyncratic skills to play their instruments. Early prototypes were not always easily sharable with other practitioners. The MIDI standard (Musical Instrument Digital Interface), established in 1983 and rapidly adopted, greatly facilitated then the modular use of different "controllers" (i.e. the physical interfaces) with different "synthesizers", i.e. sound generation units. This contributed to foster the representation of digital musical instruments as composed of a "controller/interface" and a "digital sound processor", both being changeable independently. Unfortunately, the MIDI standard froze the music interaction paradigms to a series of events triggering, using a very basic and limited model of musical events. Any more complex descriptions of gesture and sound are absent from the MIDI format. As a matter of fact, the MIDI piano keyboard, fitting this interaction paradigm, has remained for a long time the primary interface to control sound synthesis.

Nevertheless, a growing community formed of scientists, technologists and artists has explored approaches "beyond the keyboard" and MIDI representations (Miranda & Wanderley, 2006). The international conference NIME (New Interfaces for Musical Expression), started in 2001 as a workshop of the CHI conference (Bevilacqua et al., 2013), contributed to expand this community. A competition of new musical instruments also exists since 2009 held at Georgia Tech[3]. Nevertheless, the acronym NIME might be misleading, since this community, actually very heterogeneous, is not only focused on "interfaces" but is active on a broader research agenda on "musical instruments" and "interactions" (Tanaka et al., 2010).

The historical perspective we outline on electronic musical instruments should convince the reader that pioneering works in music technology often anticipated or at least offered stimulating applications of emerging technologies. We argue that music applications represent exemplary use cases to explore new challenges stimulated by advances in sciences and technology. In this chapter, we will describe the approach that we developed over ten years in the Real-Time Musical Interactions team[4] at Ircam concerning musical interfaces and interactions. By explaining both the general approach and specific examples, we aim at illustrating the links between this research and the current topics of the Human Computer Confluence research.

This review will describe design principles and concrete examples of musical interaction that are apprehended through embodied, situated and social interaction paradigms. Musical expression results from complex intertwined relationships between humans (both performing and listening) and machine capabilities. As music playing is in its essence a collective multimodal experience, musical interactions mediated by technologies provoke important research questions that parallels the challenges identified by the HCC agenda, such as "Experience and Sharing", "Empathy and Emotion", and "Disappearing computers" (Ferscha, 2013).

We will start by recalling some background and related works in Section 2, followed by our general approach in Section 3. In Section 4, we present examples of tangible interfaces and objects used in musical interactions. In Section 5, we describe the methodologies and tools to design motion-sound relationships. In Section 6, we

3 Margaret Guthman Musical Instrument Competition http://guthman.gatech.edu/

4 Since 2014, the name has changed to Sound Music Movement Interaction

briefly show how this research is naturally extended to collaborative interactions, before concluding in Section 7.

7.2 Background

We recall in this section important related works on formalizing musical interfaces and gestures. Wanderley and Depalle (Wanderley & Depalle, 2004) described a Digital Musical Instrument (DMI) as composed of an interface or gestural controller unit and a sound generation unit. These two components can be designed independently, in contrast to acoustic instruments. This representation must be completed by the mapping procedure that allows for linking sensor data to sound processor parameters, which is often represented as a dataflow chart. The mapping procedures have been formalized and recognized as a key element in the digital instrument design, with both technical and artistic challenges (Hunt & Kirk, 2000; Hunt et al., 2003). In particular, several studies, methods, and tools have been published (Wanderley & Battier, 2000; Wanderley, 2002.; Kvifte & Jensenius, 2006; Malloch et al., 2006; Malloch et al., 2007).

In parallel to the development of mapping strategies, important research has focused on musician gestures and movements. Following on early works by Gibet and Cadoz (Cadoz, 1988; Gibet, 1987; Cadoz & Wanderley, 2000), several authors formalized and categorized musical gestures (Godøy & Leman, 2009; Jensenius et al., 2009). Different gesture types involved in music playing can be distinguished: sound-producing gestures but also movements less directly involved in the sound production such as communicative gestures, sound-facilitating gestures, and sound-accompanying gestures (Dahl et al., 2009). Different taxonomies have been proposed, revealing that musical gestures cannot be reduced to simple discrete gestural control mechanisms. In particular, continuous movements, with different phases (e.g. preparation, stroke and release) and co-articulation effects must be taken into account (Rasamimanana & Bevilacqua, 2009).

Our research builds on musical gesture research as well as research in human computer interaction. For example, our approach can be related to what Baudouin-Lafon described as "Designing interaction, not interfaces" in a well-known article (Beaudouin-Lafon, 2004). While this article does not discuss music interaction *per se*, his description of “instrumental interaction”, "situated interaction" and "interaction as a sensori-motor phenomena" is particularly pertinent for our musical applications as described in the following sections.

7.3 Designing Musical Interactions

We developed over the years a holistic approach to the design of digital musical instruments, that could not be represented solely as a series of technical components chained together. Our approach is based on the concepts described below.

First, our gesture studies performed in the context of acoustic instruments (Rasamimanana & Bevilacqua, 2009; Rasamimanana et al., 2009; Schnell, 2013) and augmented instruments (Bevilacqua et al., 2006; Bevilacqua et al., 2012) helped us to formalize fundamental concepts that remain valid for digital musical instruments. We paid particular attention to the notions of *playing techniques* apprehended at high cognitive level by the performers (Dahl et al., 2009). As formalized by Rasamimanana (Rasamimanana, 2008; Rasamimanana, 2012), these can be described as action-sound units, which are constrained by the instrument acoustics, biomechanics and the musician skills.

Second, we consider the interaction between the musician, the instrument and the sound processes as "embodied" (Dourish, 2004; Leman, 2007), learned through processes described by enactive approaches to cognition (Varela et al., 1991). Playing an instrument indeed involves different types of feedback mechanisms, which can be separated in a primary feedback (visual, auditory and tactile-kinesthetic) and secondary feedback (targeted sound produced by the instrument) (Wanderley & Depalle, 2004). These feedbacks create action-perception loops that are essential to sensorimotor learning, and leads the musicians to master their instruments through practice. We consider thus the musical interaction as a process that implies various degrees of learning and that evolves over time.

Additionally, the social and cultural aspects are to be carefully considered. For example, Schnell and Battier introduced the notion of "composed instrument" (Schnell & Battier, 2002), considering both technical and musicological aspects. As a matter of fact, our research is grounded by collaborations with artists such as composers, performers, choreographers, dancers but also by industrial collaborations. In each case, the different sociocultural contexts influenced important design choices.

Figure 7.1 shows important elements we use in our digital instrument design, which are summarized below as two general guidelines that will be illustrated throughout the end of this chapter:

– Motion-sound relationships is designed from high-level description of motion and sound descriptions, using notions of objects affordances (Gibson, 1986; Tanaka, 2010; Rasamimanana et al., 2011), gestural affordances of sound (Godøy, 2009; Caramiaux et al., 2014), playing techniques (Rasamimanana et al., 2011; Rasamimanana et al., 2006), and metaphors (Wessel & Wright, 2002; Bevilacqua et al., 2013). The performers control sound parameters such as articulation and timbre or global musical parameters. In most cases we abandoned the idea that the performers control musical notes (i.e. pitches) as found in classic MIDI controllers. The motion-sound relationship should favour the building of action-perception loops that, after practicing, could be embodied. Therefore, particular attentions must be drawn to the sensori-motor learning processes involved.

– The computerized system is the *mediator* of musical interactions, which encompasses all possibilities from listening to performing. In particular, the mediation can occur between participants: musicians and/or the public. The problem is thus shifted from *human-computer interaction* to *human interactions mediated through digital technologies.*

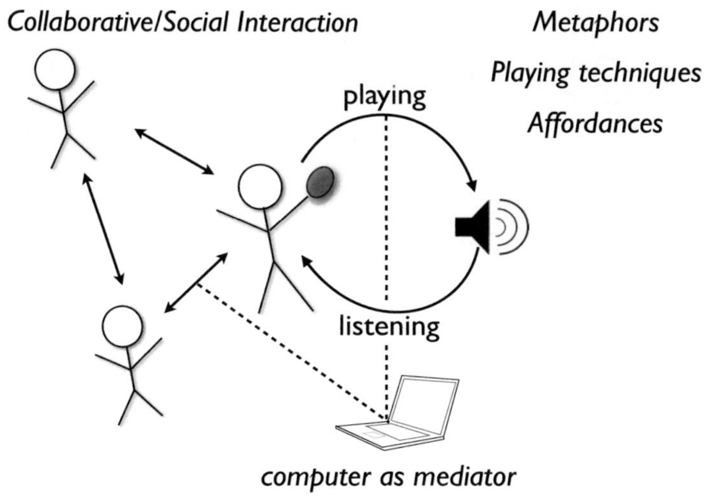

Figure 7.1: Computer-mediated musical interaction: action-perception loops (performing- listening) can be established taking into account notions such as objects affordances, playing techniques and metaphors. The collaborative and social interactions should also be taken into account

7.4 Objects, Sounds and Instruments

Music performance is traditionally associated to the manipulation of an acoustic musical instrument: a physical object that has been cautiously crafted and practiced for several years. On one hand, many digital musical instruments can be viewed in the legacy of this tradition, replacing acoustic elements by digital processes. In some cases, designing and building the controller/interface is part of an artistic endeavour (Oliver, 2010).

On the other hand, digital music practices also challenge the classical role of the instrumental gestures and the instrument in several aspects. In some cases, the performance may be limited to simple actions (e.g. buttons and sliders) that control complex music processes without requiring any particularly virtuosic motor control, which challenges traditional notions of musical virtuosity. In other case, the interface might be based on non-contact interfaces or physiological sensors that have no equivalent in acoustic instruments[5].

A great variety of interfaces emerged over the past decade, in parallel to the development of DIY ("Do It Yoursef") communities such as the community around the Arduino project[6]. Based on our different collaborations with artists and practitioners, it became evident there is a strong need for customizable motion-sensing interfaces, to support a great variety of artistic approaches.

Based on such premises, we developed the Modular Musical Objects (MO), within the Interlude project[7] conducted by a consortium composed of academic institutions (Ircam, Grame), designers (No Design), music pedagogues (Atelier des Feuillantines) and industrial partners (Da Fact, Voxler).

The general goal was to empower users to create their own "musical objects", which necessitates the customization of both tangible interfaces and software (Rasamimanana, et al., 2011). The project included the development of various scenarios based on object and sound affordances and metaphors (Schnell et al., 2011; Bevilacqua et al., 2013).

The first part of the project consisted in the design of an ensemble of hardware modules for wireless motion and touch sensing. These interfaces can be used alone or combined with existing objects or instruments. The exploration with different combinations, in particular with every-day objects, enable for the experimentation of movement-sound relationships.

From a technical point of view, the MO interfaces are based on a central unit containing an inertial measurement unit (3D accelerometer and 3 axis gyroscope). The central unit is connected wirelessly to a computer (Fléty & Maestracci, 2011). This central unit can be combined with various active accessories bridging to other sensors, passive accessories or objects. For example, a dedicated accessory connects piezo sensors to the MO (see Figure 7.2). These piezo sensors, when put on a object, allows for sensing different touch modalities (tap, scratching, etc) by directly measuring the sound wave transmitted at the surface object.

The second part consisted in creating scenarios with software modules for motion analysis and sound synthesis mostly based on recorded sounds (Schnell et al., 2011; Schnell, et al., 2009). The general design approach and scenarios have been described in several publications (Rasamimanana et al., 2011; Schnell et al., 2011; Bevilacqua et al., 2013; Schnell et al., 2011). We recall here some examples.

5 however one might argue that the role of the conductor could be similar to some non-contact interfaces

6 http://www.arduino.cc

7 http://interlude.ircam.fr, 2008–2011

A first case is the MO-Kitchen as illustrated in Figure 7.2. Here, several kitchen appliances were transformed into “musical objects”. For example a whisk with a MO attached to its top was used to control various guitar riffs, performing either small oscillatory motion or energetic strokes.

It is interesting to observe that the original affordance of the object is extended or shifted by the musical interaction. Introducing a feedback loop between the action and the perception modifies the original affordance towards an “action-sound” affordance. Similarly, associating an action to a particular sound will also modify its perception. Therefore, designing musical interactions is achieved by experimenting iteratively with objects, sounds and actions, until consistent action-sound relationships emerge.

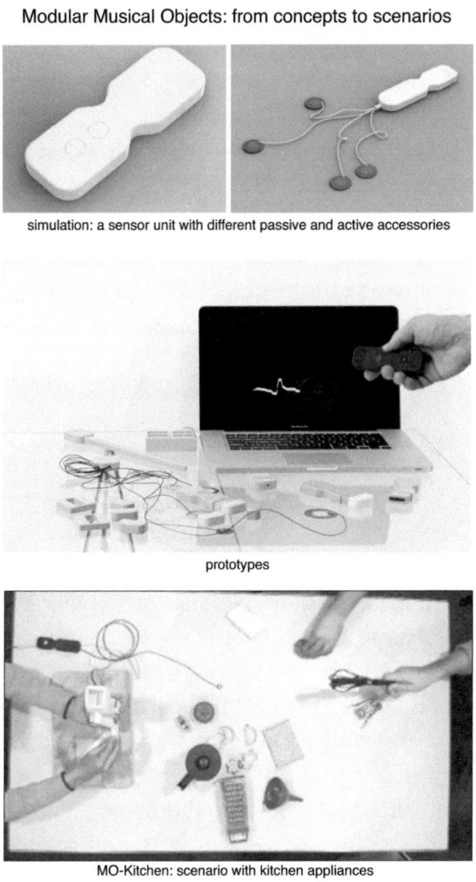

Figure 7.2: Modular Musical Interfaces by the Interlude Consortium. Top: 3D simulation of the central motion unit (top-letf) that can be modified with passive or active accessories (design: NoDesign.net, Jean-Louis Frechin, Uros Petrevski). Middle: Prototypes of the Modular Musical Objects. Bottom: MO-Kitchen scenario, illustrating the case where the MO are associated with everyday objects (Rasamimanana, Bloit & Schnell)

In another application, metaphors were used to illustrate action-sound relationships. For example, the *rainstick* metaphor was used to represent the relationship between titling an object and the simulation of "sound grains" (i.e. small sound segments) sliding virtually inside the object[8], the *shaker* metaphor was used to represent the relationship between moving energetically an object with various rhythmic patterns.

Other actions such as tracing in the air or scratching a surface were also used to control different sounds, establishing relationships between various motion characteristics (e.g. velocity and/or shape) and sound descriptors. The next section describes different strategies and tools that were developed to formalize, model and implement these cases.

7.5 Motion-Sound Relationships

Two distinct problems need to be solved to implement motion-sound interaction following the guidelines we proposed. In the first case, we wish to design movement and playing technique that match particular sounds. We describe below an approach based on what we refer to as *embodied listening*. In the second case, we aim at building interactive systems, which require programming the gesture-sound mapping procedures. We present a short overview of systems we built, using machine learning techniques.

7.5.1 From Sound to Motion

Listening to sound and music induces body movements, consciously or unconsciously. An increasing number of neuroscience studies describe the interaction occurring between listening and motor functions. For example, neurons in monkey premotor cortex were found to discharge when the animal hears a sound related to a specific action (Kohler et al., 2002). Fadiga showed that listening to specific words can produce an activation of speech motor centres (Fadiga et al., 2002). Lahav found activation in motor-related brain regions (fronto-parietal) occurring when non-musician listen to music they learned to play by ear (Lahav et al., 2007).

In the music research field, Godoy and collaborators explored different types of movement that can be performed consciously while listening, such as "mimicking" instrumental playing (Godøy et al., 2006b), or "sound tracing" that corresponds to moving analogously to some sound characteristics (Godøy et al., 2006a). Leman et al.

8 a first version was developed in collaboration with the composer Pierre Jodlowski in the European project SAME and called the Grainstick explores embodied listening by seeking correlation between musician and audience movements (Leman et al., 2009).

We found that exploring the movements induced by listening represents a fruitful approach to design movements-sound interaction. We perform experiments where subjects were asked to perform movement while listening to various sounds and short music excerpts. Different strategies are typically opted by the subjects, depending on the sound type and their cultural references. In some cases, it is possible to find a correlation between specific motion and sound parameters (Caramiaux et al., 2010). In a second study, we compared movement strategies that occur when "mimicking" sound, obtained from every day objects or obtained though digital sound processing (Caramiaux et al., 2014). We found that the users tends to mimic the action that produced the sound when they can recognize it (typically linked to every day objects), otherwise they tend to perform movement that follows acoustic sound descriptors (e.g. energy, pitch, timbral descriptors) in the case of abstract sound that cannot be associated to any every-day action.

From these experiments, we learned that, across participants, different movement strategies exist that often directly reveal which sound features the participants perceive (Tuuri & Eerola, 2012). Interestingly, a subject tends to converge after several trials to idiosyncratic movements associated to a given sound, while remaining very consistent and repeatable over time. This fact offers a very promising methodology to create user-centred approaches to specify movements-sound relationships (Caramiaux et al., 2014b).

7.5.2 From Motion to Sound

Generally two approaches for motion-to-sound mapping are generally proposed: explicit or implicit mapping. Explicit mapping refers to using mathematical relationships where all parameters are set manually. Implicit mapping procedures refer to setting relationships through implicit rules or learning procedures, typically using machine learning techniques (Caramiaux & Tanaka, 2013). Both strategies are actually complementary and can coexist in a single application (Bevilacqua, et al. 2011).

We have developed different implicit methods and an ensemble of tools (mostly in the programming environment Max/MSP[9]). First, regression techniques or dimensionality reduction (e.g. principal component analysis) (Bevilacqua, Muller, & Schnell, 2005) were implemented to allow for relationships that map, frame by frame, n input to m output. Recent works make use of Gaussian Mixture Regression (Françoise et al., 2014).

9 http://www.cycling74.com

Second, time series modelling were also implemented to take into account temporal relationships. In particular, we developed the *gesture follower* that allows for motion synchronization and recognition. It makes use of a hybrid approach between dynamic time warping and Hidden Markov Models (Bevilacqua et al. 2007; Bevilacqua et al., 2010). Working with any type of data stream input, the gesture follower allows for aligning in real-time a live performance with a recorded template. Thus, this allows for the synchronization of different temporal profiles. In this case, the motion-sound relationship is expressed in the time domain, which we denote as *temporal mapping* (Rasamimanana et al., 2009; Bevilacqua et al., 2011).

The initial gesture follower architecture was further developed into a hierarchical model (Françoise et al. 2012). For example, different movement phases such as preparation, attack, sustain, release can be taken into account. Second he extended the concept of temporal mapping using a Multimodal Hidden Markov Model (MHMM) (Françoise et al. 2013b, 2013a). In this case, both gestural and sound data are used simultaneously for training the probabilistic model. Then, the statistical model can be used to generate sound parameters based on the movement parameters.

The important point is that these machine-learning techniques allow us to build mapping *by demonstration* (similarly to some methods proposed in robotics) (Françoise et al., 2013a). Thus, these techniques can be used in the scenarios we described in the previous section, where the user's motions are recorded while listening to sound examples. These recordings are used to train the parameters that describe the motion-sound relationships. Once this is achieved, the user can explore the multimodal space that is created. Such as methodology is currently experimented and validated.

7.6 Towards Computer-Mediated Collaborative Musical Interactions

Music playing is most of the time a collaborative and social experience (Schnell, 2013). Computer-mediated communication is nowadays fully integrated in our cultural habits. Music technology started to integrate collaborative aspects in several applications, with new tools to jam, mix or annotate media collaboratively. Nevertheless, computer-mediated performance remains mainly concerned with either a single performer, or performers with their individual digital instruments. There are notable exceptions of course, such as the *reactable*, a tabletop tangible user interface that can be played collaboratively (Jordà et al 2007) , or also some examples found in laptop and mobile orchestras (Oh et al. 2010).

The different concepts and systems we described previously have been extended to collaborative playing. Figure 7.2-bottom illustrates an example where several MOs interfaces are used simultaneously. Other scenarios were explored with sport balls, inserting a miniaturized MO inside the ball. Games and sport using balls represents interesting cases that be used as starting points to invent new paradigms of music playing.

In the project Urban Musical Game[10], different scenarios were implemented. The first one was to collaboratively play music, the balls being used as instruments. Different playing-techniques (roll, throw, spin etc) were automatically linked to different digital sound processes (N. Rasamimanana et al., 2012). The second one was to focus on a game inspired by existing sports (volleyball, basketball). In this case, the sound produced by the ball motion was perceived as accompanying the game. A third class of scenarios corresponded to games driven by the interactive sound environment. In this case, the game depends on specific sound cues given to the users (see Figure 7.3).

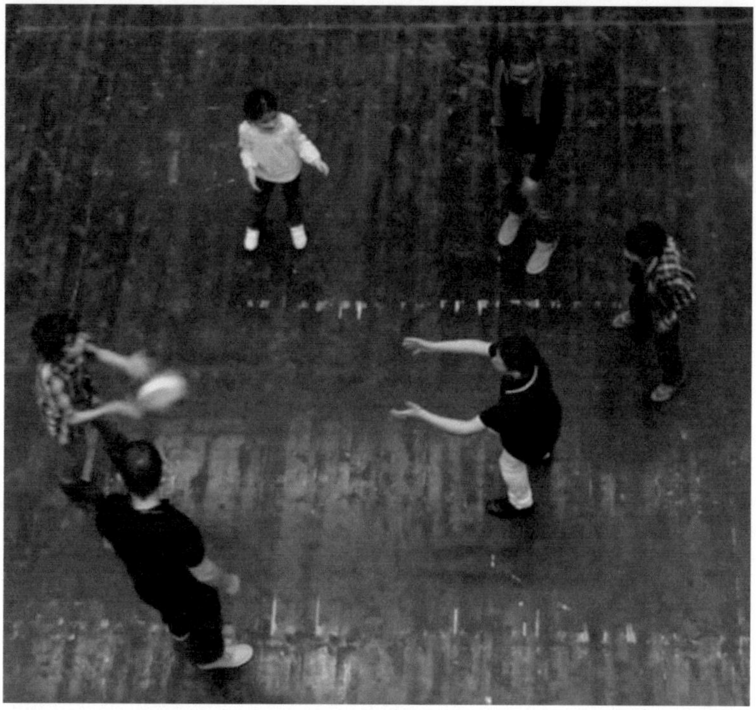

Figure 7.3: Example of one scenario of the Urban Musical Game. Participants must continuously pass the ball to the others. The person looses if she/he holds the ball when an explosive sound is heard. This moment can be anticipated by the participants by listening to evolution of the music : from the tempo acceleration and the pitch increase. Moreover, the participants can also influence the timing of the sonic cues by performing specific moves (e.g. spinning the ball)

In summary, the Urban Musical Game project allowed us to explore different roles for the sound and music in collaborative scenarios. We have just scratched the surface of important research that are necessary to develop further computer mediated collaborative interaction that will profit from the rapid growing of connected objects.

10 by Ircam-NoDesign-Phonotonic

7.7 Concluding Remarks

We presented here concepts that guided us for the development of motion-based musical interactions. While the controller/interface plays a significant role in such interactions, we argue that the important part of the design should be devoted to motion-sounds relationships. These relationships can be developed using concepts such as affordances, playing techniques and metaphors. Importantly, concepts from embodied cognition, applied in both listening and performing situation, reveal to be fruitful for designing and modelling musical interactions.

We briefly described some techniques based on machine learning to implement the musical interaction scenario, which allows designed to handle notion of movement phrases and playing techniques that can be defined by demonstration. We believe this represents a promising area of research which should eventually allow non-specialists to author complex scenarios.

We stress that the musical interactions we described can be seen as interaction *mediated* by technology. Even if tangible objects often play a central role in the presented interactions, the presence of the computer itself disappears – or at least us not perceived as such. In most of our musical applications, the computer screen is not part of the interface and hidden from the users. This allows the players to fully focus their attention on mutual interaction and collaboration keeping the designed mediation technologies in the role of supporting playing and listening.

Musical interactions can thus represent fruitful and complex use cases related to HCC research. This implies cross disciplinary projects, between scientist, technologist but also artists and designers, contributing essential elements of research and helping to shape innovative approaches.

Acknowledgements: We are indebted to all our colleagues of the Real-Time Musical Interaction team who significantly contributed to work described here, an in particular N. Rasamimanana, E. Fléty, R. Borghesi, D. Schwarz, J. Bloit, B. Caramiaux, J. Francoise, E. Boyer, B. Zamborlin. We also thanks all the people involved of the Interlude Consortium: Grame (D. Fober), NoDesign.net (J.-L Frechin and U. Petrevski), Atelier des Feuillantines (F. Guédy), Da Fact and Voxler. Special thanks to the composers A. Cera, P. Jodlowski, F. Baschet and M. Kimura. Finally, we acknowledge support of ANR and Cap Digital (Interlude ANR-08-CORD-010 and Legos 11 BS02 012), and Région Ile de France.

References

Beaudouin-Lafon, M. (2004). Designing interaction, not interfaces. In *Proceedings of the Working Conference on Advanced Visual Interfaces* (pp. 15–22). Gallipoli, Italy.

Bevilacqua, F., Baschet, F., & Lemouton, S. (2012). The augmented string quartet: Experiments and gesture following. *Journal of New Music Research* , 41 (1), 103–119.

Bevilacqua, F., Fels, S., Jensenius, A. R., Lyons, M. J., Schnell, N., & Tanaka, A. (2013). Sig NIME: music, technology, and human-computer interaction. In *CHI '13 Extended Abstracts on Human Factors in Computing Systems* (pp. 2529–2532). Paris, France.

Bevilacqua, F., Guédy, F., Schnell, N., Fléty, E., & Leroy, N. (2007). Wireless sensor interface and gesture-follower for music pedagogy. In *Proceedings of the International Conference on New Interfaces for Musical Expression* (pp. 124–129). New York, NY, USA.

Bevilacqua, F., Muller, R., & Schnell, N. (2005). MnM: a Max/MSP mapping toolbox. In *Proceedings of the International Conference on New Interfaces for Musical Expression* (pp. 85–88). Vancouver, Canada.

Bevilacqua, F., Rasamimanana, N., Fléty, E., Lemouton, S., & Baschet, F. (2006). The augmented violin project: research, composition and performance report. In *Proceedings of the International Conference on New Interfaces for Musical Expression* (pp. 402–406). Paris, France.

Bevilacqua, F., Schnell, N., Rasamimanana, N., Bloit, J., Fléty, E., Caramiaux, B., Françoise, J. & Boyer, E. (2013). De-MO: Designing action-sound relationships with the MO interfaces. In *CHI '13 Extended Abstracts on Human Factors in Computing Systems* (pp. 2907–2910). Paris, France.

Bevilacqua, F., Schnell, N., Rasamimanana, N., Zamborlin, B., & Guédy, F. (2011). Online Gesture Analysis and Control of Audio Processing. In *Musical Robots and Interactive Multimodal Systems* (pp. 127–142). Springer Tracts in Advanced Robotics (Vol. 74, pp 127–142), Springer Verlag..

Bevilacqua, F., Zamborlin, B., Sypniewski, A., Schnell, N., Guedy, F., & Rasamimanana, N. (2010). Continuous realtime gesture following and recognition. In *Lecture Notes in Computer Science* (Vol. 5934, pp. 73–84). Springer Verlag.

Cadoz, C. (1988). Instrumental gesture and musical composition. In *Proceedings of the International Computer Music Conference*, Köln, Germany.

Cadoz, C., & Wanderley, M. (2000). Gesture Music, In Trends in gestural control of music. In M. Wanderley & M. Battier (Eds.). Ircam Centre Pompidou.

Caramiaux, B., Bevilacqua, F., & Schnell, N. (2010). Towards a gesture-sound cross-modal analysis. In *Embodied Communication and Human-Computer Interaction*, Lecture Notes in Computer Science (vol 5934, pp. 158–170). Springer Verlag.

Caramiaux, B., & Tanaka, A. (2013). Machine learning of musical gestures. In *Proceedings of the International Conference on New Interfaces for Musical Expression*, Daejeon, Korea.

Caramiaux, B., Bevilacqua, F., Bianco, T., Schnell, N., Houix, O., & Susini, P. (2014a). The Role of Sound Source Perception in Gestural Sound Description. *ACM Transactions on Applied Perception*. 11 (1). pp.1–19.

Caramlaux, B., Francolse, J., Schnell, N., Bevilacqua, F. (2014b). Mapping Through Listening, *Computer Music Journal*, 38, 34–48.

Dahl, S., Bevilacqua, F., Bresin, R., Clayton, M., Leante, L., Poggi, I., & Rasamimanana, N. (2009). Gestures in performance. In Leman, M. and Godøy, R. I., (Eds.), *Musical Gestures. Sound, Movement, and meaning,* (pp. 36–68). Routledge.

Dourish, P. (2004). *Where the action is: the foundations of embodied interaction*. The MIT Press.

Fadiga, L., Craighero, L., Buccino, G., & Rizzolatti, G. (2002). Short communication: Speech listening specifically modulates the excitability of tongue muscles: A TMS study. *European Journal of Neuroscience*, 15, 399–402.

Ferscha, A. (Ed.). (2013). *Human Computer Confluence: The Next Generation Humans and Computers* Research Agenda. Linz: Institute for Pervasive Computing, Johannes Kepler University Linz. ISBN: 978-3-200-03344-3. Retrieved from http://smart.inf.ed.ac.uk/human_computer_confluence/.

Fléty, E., & Maestracci, C. (2011). Latency improvement in sensor wireless transmission using IEEE 802.15.4. In A. R. Jensenius, A. Tveit, R. I. Godøy, & D. Overholt (Eds.), *Proceedings of the International Conference on New Interfaces for Musical Expression* (pp. 409–412). Oslo, Norway.

Françoise, J., Caramiaux, B., & Bevilacqua, F. (2012). A hierarchical approach for the design of gesture-to-sound mappings. *Proceedings of the 9th Sound and Music Conference* (SMC), Copenhague, Danemark.

Françoise, J., Schnell, N., & Bevilacqua, F. (2013a). Gesture-based control of physical modeling sound synthesis: a mapping-by-demonstration approach. In *Proceedings of the 21st ACM International Conference on Multimedia* (pp. 447–448). Barcelona, Spain.

Françoise, J., Schnell, N., & Bevilacqua, F. (2013b). A multimodal probabilistic model for gesture – based control of sound synthesis. In *Proceedings of the 21st ACM International Conference on Multimedia* (pp. 705–708).

Françoise, J., Schnell, N., Borghesi, R., Bevilacqua, F. (2014). Probabilistic Models for Designing Motion and Sound Relationships. In *Proceedings of the 2014 International Conference on New Interfaces for Musical Expression* (NIME'14). London, UK.

Gibet, S. (1987). Codage, représentation et traitement du geste instrumental: application à la synthèse de sons musicaux par simulation de m écanismes instrumentaux. PhD Dissertation, Institut National Polytechnique, Grenoble.

Gibson, J. J. (1986). *The ecological approach to visual perception*. Routledge.

Godøy, R. I. (2009). Gestural affordances of musical sound. In R. I. Godøy & M. Leman (Eds.), *Musical gestures: Sound, movement, and meaning* (pp 103–125). Routledge.

Godøy, R. I., Haga, E., & Jensenius, A. R. (2006a). Exploring music-related gestures by sound-tracing- a preliminary study. In *Proceedings of the COST287 ConGAS 2nd international symposium on gesture interfaces for multimedia systems*, (pp. 27–33). Leeds, UK.

Godøy, R. I., Haga, E., & Jensenius, A. R. (2006b). Playing "air instruments": Mimicry of sound-producing gestures by novices and experts. In *Lecture Notes in Computer Science*. (Vol. 3881, pp 256–267). Springer-Verlag.

Godøy, R. I., & Leman, M. (Eds.). (2009). *Musical gestures: Sound, movement, and meaning.* Routledge.

Hunt, A., & Kirk, R. (2000). Mapping Strategies for Musical Performance. In M. M. Wanderley & M. Battier (Eds.), *Trends in gestural control of music* (pp. 231–258). Ircam Centre Pompidou.

Hunt, A., Wanderley, M. M., & Paradis, M. (2003). The importance of parameter mapping in electronic instrument design. *Journal of New Music Research*, 32(4), 429–440.

Jensenius, A. R., Wanderley, M., Godøy, R. I., & Leman, M. (2009). Musical gestures: concepts and methods in research. In R. I. Godøy & M. Leman (Eds.), *Musical gestures: Sound, movement, and meaning*. (pp. 12–35). Routledge.

Jordà, S., Geiger, G., Alonso, M., & Kaltenbrunner, M. (2007). The reacTable: exploring the synergy between live music performance and tabletop tangible interfaces. In *Proceedings of the 1st international conference on Tangible and Embedded Interaction* (pp. 139–146). ACM.

Kohler, E., Keysers, C., Umilta, M. A., Fogassi, L., Gallese, V., & Rizzolatti, G. (2002). Hearing sounds, understanding actions: action representation in mirror neurons. *Science*, 297(5582), 846–848.

Kvifte, T., & Jensenius, A. R. (2006). Towards a coherent terminology and model of instrument description and design. In *Proceedings of the Conference on New Interfaces for Musical Expression* (pp. 220–225). Paris, France.

Lahav, A., Saltzman, E., & Schlaug, G. (2007). Action representation of sound: Audiomotor recognition network while listening to newly acquired actions. The *Journal of Neuroscience*, 27 (2), 308–314.

Leman, M. (2007). *Embodied music cognition and mediation technology*. Cambridge, Massas-suchetts: The MIT Press.

Leman, M., Desmet, F., Styns, F., Van Noorden, L., & Moelants, D. (2009). Sharing musical expression through embodied listening: A case study based on Chinese Guqin music. *Music Perception*, 26(3), 263–278.

Malloch, J., Birnbaum, D., Sinyor, E., & Wanderley, M. (2006). Towards a new conceptual framework for digital musical instruments. In *Proceedings of the Digital Audio Effects Conference* (DAFx). Montreal, Canada.

Malloch, J., Sinclair, S., & Wanderley, M. M. (2007). From controller to sound: Tools for collaborative development of digital musical instruments. *Proceedings of the 2007 International Computer Music Conference*, Copenhagen, Denmark.

Miranda, E., & Wanderley, M. (2006). *New digital musical instruments: Control and interaction beyond the keyboard*. A-R Editions.

Oh, J., Herrera, J., Bryan, N. J., Dahl, L., & Wang, G. (2010). Evolving the mobile phone orchestra. In *Proceedings of the International Conference on New Interfaces for Musical Expression* (pp. 82–87). Sydney, Australia

Oliver, J. (2010). The MANO controller: A video based hand tracking system. In *Proceedings of the International Computer Music Conference*. New York, USA.

Rasamimanana, N. (2012). Towards a conceptual framework for exploring and modelling expressive musical gestures. *Journal of New Music Research* , 41 (1), 3–12.

Rasamimanana, N., Bevilacqua, F., Bloit, J., Schnell, N., Fléty, E., Cera, A., Petrevski, U., & Frechin, J.-L. (2012). The Urban Musical Game: Using sport balls as musical interfaces. In *CHI '12 Extended Abstracts on Human Factors in Computing Systems* (pp. 1027–1030). .

Rasamimanana, N., Bevilacqua, F., Schnell, N., Guedy, F., Flety, E., Maestracci, C., Petrevski, U., & Frechin, J.-L. (2011). Modular musical objects towards embodied control of digital music. In *Proceedings of the fifth International Conference on Tangible, Embedded, and Embodied Interaction* (pp. 9–12). Funchal, Protugal.

Rasamimanana, N. H. (2008). *Geste instrumental du violoniste en situation de jeu : analyse et modélisation*. PhD dissertation, Université Pierre et Marie Curie..

Rasamimanana, N. H., & Bevilacqua, F. (2009). Effort-based analysis of bowing movements: evidence of anticipation effects. *The Journal of New Music Research*, 37(4), 339–351.

Rasamimanana, N. H., Fléty, E., & Bevilacqua, F. (2006). Gesture analysis of violin bow strokes. In *Gesture in human-computer interaction and simulation* (Vol. 3881, pp. 145–155). Springer Verlag.

Rasamimanana, N. H., Kaiser, F., & Bevilacqua, F. (2009). Perspectives on gesture-sound relationships informed from acoustic instrument studies. *Organised Sound*, 14(2), 208–216.

Schnell, N. (2013). *Playing (with) sound – Of the animation of digitized sounds and their reenactment by playful scenarios in the design of interactive audio applications*. PhD dissertation, Institute of Electronic Music and Acoustics, University of Music and Performing Arts Graz.

Schnell, N., & Battier, M. (2002). Introducing composed instruments, technical and musicological implications. In *Proceedings of the 2002 Conference on New Interfaces for Musical Expression* (pp. 1–5). Dublin, Ireland.

Schnell, N., Bevilacqua, F., Guédy, F., & Rasamimana, N. (2011). Playing and replaying – sound, gesture and music analysis and re-synthesis for the interactive control and re-embodiment of recorded music. In H. von Loesch & S. Weinzierl (Eds.), *Gemessene interpretation computergestützte aufführungsanalyse im kreuzverhör der disziplinen, klang und begriff*. Schott Verlag.

Schnell, N., Bevilacqua, F., Rasamimana, N., Bloit, J., Guedy, F., & Fléty, E. (2011). Playing the "MO" – gestural control and re-embodiment of recorded sound and music. In the *Proceedings of the International Conference on New Interfaces for Musical Expression* (pp. 535–536). Oslo, Norway.

Schnell, N., Röbel, A., Schwarz, D., Peeters, G., & Borghesi, R. (2009). MuBu and friends: Assembling tools for content based real-time interactive audio processing in Max/MSP. In *Proceedings of the International Computer Music Conference (ICMC)*. Montreal, Canada.

Tanaka, A., (2010). Mapping out instruments, affordances, and mobiles. In *Proceedings of the 2010 New Interfaces for Musical Expression* (pp. 88–93), Sydney, Australia.

Tuuri, K., & Eerola, T. (2012, June). Formulating a Revised Taxonomy for Modes of Listening. *Journal of New Music Research*, 41(2), 137–152.

Varela, F., Thompson, E., & Rosch, E. (1991). *The Embodied Mind: Cognitive Science and Human Experience*. Cambridge, USA: Massachusetts Institute of Technology Press.

Wanderley, M.M. (2002). Mapping Strategies in Real-time Computer Music. *Organised Sound*, 7(2).

Wanderley, M., & Battier, M. (Eds.). (2000). *Trends in gestural control of music*. Ircam.

Wanderley, M., & Depalle, P. (2004). Gestural control of sound synthesis. In *Proceedings of the IEEE* (Vol. 92, p. 632–644).

Wessel, D., & Wright, M. (2002, September). Problems and Prospects for Intimate Musical Control of Computers. *Computer Music Journal*, 26(3), 11–22.

Fivos Maniatakos

8 Designing Three-Party Interactions for Music Improvisation Systems

Abstract: For years, a major challenge among artists and scientists has been the construction of music systems capable of interacting with humans on stage. Such systems find applicability in contexts within which they are required to act both as independent, improvising agents and as instruments in the hands of a musician. This is widely known as the player and the instrument paradigm.During the last years, research on Machine Improvisation has made important steps towards intelligent, efficient and musically sensible systems that in many cases can establish an interesting dialog with a human instrument player. Most of these systems require, or at the very least encourage, the active participation not only of instrument players but also of computer users-operators that conduct actions in a certain way. Still, very little has been done towards a more sophisticated interaction model that would include not only the instrument player and the machine but also the computer operator, who in this case should be considered as a computer performer.In this paper we are concerned with those aspects of enhanced interactivity that can exist in a collective improvisation context. This is a context characterized by the confluent relationship between instrument players, computers, as well as humans that perform with the help of the computer, onstage. The paper focuses on the definition of a theoretical as well as a computational framework for the design of modern machine improvisation systems that will leave the necessary space for such parallel interactions to occur in real-time. We will study the so-called three party interaction scheme based on three concepts: first, with the help of the computer, provide an active role for the human participant, either as an instrument player or as a performer. Secondly, create the framework that will allow the computer being utilized as an augmented, high-level instrument. Lastly, conceive methods that will allow the computer to play an independent role as an improviser-agent who exhibits human music skills.

Keywords: Machine Improvisation, Computer Aided Improvisation, Three Party Interaction, Automata

8.1 Introduction

A major aspect of the computer's contribution to music is reflected in interactive systems. These are computer systems meant to perform together with human performers on stage. It seems that there are at least two a priori reasons for such systems to exist and they are both straightforward to understand: sound synthesis and algorithmic processing. By expanding the acoustic instruments with a supplementary layer, interactive systems added a completely new dimension to the way music is generated and perceived onstage. On the other hand, the computers efficiency in executing complex algorithms, otherwise impossible to test manually, has allowed the introduction of computational paradigms into the world of composition and improvisation. These two concepts are known as the instrument and the player paradigm respectively. With musical demands increasing over the years, interactive systems have come on age, only to be constrained by the limitations imposed by both the theoretical background and the technically plausible.

Machine musicianship (see (Rowe, 1992)) is regarded as the key to the success of interactive systems. The first reason for this is straightforward: due to their apparent association with human skills, computer skills have to be advanced enough so as to substantiate the computer's raison d'être in the music field. The second reason is perhaps the most important: making the computer more musically intelligent can help people engage with music. Consequently, through a human-oriented approach, machine musicianship can be seen as a means of improving audiation, which, according Gordon in (Gordon, 1980), is "an individual's ability to communicate through music". Machover (Oteri, 1999) has wonderfully expressed the computer's role in enhancing musical sociability: the deployment of computers as a way of reducing practical inconveniences and of increasing the level of communication that can be achieved through music, combined with a vision of engaging more people in music regardless of their dexterity level, makes it nothing less that appealing. In (Rowe, 2001), Rowe expresses a similar thought: "… Interactive systems require the participation of humans making music to work. If interactive music systems are sufficiently engaging as partners, they may encourage people to make music at whatever level they can."

These ideas are also discernible in the history of machine improvisation systems. In the beginning, research seemed to focus more on the development of autonomous, self-contained virtual improvisers and composers (Mantaras & Arcos, 2002). Algorithmic composition of melodies, adaptation to harmonic background, stochastic processes, genetic co-evolution, dynamic systems, chaotic algorithms, machine learning and natural language processing techniques were a few of the approaches that were followed and that one can still find in machine improvisation. However, most of these machine improvisation systems, even with interesting sound results either in a pre-defined music style or in the form of free- style computer synthesis, did not adequately refer to the part of interaction with humans.

Nowadays, the incorporation of human participants in the process is almost non-negotiable. During the last years, research on Machine Improvisation has made important steps towards intelligent, efficient and musically sensible systems, based on the instrument or the player paradigm, or both. In many cases, such improvisation systems manage to establish an interesting dialog with a human instrument player and, in many cases, encourage the active participation of a computer user that conducts actions in a certain manner.

Still, very little has been done towards a more sophisticated interaction model that would include not only the instrument player and the machine but also the machine operator (computer user or performer). Do modern computer improvisation systems really manage to utilize the potential of this new form of interactivity, that is, between the computer and its user? And what would be the theoretical framework of such an approach that would permit a double form of interactivity between (a) the computer and instrument player (b) the computer and the performer?

In this work we are concerned with those aspects of enhanced interactivity that can exist in a modern music improvisation context. This is a context characterized by the presence of instrument players, computers, as well as humans that perform with the help of the computer. It is therefore the focus of this paper to define a theoretical as well as a computational framework that will leave the necessary space for such interactions to occur in real-time. In the next sections we will study the so-called three party interaction scheme and the architecture of GrAIPE (Graph Aided Interactive Performance Environment) improvisation system that is based on three basic concepts: first, with the help of the computer, provide an active role for the human participant, either as an instrument player or as a performer. Secondly, create the framework that will allow the computer to be utilized as an augmented, high-level instrument. Lastly, conceive methods that will allow the computer to play an independent role as an improviser-agent who exhibits human music skills.

8.2 Interactive Improvisation Systems

8.2.1 Compositional Trends and Early Years

The exploration of random processes for music composition has been of great interest to many composers of the last century. Cage is one of the first composers to underline, through his compositional work, the importance not so much of the resulting sound but of the process necessary for its creation. It was as early as 1939 with his work Imaginary Landscape that he detached himself from the musique concrete paradigm of sound transformation in controlled environments, thus stressing the importance of both the creation process and the randomness that occurs in less controlled performance contexts. It is precisely this trend that we come across in his later works, such as William's Mix (1953) and Fontana Mix (1958) as well as in studio works of other composers of the time, such as Reich's Come Out (1966) and Eno's Discrete Music (1975) and in live performance projects by both Cage and Tudor, namely Rainforest and Variations V (see (Eigenfeldt, 2007)) for more details on the above compositional works).

While algorithmic composition has placed the composition process at the centre of attention, it was the "complexification" of this process that was indented to become the basic constituent of what was identified as interactive composition. Interactive composition focused on how to make the composition process complex enough so as to assure the unpredictability of the result. This paradigm, first introduced by Joel Chadabe (see (Chadabe, 1984)), grounded the computer as an indispensable component of the composition process and as the medium to achieve “creative” randomness through algorithmic complexity. The basic idea found behind interactive composition is the one of a sophisticated “instrument” whose output exceeds the one-to-one relationship with the human input by establishing a mutually influential relationship between the performer and itself. The partial unpredictability of information generated by the system, combined with the partial control of the process from the part of the performer, creates a mutually influential relationship between the two, thus, placing both into an interactive loop.

8.2.2 Interacting Live With the Computer

Interactive composition has signalled the beginning of a new era in computer music systems, providing a new paradigm for human computer interaction in music composition and performance.

The Voyager interactive musical environment is a personal project by trombonist and composer George Lewis (Lewis, 2000). The software, first written in Forth language at the early 1980s, was intended as a companion for onstage trombone improvisation, by guiding automatic composition through real-time analysis of the various aspects of the trombone players performance. According to Lewis, Voyager follows the player paradigm in Rowe’s taxonomy, in the sense that it is designed to generate complex responses through internal processes thus humanizing its behaviour.

Rowe’s Cypher system (1990) reflected the motivation to formalize concepts on machine musicianship for the player paradigm (see (Rowe, 1992, 2001, 1999)). This system can be regarded as a general set of methods that cope with four basic areas of machine musicianship: analysis, pattern processing, learning, and knowledge representation. Rowe’s ideas have had major influence on machine improvisation systems of the last decade. A typical example of such systems are those employing Lexicography-based methods, such as suffix trees, while there are also other, non pattern-based systems that may produce similar results. Thom with her BAND-OUT-OF-A-BOX (BOB) system (Thom, 2000) addresses the problem of real-time interactive improvisation between BOB and a human player. In other words, BOB is a “music companion for real-time improvisation. Thom proposes a stochastic model based on a greedy search within a constrained space of possible notes to be played. Her system learns these constraints -hence the stochastic model- from the human player by means of an unsupervised probabilistic clustering algorithm. Its approach is more performer than designer based, as it adapts to the playing of the instrument player. Furthermore, the system has a high degree of autonomy, using exclusively non-supervised methods.

An interaction paradigm which is of major interest is the one of "stylistic reinjection", employed by the OMax system (Assayag & Bloch, 2007; Assayag, Bloch, Chemillier, Cont, & Dubnov, 2006). OMax is a real-time improvisation system which use on the fly stylistic learning methods in order to capture the playing style of the instrument player. OMax learning mechanism is based on the Factor Oracle (FO) automaton (introduced in (Allauzen, Crochemore, & Raffinot, 1999)). OMax provides a role for the computer user as well, in the sense that during a performance, the user can change on the fly a number improvisation parameters. The capacity of OMax to adapt easily to different music styles without any preparation, together with its ability to treat audio directly as an input through the employment of efficient pitch tracking algorithms, make it an attractive environment for computer improvisation.

Another system worth mentioning is The Continuator (Pachet, 2002). Based on suffix trees, the system's purpose was to fill the gap between interactive music systems and music imitation systems. Given a mechanism that assures repositioning from a leaf to somewhere inside the tree, generation can be seen as the concatenated outcome of edge labels, called "continuations", emitted by the iterated navigation down the branches of the tree. Tests with jazz players, as well as with amateurs and children confirmed the importance of the system for the instrument player – computer interaction scheme. In (Pachet & Roy, 2011) the authors exploit the potential of integrating general constraints into Markov chains. Moving towards this direction, they reformulate the Markov probability matrix together with constraint satisfaction practices so as to generate steerable Markovian sequences.

Schwarz's CataRT project is an efficient, continuously evolving real-time concatenative sound synthesis system, initially conceived in the cadre of the instrument paradigm. After five years of continuous development, CataRT in now capable of dealing with the problem of finding continuations. It has also recently started challenging the CSS's potential to function as an improvisation companion in the cadre of the player paradigm (Schwarz & Johnson, 2011).

8.3 Three Party Interaction in Improvisation

We use the term three-party interaction to refer to the ensemble of interactions arising from a modern, collective improvisation context. In Figure 8.1, one can see the basic concepts of the three party interaction scheme. The participants in this scheme are: the musician, the machine (computer) and the computer performer. Communication among the three is achieved either directly, such as in the case between the performer and the computer, or indirectly through the common improvisation sound field. During an improvisation session, both musician and performer receive a continuous stream of musical information, consisting of a melange of sounds coming from all sources and thrown into the shared sound field canvas. Incoming information is then interpreted through human perceptual mechanisms. This interpretation involves the separation of the sound streams and the construction of an abstract internal representation inside the human brain on the low and high level parameters of each musical flux, as well as on the dynamic features of the collective improvisation. During a session, the musician is in a constant loop with the machine. She/he listens to its progressions and responds accordingly. The human, short-time memory mechanisms make it able for her/him to continuously adapt to the improvisation decisions of the machine and the evolution of the musical event as a group, as well as to react to a sudden change of context.

At the same time, the machine is listening to the musician and constructs a representation on what she/he has played. This is one of the standard principles for human machine improvisation. Furthermore, the machine potentially adapts to the mid-term memory properties of the musician's playing, thus re-injecting stylistically coherent patterns. During all these partial interaction schemes, the performer behind the computer, as a human participant, is also capable of receiving and analyzing mixed-source musical information, separating sources and observing the overall evolution.

The novelty of our architecture relies mainly on the concepts hidden behind the communication between performer and machine. Instead of restricting the performer's role to a set of decision making actions, our approach aims at putting the performer in a position where she/he is in a constant dialog with the computer. This means, instead of taking decisions, the performer 'discusses' his intentions with the computer; the computer, in its turn, makes complex calculi and proposes certain solutions to the performer. The latter evaluates the computer's response and either makes a decision or lances a new query to the machine. Conversely, the machine either executes the performer's decision or responds to the new query. This procedure runs continuously and controls the improvisation.

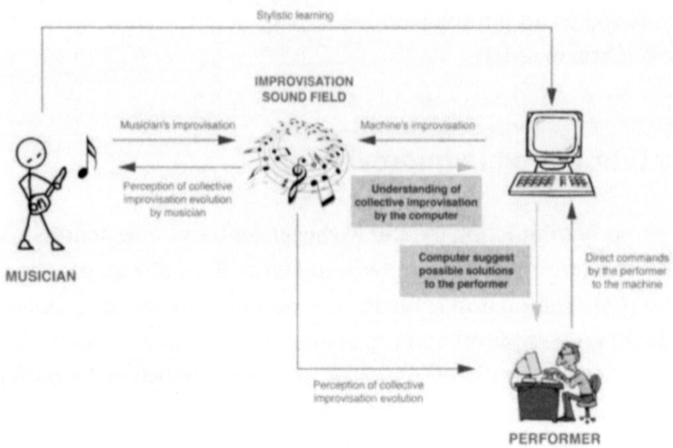

Figure 8.1: Three-Party Interaction Scheme for collective improvisation. In yellow the interactions held according to the human and the instrument paradigm

The second concept concerns the computer's understanding of improvisation. This necessity derives from the fact that even though the computer is able to learn, at least to a certain extent, the stylistic features of the musicians playing, still the understanding of the overall improvisation process remains beyond its grasp. Therefore, there has to be a dedicated mechanism that will assure the interaction between the machine and each of the participants of the improvisation. Moreover, such a mechanism can prove to be beneficial for the performer – machine interaction as well, as it can make the computer more 'intelligent' in its dialog with the performer.

As mentioned in Section 1, building frameworks with the intelligence to tackle simultaneously all issues arising from three party interaction is not straightforward. Most systems are based on just one method and, although they adapt well to a restricted subset of requirements, they usually fail to provide a complete framework for dealing with the musicianship of improvisation agents. For instance, a system may show increased accompaniment and solo improvisation skills for a particular music style, whilst at the same time fail to adapt to other musical styles.

On the other hand, hybrid systems that use different modules in parallel -each based on a different approach- failed to provide clear answers to the problem. Tackling a variety of problems demands heteroclite actions arising from distinct methods and representations. Dispersing resources to numerous, distinct strategies simultaneously, increases the computational cost. As the whole system has to make everything work together in real-time, the computational cost may be prohibitive. One way towards a universal framework for machine improvisation agents is to find common elements among the different approaches and bring them together. Nevertheless, the main reason for the difficulty for these heuristics to work together and cooperate for achieving solutions to composite problems, is the lack of a universal, music-dedicated representation. Such a representation would allow all different methods to be regrouped and work in reduced memory cost.

Thus, the technical requirements of this representation framework should be the following:

- It should provide tools for sequence generation coherent to the stylistic features of the improvisation as established by the ensemble of the participants,
- It should entail mechanisms to detect modes of playing of each of the participants during improvisation, to detect the short-term, expressive features and be capable of responding accordingly,
- It should have mechanisms allowing human-driven, stylistically coherent sequence generation, in order to interact with the performer,
- It should be computationally efficient, fully customizable and expandable with respect to the different types of interaction that it can establish either with the instrument player or with the human operator.

8.4 The GrAIPE Improvisation System

GrAIPE is a software built to support the previously mentioned requirements for improvisation in the three party interaction context. “GrAIPE” stands for Graph Assisted Interactive Performance Environment. GrAIPE is a data-driven system, in the sense that it does not need any a priori knowledge to improvise, but learns directly from the content. Its mechanism is based on the simple principle of detecting and representing similarities of musical motifs inside the sequences, fed to the system during the learning process. With the help of this representation, the system is then capable of detecting musically meaningful continuations between non-contiguous motifs inside the sequence. When in improvisation mode, the system navigates inside this representation either linearly or non-linearly. In the first case, it reproduces exactly a part of the original sequence, whereas in the second, it jumps (reinjects) to a distant point of the sequence, thus producing a musical motif that is musically interesting even though it does not exist in the original sequence. By balancing these two navigation modes, GrAIPE manages to produce novel music material by meaningfully recombining motifs of the original sequence.

What is new about GrAIPE in comparison with conventional improvisation systems is the mechanism for controlling interaction in improvisation. This mechanism is based on the representation structure that lies beneath GrAIPE, the Music Multi Factor Graph (MMFG) introduced in (Maniatakos, 2012). The MMFG is a graph-like structure for representing musical content. It contains a number of nodes equal to the number of successive musical events that occur in the given sequence, as well as weights that determine possible reinjections.

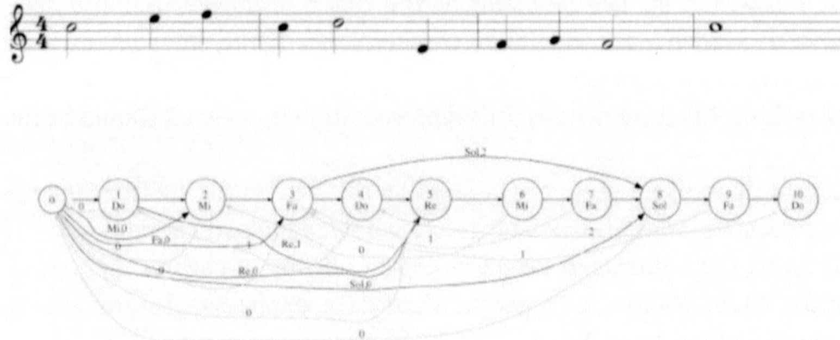

Figure 8.2: Top: Music sequence: S = [Do,Mi,Fa,Do,Re,Mi,Fa,Sol,Fa,Do]. Bottom: MFG-Cl for sequence S. There is one-to-one correspondence between the notes and the states of the MFG (each note event is exactly one state). Arrows in black and grey color represent transitions (factors) and suffix links respectively

The key behind MMFG’s novelty is its double identity, being simultaneously a Repeat Non-Linear (RNL) graph and a Multi Factor Graph (MFG) automaton (for both see

(Maniatakos, 2012)). Due to its identity as a RNL graph, it manages to exhaustively detect all possible continuations inside a learned sequence, sort them according to their musical quality and schedule reinjections through time. By being a MFG automaton, MMFG provides the tools for finding a given pattern inside a sequence with minimal computational cost. Furthermore, as shown in (Maniatakos, 2012), MMFG is the result of merging the two structures together by taking advantage of their common properties as structures. Building MMFG is accomplished at almost no additional memory cost than the one needed for RNL and, in any case, far less than building the graph and the automaton separately.

With the help of MMFG, it is possible to resolve not only problems for pattern matching and sequence scheduling but also composite problems that arise when combining the two categories of problems together. GrAIPE allows the user to declare a number of constraints relating to the improvisation and, by employing a number of algorithms called "primitives", proposes improvisation scenarios compliant with the user's constraints.

The table of Figure 8.3 illustrates the steps of the scheduling process for music sequence generation with the help of MMFG's primitives. MMFG provides a variety of strategies for declaring the source, the destination and the generation parameters. Concerning the designation of the source, this can be done through pure temporal parameters, such as in absolute terms or at a specified time interval. Alternatively, it can also be done by declaring a source state locally, or by satisfying the condition that a specific pattern (chroma, rhythmic, or timbral) is recognized. In a similar manner we can declare the target of the scheduled sequence, with the help of explicit (state) or implicit local parameters (for example, at a certain motif inside the sequence). A number of different configurations can be performed to specify the temporal parameters connected to the target. For instance, one can ask the system to go to a specific target "immediately" (by forcing the transition to the target state), to transit smoothly towards a specified target "as quickly as possible", or in terms of absolute time or in a time interval (i.e improvise smoothly and arrive to a target t within 5 seconds). Finally, there can also be many other possible parameters in order to specify the characteristics of the generation process. These parameters rely on filtering transitions from/to a state according to quality parameters, or by applying quality constraints to the entire path. In the table of Figure 8.3 there are also methods for balancing the tradeoffs of stylistic coherency vs. novelty and looping vs. originality.

This parameterization of the scheduling process with the help of MMFG provides a framework of large-scale control over the generation process. The great advantage of this approach is the fact that, once the scheduling parameters are defined, generation can then be done automatically without any additional intervention from the part of the user. By declaring long-term goals and leaving the note-level generation -according to a set of rules- to the computer, it is possible to achieve precise control on the temporal aspects of generation. This facilitates generation in the improvisation context, where precise temporal control is indispensable, but not straightforward to achieve through conventional methods.

From		To		How			
where	when	where	when	q quality constraints	Q quality constraints	coherency vs novelty	domain constraints
at state s	at moment T	to state t	immediately	bounded below		$P=\frac{non-lin}{linear}$	repeating contin- uations (looping)
at the ac- tual state	in ΔT time	to pattern q	as quickly as possible	bounded above	$L_1 \leq \sum q \leq L_2$	γ linear transitions every 1 non-linear	limited repetitions
at pattern p	at event e	to rhyth- mic pat- tern q_r	at second T	double bounded			unique continua- tions
at rythmic pattern p_r			at approxi- mately ΔT time				

Figure 8.3: Panorama of control parameters for generation. The scheduling process is divided into 3 basic steps: source, target and path (from, to, how). Both source and target can be implied either through local (state) or contextual (pattern) parameters. The scheduled path is described with the help of constraints, which can be local (intra-state) and global (interstate), or may concern information about coherency/novelty tradeoff and the rate of repeated continuations. Problems of different classes can be combined, each time giving a different generation method

8.5 General Architecture for Three Party Improvisation in Collective Improvisation

The internal architecture of GrAIPE is shown in Figure 8.4. This architecture consists mainly of six modules which can act either concurrently or sequentially. On the far left we consider the musician, who feeds information into two modules: the pre-processing module and the short-term memory module. The pre-processing module is responsible for the symbolic encoding of audio information and stylistic learning. On the far right side of the figure we see the renderer, the unit that sends generated audio out to the environment.

The MMFG structure lies inside the Multiple representation module, and entails the long and short-term stylistic features of the learned material. This material can be either pre-learned sequences or the improvisation flows of the instrument players that the systems learns on-the-fly.

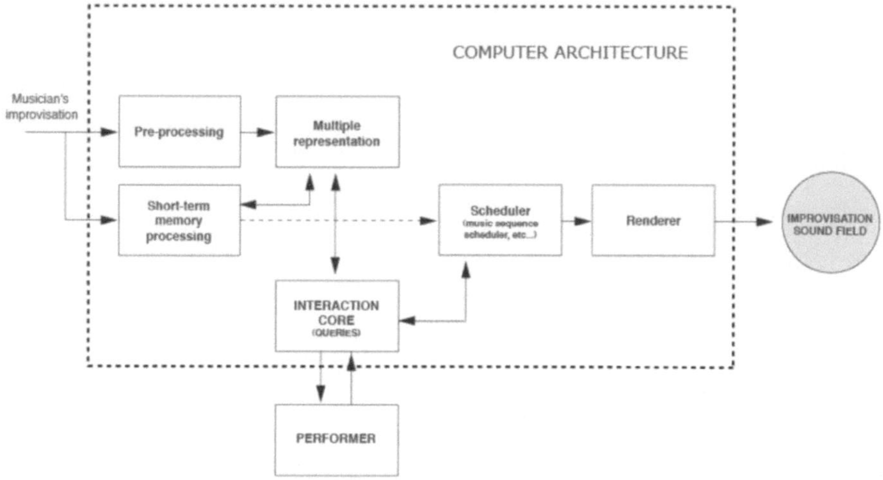

Figure 8.4: Overall Computer Architecture of GrAIPE

The short-term memory processing module is responsible for detecting the short-term memory features of the overall improvisation. In order to internally reconstruct a complete image for the improvisation's momentum, this module gathers information both from the representation module and the scheduler; from the first in order to know what is being played by the musician and from the second so as to monitor the computer's short-term playing.

In the lower side of Figure 8.4 one can find the interaction core module. This core consists of a part that is responsible for interfacing with the performer and a solver that responds to her/his questions. The performer lances queries under the form of musical constraints. She/he can ask, for instance, about the existence of navigation paths -a.k.a generated sequences- according to a certain target state, which are subject to a combination of a number of global and local constraints (see Figure 8.3). In order to respond, the solver attires information from the representation module. The minute the performer takes a decision, information is transmitted to the scheduler.

The Scheduler is an intelligent module that accommodates commands arriving from different sources. For instance, a change-of-strategy command by the performer arrives via the interaction core module to the scheduler. The scheduler is responsible for examining what was supposed to be scheduled according to the previous strategy and organizes a smooth transition between the former and the current strategy. Sometimes, when contradictory decisions nest inside the scheduler, the last may commit a call to the core's solver unit in order to take a final decision. It is worth mentioning that the dotted-line arrow from the short-term memory processing module towards the scheduler introduces the aspect of reactivity of the system to emergency situations: when the first detects a surprise event, instead of transmitting information via the representation module -and thus not making it accessible unless information reaches the interaction core-, it reflects information directly to the scheduler in the form of a 'scheduling alarm'. Hence, via this configuration, we leave open in our architecture the option for the system to take autonomous actions under certain criteria. The last, in combination with what has been mentioned earlier in this section, establishes in full the three party interaction in a CAI context.

8.6 Interaction Modes

8.6.1 GrAIPE as an Instrument

The interaction core encloses all stylistic generation schemes relative to the instrument paradigm. The computer user-performer can combine all different methods and approaches discussed in Section 4 to interact with material learned before or during the improvisation session and control a stylistically-coherent improvisation. The dialogue with the computer is supported with methods based on the recognition of patterns and sequence scheduling, through the use of musical constraints (time-to-target, path constraints, etc.). There exist an infinite number of different possible configurations for such an interaction to occur. Here, we present two basic tracks: one for graphic and one for physical interfaces.

A very simple but efficient graphical interface is built on the concept shown in Figure 8.5. The vertical axis represent the "reference time" of the sequence modelled by MMFG, with the possibility that the size of the last will gradually increase from the right during the improvisation. The horizontal axis represents the "improvisation time", which is the time elapsed from the beginning of the improvisation. Consequently, each point of this field corresponds to one moment of the improvisation time, as well as to a position inside the MMFG. Due to the axis configuration, a linear navigation without any continuations would graphically result in a linear function $y(x) = x + b$. Programming time goals, with the help of such a graphical interface, is straightforward. Just by selecting a point in the field, the scheduling parameters of "where" and "when" for the target state get instantly defined. The advantage of this approach is that it allows for an overview of the entire improvisation time with respect to the regions of MMFG that have already been used for improvisation, as well as for a view of linearity vs. non-linearity and thus coherency vs. novelty. A generalized interaction would consist in defining a number of points from which the generation should pass in the future. Finally, by attaching more information at each point or in between points, it is possible to further refine the generation process with additional constraints.

The integration of a physical instrument-like interface may also result in interesting human-computer interactions. Let's take, for instance, the case of a midi piano. Such an instrument facilitates the insertion of patterns into the generation system. We could then use these input patterns as a guide for automated generation. By using the "as quick as possible" primitive of 1 we could imagine a scenario where the user indicates only the target patterns and the computer tries to rapidly assign to these patterns by generating the rest of the material while either keeping, or not, the stylistic features of the sequence. By generalizing the above approach, it is easy to imagine various interactions based on the augmented instrument paradigm. These interactions are based on the principle that the user provides note input that is not played as is, but it is used as first material for the computer to generate stylistically coherent content. Such an approach could be of interest to people that are not experts or have not reached the end of their learning curve for a particular music style. By implying their musical ideas in the form of a sketch, and with the help of the computer, they are able to participate, at least to a certain degree, in a collaborative improvisation context and enjoy making music with other people.

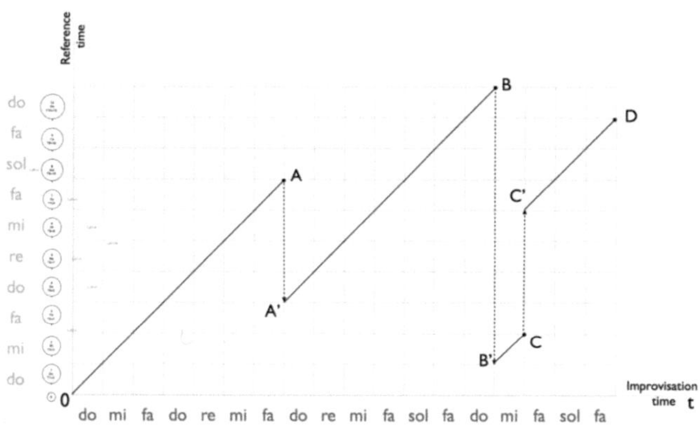

Figure 8.5: Graphical Interface for the interaction core. The vertical and the horizontal axis represent the reference and the improvisation time respectively. We suppose that the system has learned the sequence S of Figure 8.2 through the MMFG (on the vertical axis). Linear improvisation corresponds to the linear function $y(x) = x + b$ (vectors [0, A], [A′, B], [B′, C], [C′, D]). Continuations through external transitions correspond to vectors [A,A′], [B,B′], [C,C′] and are due, each time, to the structure of MMFG. A point in this 2–D plane specifies the "where" (reference time at the vertical axis) and the "when"(improvisation time at the horizontal axis). The user can guide the improvisation process by setting points -thus Q constraints- in this 2–D plane. In the case shown in the figure, we may consider that the user, at time 0, selected the point D. This means that the system should improvise in such way so as to find itself after 17 notes at note fa. The path 0AA′BB′CC′D shows the sequence that has been selected by the computer in order to fulfil the constraints set by the user. The produced sequence is the one shown in the figure below the horizontal axis

8.6.2 GrAIPE as a Player

The reactive component includes strategies inspired from the player paradigm. It consists of methods that assign autonomy to the system so as to participate as an independent agent. It is implemented inside the interaction core and the scheduler module.

Nonetheless, in order for such an autonomous agent to exist, the last needs to perform a thorough understanding of the improvisation environment. In terms of stylistic generation, this is translated as the capacity to build internal representations and detect events arising from every flow in the improvisation context. Methods for representation of multiple flows and with respect to various music parameters, as well as methods for detection of patterns, are both natively supported by MMFG through the strategies described in (Maniatakos, 2012). With the help of these methods, it is then possible to envisage strategies for programming general modes of interactions in the musical level that this agent should apply. For example, it is possible to schedule general responses of the system that are triggered by detected events. In this sense, control methods of 1 can serve as the means by which to design one or more behaviors and interactions modes, that the system will eventually apply depending on the evolution of the improvisation.

Another useful approach arises from a predictive utilization of the recognition component. By using a memory window for the recent past of the instrument players' flows, one can use the results of the pattern detection of the MMFG to predict future events. Then, by combining the last with the above strategies of detect and act, it is possible to anticipate future behaviors of the agent by associating future scenarios to predictions.

Of particular interest in the design of the reactive component are the methods for combining material occurring from different sequences. The capacity of a system to combine material arising from different participants of the improvisation, as well as the capacity to retrospect its own improvisation, are crucial for the complexification of the agent's behaviour. In a context of an improvisation of more than one instrument players, the system analyzes in parallel the multiple flows and can improvise according to heuristics for balancing the generated material among the different flows learned.

8.7 Conclusion

The interest in the present study of the three-party interaction context for modern improvisation arose from the double role of the computer operating, on occasion, as an independent improvisation agent and as an instrument- depending on the type of human intervention -as an instrument player or a computer performer. This resulted in a large number of potential interactions that can simultaneously occur among the improvisation participants. By relying on the MMFG structure, we establish a set of tools and methods for dealing with the two paradigms: the one of the computer as an independent agent and the second as a high-level musical instrument.

Similarly to former sequential models for sequence generation, MMFG-based generation is the result of navigating inside the graph-like representation provided by the MMFG. The novelty of our approach lies in our successful effort to provide a complete set of tools in order to control the musical result of these heuristics and methods. The conception of these toolset follows a bottom-up arrangement, in the sense that simple tools (primitives) are defined, in a first place, in the form of queries over the MMFG representations, and more complex ones arise from the combination of the former.

References

Allauzen, C., Crochemore, M., & Raffinot, M. (1999). Factor oracle: a new structure for pattern matching.

Assayag, G., & Bloch, G. (2007). Navigating the oracle: a heuristic approach. *In International computer music conference ICMC'07,Copenhagen.*

Assayag, G., Bloch, G., Chemillier, M., Cont, A., & Dubnov, S. (2006). Omax brothers : a dynamic topology of agents for improvisation learning. In Workshop on audio and music computing for multi- media, ACM multimedia 2006. Santa Barbara, USA.

Chadabe, J. (1984). Interactive composing: an overview. *Computer Music Journal,* 8, 22–27.

Eigenfeldt, A. (2007). Real-time composition or computer improvisation? A composer's search for intelligent tools in interactive computer music. *In proceedings of EMS 2007: Electroacoustic music studies network-de mont- fort/leicester.*

Gordon, E. (1980). *Learning sequences in music: skill, content, and patterns.* G.I.A. Publications.

Lewis, G. (2000). Too many notes: Computers, complexity and culture in voyager. *Leonardo Music Journal,* 10, 33–39.

Maniatakos, F. (2012). Graphs and Automata for the Control of Interaction in Computer Music Improvisation. PhD Thesis, University of Pierre and Marie Curie (UPMC), Paris.

Mantaras, R. D., & Arcos, J. (2002). AI and music. from composition to expressive performance. *AI Magazine,* 23(3).

Oteri, F. J. (1999).: *Interview with todd machover: Technology and the future of music.* NewMusicBox.

Pachet, F. (2002, September). The continuator: Musical interaction with style. *In ICMA (Ed.), Proceedings of ICMC* (p. 211–218). Goeteborg, Sweden: ICMA. (best paper award)

Pachet, F., & Roy, P. (2011, March). Markov constraints: steerable generation of markov sequences. *Constraints,* 16(2), 148–172.

Rowe, R. (1992). Interactive music systems: Machine listening and composing. *Cambridge, MA, USA: MIT Press.*

Rowe, R. (1999). Incrementally improving interactive music systems. *Contemporary Music Review,* 13(2), 47–62.

Rowe, R. (2001). *Machine musicianship.* Cambridge, MA, USA: MIT Press.

Schwarz, D., & Johnson, V. (2011). Corpus-based improvisation. *In (re)thinking improvisation. Malm, Sweden.*

Thom, B. (2000). Articial intelligence and real-time interactive improvisation. *In AAAI-2000 music and ai workshop. AAAI Press.*

Doron Friedman and Béatrice S. Hasler

9 The BEAMING Proxy: Towards Virtual Clones for Communication

Abstract: Participants of virtual worlds and video games are often represented by animated avatars and telerobotics allows users to be remotely represented by physical robots. In many cases such avatars or robots can also be controlled by fully-automated agents. We present a conceptual framework for a communication proxy that unifies these two modes of communication. The users can communicate via their avatar or robotic representation, an autonomous agent can occasionally take control of the representation, or the user and the autonomous agent can share the control of the representation. The transition between modes is done seamlessly throughout a communication session, and many aspects of the representation can be transformed online, allowing for new types of human computer confluence. We describe the concept of the communication proxy that has been developed and explored within the European Union BEAMING project, and describe one of the studies involving the proxy, in which the experimenter was perceived as both a man and a woman simultaneously.

Keywords: Avatars, Intelligent Virtual Agents, Autonomous Agents, Teleoperation, Mixed Initiative, Adjustable Autonomy

9.1 Introduction

What would it be like to have a digital clone that looks like you, behaves like you, and represents you in events that you cannot attend? What would it be to be perceived by others to be a man and a woman at the same time? These days we hold many personal and professional meetings that do not take place face to face, but are mediated through communication technologies, such as mobile phones, video conference systems, social networks, online virtual worlds, and more. This opens the possibility that our representation in the communication medium would be controlled by autonomous software rather than by ourselves. We are by now accustomed to simple automated responses such as voice answering machines and automated email replies. In this chapter we describe a communication proxy that takes this concept further into a more sophisticated representation of the user that can engage others in lengthy events, opening possibilities of novel human computer confluence scenarios.

The proxy is part of the BEAMING[11] project, which deals with the science and technology intended to give people a real sense of physically being in a remote location

11 http://beaming-eu.org

with other people, and vice versa – without actually traveling (Steed et al., 2012). We explore the concept of the proxy in the context of several applications: remotely attending a business meeting, remote rehearsal of a theater play, remote medical examination, and remote teaching. In such applications it is useful to have a digital extension of yourself that is able to assist you while communicating with others or replace you completely, either for short periods of a few seconds, due to some interruption, or even for a complete event. Our approach is to see the proxy as an extension of our own identity, and allow a seamless transition between user control and system control of the representation.

The communication proxy operates in three modes of control: if the proxy is in autonomous (foreground) mode, its purpose is to represent its owner in the best way possible. To that purpose, the proxy has to be based on models of the owner's appearance and behavior, and to be aware of its owner's goals and preferences. When the proxy owner is using the telepresence system himself then the proxy is in background mode; the proxy is idle but can record data and is ready to automatically take control of the avatar representation. In addition, the proxy can operate in mixed mode; in this case the owner controls some aspects of the communication and the proxy controls other aspects, both at the same time.

We are interested in the proxy not only as a technological challenge but also conceptually, as a possible future inhabitant of society. Proxies could be physical humanoid robots, but since we spend increasing amounts of our time in digital spheres they could also be virtual agents. Most of us can think of cases where they would have loved to have someone replace them in annoying, boring, or unpleasant events. However, in what contexts will proxies be socially acceptable? What are the legal and ethical implications? In this chapter we focus on these conceptual issues that came up from our work; for a more technical overview see (Friedman, Berkers, Salomon, & Tuchman, 2014).

9.2 Background

9.2.1 Semi-Autonomous Virtual Agents

The proxy is a specific type of an intelligent virtual agent. Such agents have been studied widely, mostly as autonomous entities (e.g., see (Prendinger & Ishizuka, 2004; Swartout et al., 2006). There has been a lot of research on believability (starting from (Bates, 1994) and expressiveness of virtual agents (e.g., (Pelachaud, 2005), multi-modal communication, and the role of nonverbal behavior in coordinating and carrying out communication (e.g., (Vinayagamoorthy et al., 2006).

Semi-autonomous avatars were first introduced by Cassell, Vilhjlmsson and colleagues (Cassell, Sullivan, Prevost, & Chrchill, 2000; Cassell & Vilhjálmsson, 1999; Vilhjlmsson & Cassell, 1998). Their system allowed users to communicate via text while their avatars automatically animated attention, salutations, turn taking, back-channel feedback, and facial expression. This is one of the main interest points in the shared control spectrum, in which the verbal communication is handled by the human and the nonverbal behavior is automated, but we will see additional motivations for shared control below.

Others have discussed and demonstrated semi-autonomous avatars, mostly addressing the same goal: automating non-verbal behavior. Penny et al. (Penny, Smith, Sengers, Bernhardt, & Schulte, 2001) describe a system incorporating avatars with varying levels of autonomy: *Traces*, a Virtual Reality system in which a user's body movements spawn avatars that gradually become more autonomous. Graesser et al. (Graesser, Chipman, Haynes, & Olney, 2005) presented an educational mixed-initiative intelligent virtual agent focusing on natural-language dialogue. Gillies et al. (Gillies, Ballin, Pan, & Dodgson, 2008) provide a review and some examples of semi-autonomous avatars. They raise the issue of how the human communicates with his semi-autonomous avatar, and enumerate several approaches.

9.2.2 Digital Extensions of Ourselves

Science fiction themes often portray autonomous artificial humans (such as in the movie Bladerunner[12]) or remote control of a virtual or physical representation (such as in the movie Surrogates[13]). Some of these entities are reminiscent of our proxy; for example, in the book series Safeload the writer David Weber introduces the concept of a personality-integrated cybernetic avatar (commonly abbreviated to PICA): this is a safe and improved physical representation of yourself in the physical world, and you can also opt to "upload" your consciousness into it. Such concepts are penetrating popular culture; for instance, the recent appearance of digital Tupac at the Coachella festival in 2012, which provoked much discussion of the social implications and ethical use of digital technology (the original Tupac was a rap musician killed in 1996). Artstein et al. (Artstein et al., 2014) have implemented such an interactive virtual clone of a holocaust survivor, focusing on photorealistic replication.

Clarke (Clarke, 1994) introduced the concept of a digital persona, but this was a passive entity made of collected data, rather than an autonomous or semi-autonomous agent. Today we see such virtual identities in online social networks, such as Facebook profiles, but these are passive representations. Ma et al. (Ma, Wen, Huang, & Huang, 2011) presented a manifesto of what they call a cyber-individual, which is "a comprehensive digital description of an individual human in the cyber world" (p. 31). This manifesto is generic and is presented in a high level of abstraction, and it

12 http://www.imdb.com/title/tt0083658/
13 http://www.imdb.com/title/tt0986263/

is partially related to our more concrete concept of the proxy as described here. The notion that computers in general have become part of our identity in the broadest sense is being discussed by psychologists (Turkle, 1984, 1997) and philosophers (e.g., as in the extended mind theory (Clark & Chalmers, 1998). In this project, we take a step in making these ideas concrete, towards merging the identity of the person with his avatar representation.

9.2.3 Semi-Autonomous Scenarios in Robotic Telepresence

Shared control was explored extensively in the context of teleoperation, in order for robots and devices to overcome the delay that is often introduced by telecommunication (Sheridan, 1992). There is a distinction among several modes of operation: i) master-slave: the robot is completely controlled by the operator, ii) supervisor-subordinate: the human makes a plan and the robot executes it, iii) partner-partner: responsibility is more or less equally shared, iv) teacher-learner: the robot learns from a human operator, and v) fully autonomous. This taxonomy is geared towards teleoperation and task performance, whereas we are interested in the remote entity as a representation of the operator, mostly in social contexts. Thus, our taxonomy is somewhat different. Master-slave is equivalent to the background mode of the proxy, and the proxy can also learn during this mode (similar to the teacher-learner mode). In terms of controlling a representation there is little difference between the supervisor-subordinate mode and our proxy's foreground mode. Finally, we are left with the partner-partner mode, which we call the mixed mode proxy, and that is the territory that we wish to further explore.

Telerobotics has also been used for social communication. Paulos and Canny (Paulos & Canny, 2001) describe personal roving presence devices (PRoPs) that provide a physical mobile proxy, controllable over the Internet to provide tele-embodiment. These only used teleoperation (or the master-slave mode). Venolia *et al.* (Venolia *et al.*, 2010) have come up with the concept of the embodied social proxy and have evaluated it in a real-life setting. The goal was to allow remote workers to be more integrated with the main office. Their setup evolved to include an LCD screen, cameras and a microphone – all mounted on a mobile platform. The live communication included video conference and when away the display showed abstract information about the remote person: calendar, instant-messaging availability, and connectivity information. Thus, there is an overlap between this concept and our proxy in terms of motivation. However, the representation of the users when they are away is minimal and iconic, whereas our goal is to provide a rich representation in such cases. Additionally, this concept does not include a mixed mode of shared control. Telepresence robots have recently been made available for hire on a commercial basis by several companies.

Ong et al. (Ong, Seet, & Sim, 2008) describe a telerobotic system that allows seamless switching between foreground and background modes, but it is also geared at teleoperation and task performance rather than communication. More recently, there have been demonstrations of robotic telepresence with shared control: Lee et al. describe a semi-autonomous robot for communication (Lee, Toscano, Stiehl, & Breazeal, 2008), designed as a teddy bear. The robot is semi-autonomous in that it can direct the attention of the communicator using pointing gestures.

9.3 Concept and Implications

9.3.1 Virtual Clones

There are many aspects of a person that we may wish to capture in the proxy: appearance, non-verbal behavior, personality, preferences, professional knowledge, social network of friends and acquaintances, and more. In designing the proxy we distinguish between two relatively independent goals: i) appearance: the proxy has to pass as a recognizable representation of its owner, and ii) goals: the proxy has to represent the interests of its owner.

Appearance is dealt with by the computer graphics and image processing communities; clearly, progress in these communities can lead to highly photorealistic communication proxies. Creating a 3D look-alike of a person is now possible with off-the-shelf products, and humanoid robotic look-alikes have also been demonstrated (Guizzo, 2010). Personal characteristics in other modalities can also be replicated with various degrees of success: sound, touch, and non-verbal communication style. We have shown previously how the social navigation style of the owner can be captured by the proxy using a behavioral-cloning approach (Friedman & Tuchman, 2011): we capture the navigation style of users in a virtual world when they are approaching a new user, and construct a behavioral model from this recorded data that may be used when the proxy is in foreground mode.

It is important that the proxy's "body language," mostly gestures and postures, will be similar to its owner's. In a relevant study, Ibister and Nass (Isbister & Nass, 2000) separated verbal from non-verbal cues in virtual characters: they exposed users to virtual humans whose verbal responses came from one person and whose non-verbal behavior came from another person. Consistent characters were preferred and had greater influence on people's behaviors.

We see digital proxies as an important part of the everyday life in the rest of the 21st century. We spend a lot of time in cyberspace, and virtual proxies are natural candidates. Our first-generation proxy inhabited the 3D virtual world SecondLife[14] (SL).

14 http://www.secondlife.com

It is based on our SL bot platform, which allows bots to perform useful tasks, such as carrying out automated survey interviews in the role of virtual research assistants (Béatrice S Hasler, Tuchman, & Friedman, 2013). We have prepared the SL proxy for the co-author of this chapter to give a talk inside SL as part of a real-world conference (Figure 9.1): a workshop on Teaching in Immersive Worlds, Ulster, Northern Ireland, in 2010. The appearance of the proxy was canceled on the day of the event due to audio problems in the conference venue, but a video illustrates the vision and concept[15].

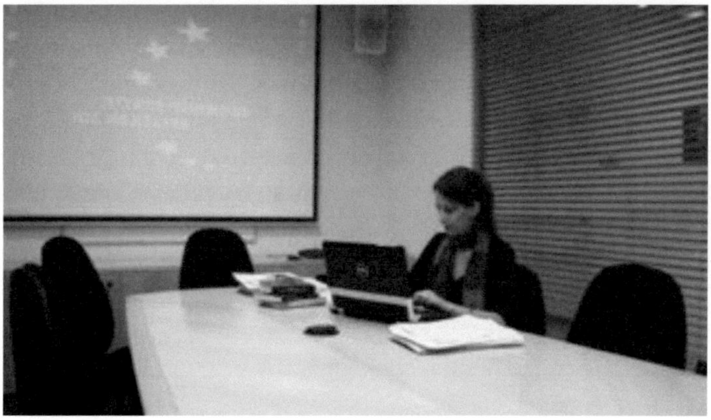

(a)

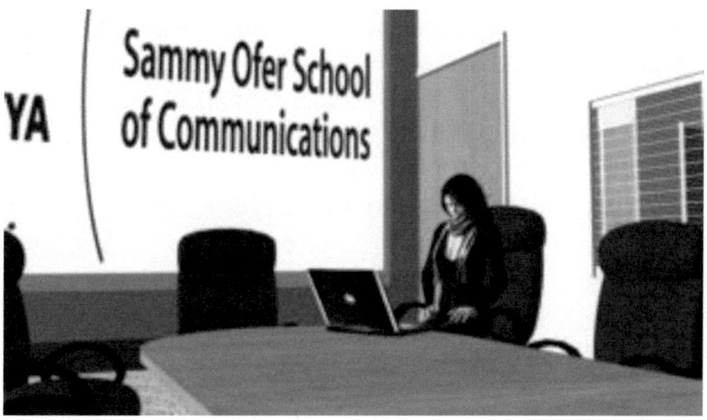

(b)

Figure 9.1: (a) The co-author of this chapter at work. (b) The virtual-world avatar, used as her proxy

15 Video: http://y2u.be/1R4Eo3UDT9U

9.3.2 Modes of Operation

The proxy works in several modes of operation along the control spectrum and is able to switch smoothly between modes during its operation:

- Background mode (Figure 9.2a): When the user is in control of the avatar, the proxy is in background mode. During a communication session, the proxy owner may be distracted: have someone enter their office, receive a phone call, or they need a coffee break. The proxy is able to automatically detect these situations and proactively switch to foreground (or mixed) mode (e.g., when the owner is tracked and decides to leave the room). Alternatively, the owner can initiate the transition. During background mode, the owner's behavior is recorded; this is expected to be the main source for behavioral models for the proxy. Typically, we record the proxy owner's non-verbal behavior; the skeleton data is tagged with metadata regarding the context, and this data is used in mixed and foreground mode to allow the proxy to have its owner's "body language."
- Foreground mode (Figure 9.2b): When the owner is away, the proxy is in foreground mode. The proxy should know when to take control of the remote representation (i.e., switch to foreground mode), and when to release control back to the user (i.e., switch back to background mode). This "covering up" for the owner may be necessary for short interruptions of several seconds, or for the whole duration of events. If the proxy merely replaces the owner for a short while then its behavior can be very basic; for some applications it may be useful only to have the proxy display reactive body language. For longer sessions of communication it is highly useful for a proxy to be able to answer some informational questions on behalf of its owner, and to have some understanding of the owner's goals. Ideally, the proxy would be able to learn this information implicitly from observing the user (while in background mode), or from user data. For example, our proxy can have access to its owner's calendar and location (based on the owenr's smartphone location), and access to additional inputs can be conceived.
- Mixed mode (Figure 9.2c): When the proxy owner and the proxy both control the same communication channel at the same time, we say that the proxy is in mixed mode. In this case the owner would control some of the functionality and the proxy would control the rest. The challenge becomes to allow for a fluent experience to the owner.

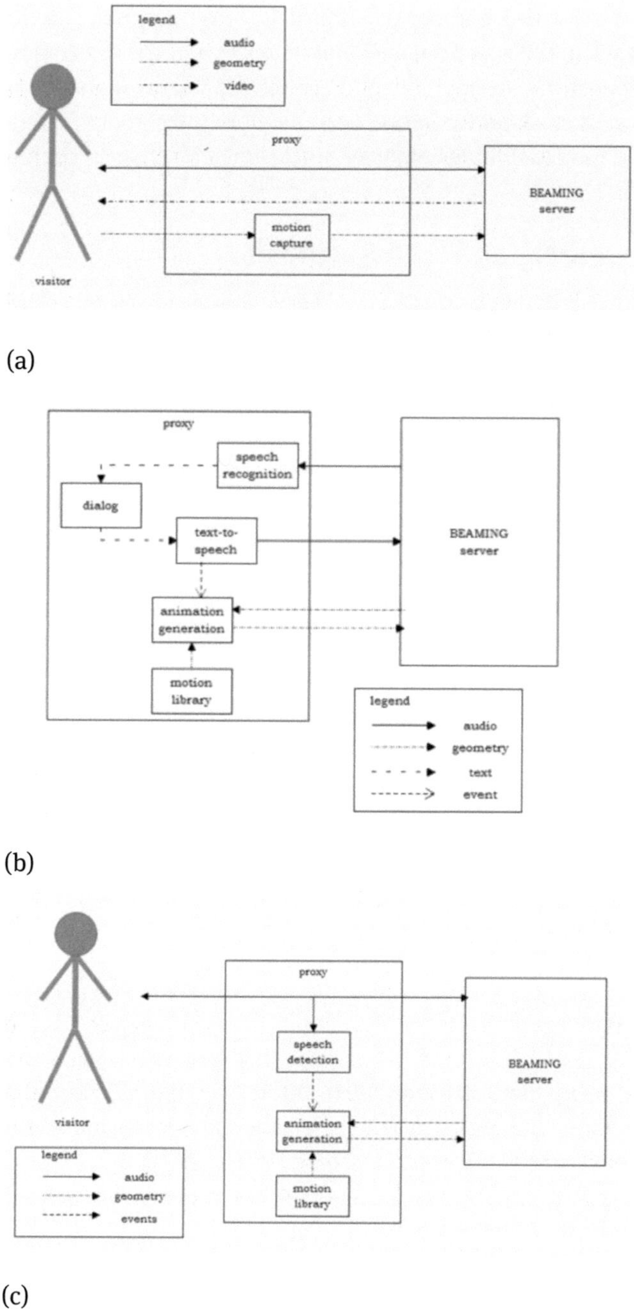

Figure 9.2: Schematic network diagrams of the proxy configured in three modes: (a) background, (b) foreground, and (c) mixed mode. The diagrams are deliberately abstracted for simplification. Full lines denote continuous data streams, and dotted lines denote discrete events. Different colors denote the different modalities

The spectrum between user control and agent control is often described as in Figure 9.3. However, this view of the spectrum does not help us chart the interesting space in the middle of the spectrum. As mentioned in Section 2.3, the taxonomy from teleoperation is geared towards task performance, and therefore there are not many lessons to be learned about the possibilities of mixed mode when it comes to shared control of a representation.

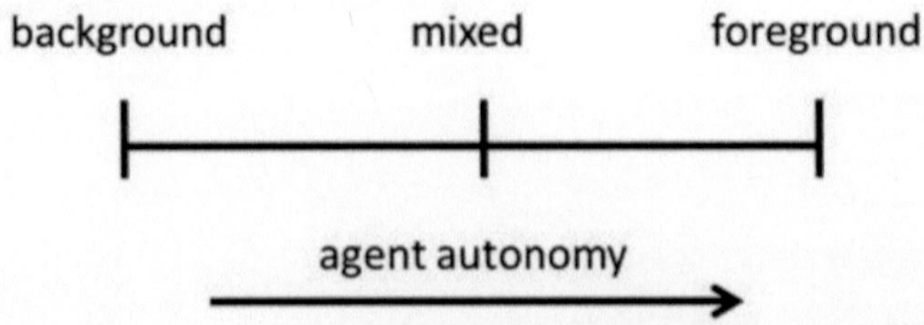

Figure 9.3: The spectrum from full agent autonomy (foreground mode) on the one side to full human autonomy (background mode) on the other, with mixed mode in the middle.

Therefore, we suggest a conceptualization based on functional modules. From a technical point of view, the proxy operates as a network of interconnected modules (Friedman et al., 2014). In principle, the functionality of each module can be carried out by both the software agent or by the human. For example, the decision of what to say can be dictated either by a human or by a natural language generation component, and this is independent of voice generation (e.g., in principle we can have a text generated by a chatbot read out loud by the proxy owner). Thus, we suggest that the human-agent shared control spectrum can be defined by the set of possible configurations of modules; if the number of components is N then the number of shared control modes is 2^N.

9.3.3 "Better Than Being You"

Presence has been coined "being there" (Heeter, 1992). Our expectation is that when advanced telecommunication technologies are deployed they may even provide a "better-than-being-there" experience, at least under some circumstances and in some respects. Similarly, an interesting opportunity presents itself: the proxy can be used to represent the owner better than the owner would represent him- or herself. For example, you may consider a proxy that is based on your appearance with a beautifier transformation applied (Looks, Goertzel, & Pennachin, 2004). Analogically, we have demonstrated the possibility of a proxy that extends your vocabulary in foreign non-verbal gestures (Béatrice S Hasler, Salomon, Tuchman, Lev-Tov, & Friedman, 2013): The proxy can be configured to recognize that the owner has performed culture-specific gestures and replace these gestures, online, with the equivalent gestures in the target culture's vocabulary[16]. In another study we have used the proxy system's ability for automated generation of non-verbal communication to use imitation in order to increase intergroup empathy (B. S. Hasler, Hirschberger, Shani-Sherman, & Friedman, 2014).

One of the applications of the proxy is allowing a person to take part in multiple events at the same time. For example, the proxy owner can be located at his home or in her office, remotely attend one event in one location using telepresence, while her proxy fills in for her in a second event (in a third physical location). The proxy owner can switch between the two events back and forth, such that at each moment her attention is given to one event while the proxy replaces her in the other event. Such a scenario requires the operation of two different configurations of the proxy working in synchrony; technically, this involves running two clones of the proxy (which itself is a clone of the individual human) simultaneously.

Another advantage of the proxy over its human owner is that the proxy can have what we refer to as online sensors. Just like the proxy handles input streams, such as video and audio in ways that are analogous to human senses it can also be configured to receive input streams from the online world. Our proxy is integrated with Twitter, Skype, and with a smartphone: using an iPhone application we allow the proxy to receive a continuous stream of information about the owner's smartphone location, and the proxy also has access to its owner's calendar. Currently this allows the proxy to answer simple queries about its owner's whereabouts and schedule, but more sophisticated applications of these data streams can be imagined.

9.3.4 Ethical Considerations

We envision that in the not-too-far future our society may be swarming with various kinds of proxies, and specifically communication proxies. Thus, we provide here a preliminary ethical discussion. For a legal analysis of the proxy's implications on contractual law and some recommendations, see the BEAMING legal report (Purdy, 2011) (specifically, see pages 68–77 that refer to the proxy).

De'Angeli (De'Angeli, 2009) discusses the ethical implications of autonomous conversational agents, suggesting a critical rhetoric approach that tries to shift the focus from the engineering of the agents to their psychological and social implications, mostly based on findings that virtual conversations can at times encourage disinhibited and antisocial behavior. Whitby (Whitby, 2008) discusses the risks of abusing artificial agents, and in particular robots, for example, in that the abuse might desensitize the perpetrators. These discussions are relevant, but our concept of

16 http://y2u.be/Wp6VPb2EaFU

the proxy introduces additional issues, since we focus on the proxy as an extension of its owner, rather than as a separate entity.

One of the key issues is the ethics of deception. There is a general consensus in human societies that we need to know who we are really dealing with in social interactions. In general, we can expect people to notice whether they are interacting with the person or the proxy, especially with current technologies. But assume that the proxy takes over just for a few seconds to hide the fact that your colleague decided to respond to a mobile phone call. Is this socially acceptable if you are not aware that your colleague's proxy took over? In fact, this deception already takes place in online chat support systems, where support staffs switch between typing themselves and using automated chatbots back and forth. The fact that these services exist indicates that people can accept these unclear transitions, at least in some contexts.

Legal and ethical issues are hard to disentangle from technical issues. For example, a proxy owner may explicitly instruct their proxy to avoid taking responsibility for any assigned tasks. However, assume that during a session everyone is seated, and the boss says: "those who wish to be responsible for this task please remain seated." Since we do not expect the proxy to be able to understand such spoken (or even typed) text (at least not with high certainty), there is a fair chance that the proxy would remain seated. Does this now make the proxy's owner committed? This may be especially tricky if the proxy remained seated while in mixed mode.

9.4 Evaluation Scenarios

One evaluation study was conducted in the context of a real classroom, and the proxy replaced the lecturer during class[17]. This study was intended as a technical evaluation of the system as well as obtaining feedback on the concept of the proxy; the results are described in detail in a separate paper (Friedman, Salomon, & Hasler, 2013) (Figures 9.6, 9.7). In this chapter we describe, in detail, another study, which aims to illustrate how the concept and architecture of our proxy can be used in an unconventional novel fashion.

17 http://y2u.be/43l739kKFfk

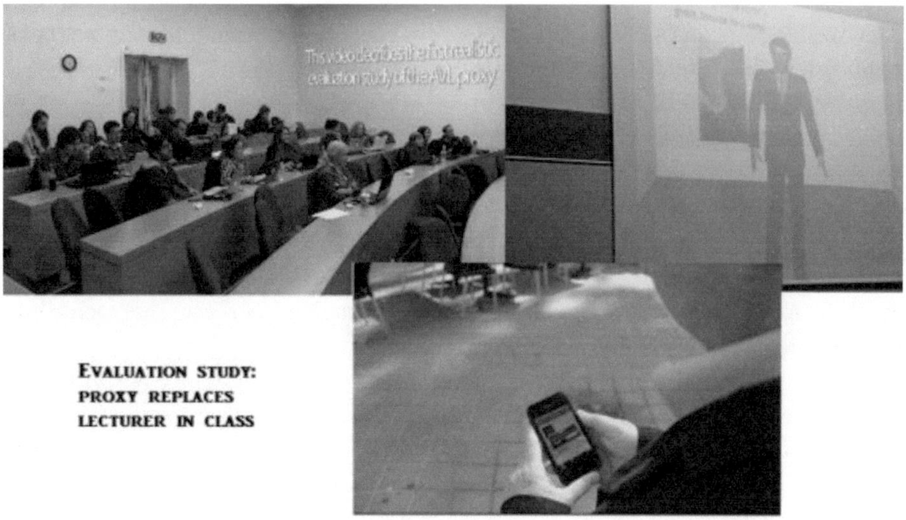
EVALUATION STUDY:
PROXY REPLACES
LECTURER IN CLASS

Figure 9.6: Screenshots from the case study. Top left: the classroom. Top right: the proxy representation as projected in class. Bottom: the proxy owner receiving a Skype call from the proxy

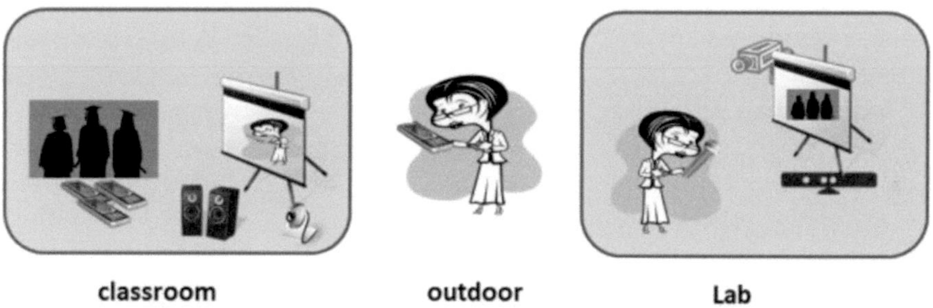
classroom
outdoor
Lab

Figure 9.7: A schematic diagram of the study setup, showing the proxy owner in the lab presented as an avatar on the screen in the classroom. The students communicate with the proxy using mobile devices. During the experiment the proxy owner was also outdoors and communicated with the class in mixed mode

9.4.1 The Dual Gender Proxy Scenario

Telepresence provides an opportunity to introduce a "better than being there" experience. For example, Bailenson et al. introduced the transformed social interactions (TSI) paradigm (Bailenson, Beall, Loomis, Blascovich, & Turk, 2004), which explains how the unique characteristics of collaborative virtual environments may be leveraged to provide communication scenarios that are better than face to face communication. In this section we show how the proxy concept can be naturally extended to include the TSI paradigm.

The study consisted of a business negotiation scenario: in each session two participants of mixed gender were given background information about a business decision, and were asked to reach an agreement within 20 minutes. The participants were told that they would hold the discussion using video conference and that there would be a mediator, represented by an avatar, whose role is to help them reach an agreement in the allotted time. The instructions were provided in a way that would not disclose the gender of the mediator.

In each session the two participants were placed in two separate meeting rooms, in front of a large projection screen, and were provided with a microphone for speaking. Both participants watched a split screen: most of the screen showed the mediator avatar, in our custom application, and a small portion of the screen, in the top right corner, showed a live video feed of the other participant in the other room, using Skype (Figures 9.8, 9.9). The mediator controlling the mediator avatar was a confederate, sitting in a third room. Using our proxy program the confederate received the live video and audio session from Skype, and could type responses in a text window. The text was immediately converted into speech and was delivered by the proxy avatar simultaneously to both participants. The confederate used a structured template of a discussion in order to keep the intervention as close as possible in all the experimental sessions. In all sessions the confederate avatar was controlled by the same female experimenter.

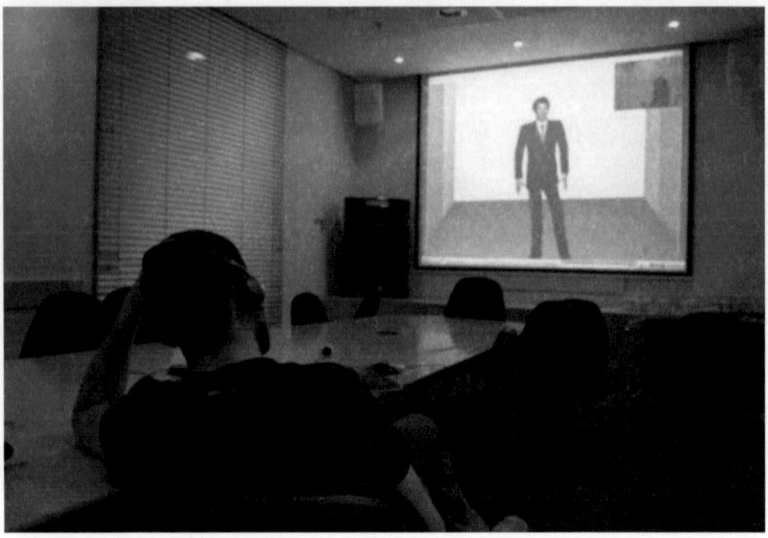

Figure 9.8: A screenshot of one of the participants in front of a projection screen, showing the mediator and the live video feed

Eighteen participants (ages 22–28) were recruited on campus and participated in the study for academic credit. The study included three conditions, with three different couples in each condition: i) MM – both participants experienced a male mediator, ii) FF – both participants experienced a female mediator, and iii) MF – the male participant experienced a male mediator and the female participant experienced a female mediator (Figure 9.10). All couples were mixed: a male and a female.

The hypothesis was that the participants would perceive a mediator of the same gender as themselves to be "on their side." Therefore, a further hypothesis is that the mediator would play its role more effectively in the dual gender (MF) condition. At the end of the session each participant went through a semi-structured interview, with a fixed set of questions. The interview started with general questions about the negotiation session and about the experience with the technical setup. This was followed by two questions about the mediator and his/her perceived contribution. Only the last question explicitly asked the participants about the mediator's gender and how this played a part in the mediation process. The interviews were videorecorded and transcribed for analysis.

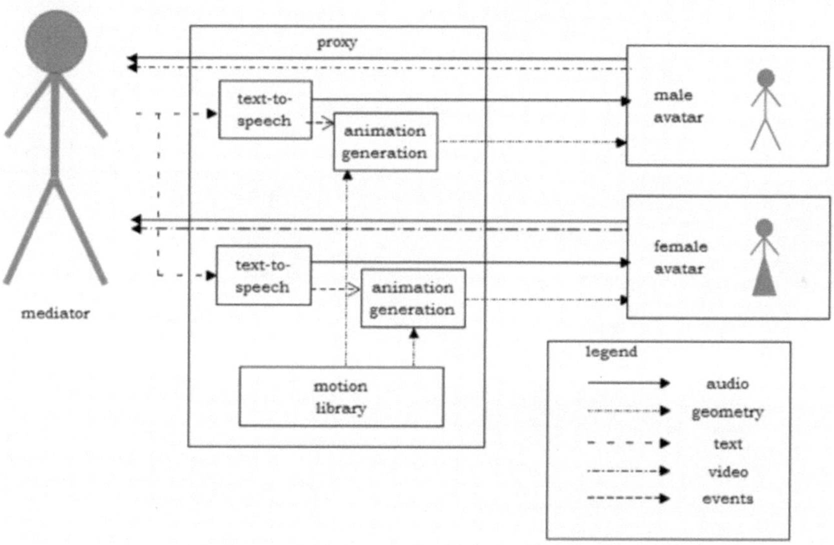

Figure 9.9: A simplified diagram of the proxy setup used in this study. The diagram shows the generic components connected by arrows for continuous streams and by dotted arrows for discrete events

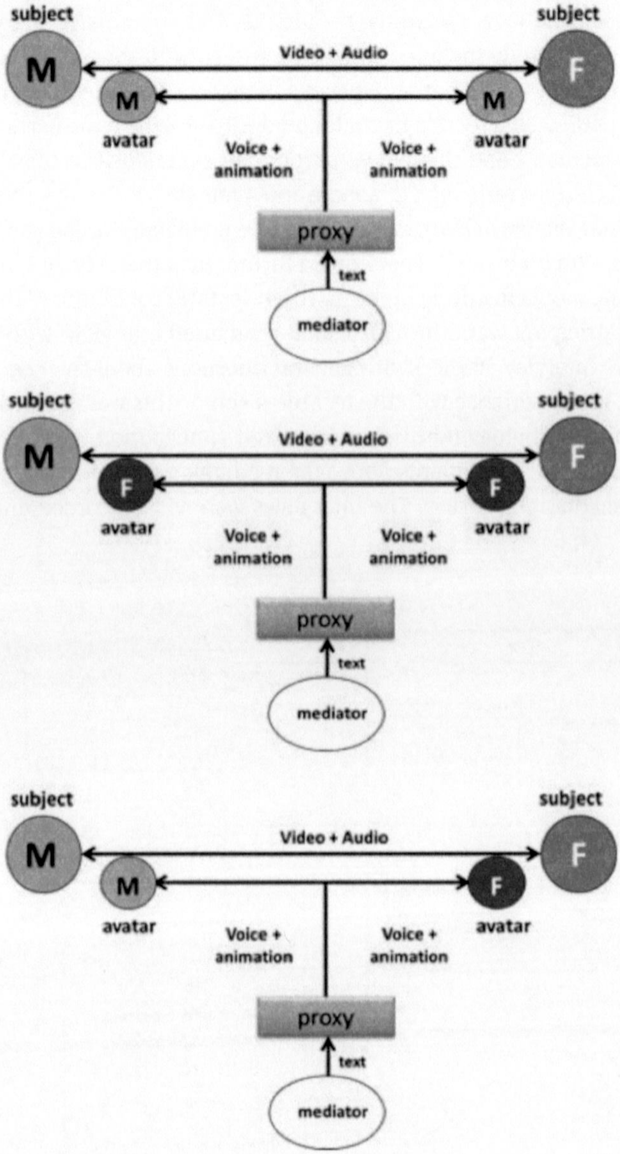

Figure 9.10: The three conditions in the study: top: MM – both participants experience a male avatar, middle: FF – both participants experience a female avatar, bottom: MF – the male participant experiences a male avatar and the female participant experiences a female avatar

9.4.2 Results

Since the number of sessions in each of the three conditions was small (three sessions each) we could not perform a quantitative analysis. One out of three in the MM condition reached an agreement in the allotted time, one out of three in the FF condition, and two out of three in the MF mixed gender condition; this provides preliminary support for our research assumptions but could be anecdotal.

The subjective reports further support our assumptions. Even when the participants did not explicitly refer to the gender of the mediator, their comments reveal that the gender of the mediator may have been significant to the experience. In the MM condition the participants referred to the mediator's gender several times. Participant F1 (age 23) commented: "I would advise to think about a solution that would make the mediator more useful," whereas a male participant (M2, age 24) commented: "despite the slight delay he [the mediator] promoted us and encouraged us to reach an agreement." One of the female participants explicitly commented (F3, 26): "the mediator wasn't fair. Every sentence he uttered was biased towards the other side. In negotiation the mediator is supposed to be unbiased and not so aggressive as was the case here."

The subjective reports further confirmed our hypothesis in the FF condition. For example, one of the male participants (M5, 22) commented: "the mediator was too gentle. Although she intervened frequently she was notable to narrow the wide gaps, and even damaged the negotiation. I think the mediator needs to be a man who will take control of the negotiation from start to finish."

In the dual gender condition, further comments reinforce our expectations; participant F8 (25): "I think the mediator helped us move forward, no doubt the gentle and positive female character assisted the negotiation." Participant M9 (27): "in 2–3 more minutes we would have reached agreement; the mediator helped me and was on my side." Participant F9 (26): "The mediator was efficient. Even though we started with large gaps she helped us move forward and we were very close to agreement. I have no doubt that her presence accelerated the process."

9.5 Conclusions

We have introduced the concept of a communication proxy, which is able to replace a human in a telepresence session and seamlessly switch among several control modes of the human-machine control spectrum, and transform various aspects of the communicator online. We have described an implemented system, which allowed us to explore various configurations and modes of communication with a shared set of modules.

For many of us it would be convenient to use proxy replacements. However, would we want to live in a society where others are often represented by proxies?

As mentioned in (Friedman et al., 2013) there was a significantly higher acceptance of the concept of a proxy by male participants than female participants, but a vast majority of both genders would be happy to use a proxy. Based on these preliminary findings we conclude that we are likely to see various kinds of communication proxies gradually deployed. We encourage the developers of such autonomous intelligent agents to be aware of the social, ethical, and legal implications while pushing the technology further.

Acknowledgements: BEAMING is supported by the European Commission under the FP7 ICT Work Program; see www.beaming-eu.org for more information. We would like to thank Oren Salomon, Peleg Tuchman, and Keren-Or Berkers for programing several parts of the proxy. The case studies were produced by undergraduate students of the Sammy Ofer School of Communication in the Interdisciplinary Center (IDC), Herzliya (Israel). The teaching scenario was produced by IDC students, Jonathan Bar and Jonathan Kaplan. The dual gender scenario was produced by IDC students, Ori Fadlon, Lee Chissick and Daniel Goldstein.

References

Artstein, R., Traum, D., Alexander, O., Leuski, A., Jones, A., Georgila, K., . . . Smith, S. (2014). *Time-offset interaction with a holocaust survivor.* Paper presented at the Proceedings of the 19th international conference on Intelligent User Interfaces.

Bailenson, J. N., Beall, A. C., Loomis, J., Blascovich, J., & Turk, M. (2004). Transformed Social Interaction: Decoupling Representation from Behavior and Form in Collaborative Virtual Environments. *Presence: Teleoperators and Virtual Environments,, 13*, 428–441.

Bates, J. (1994). The role of emotion in believable agents. *Communications of the ACM, 37*(7), 122–125.

Cassell, J., Sullivan, J., Prevost, S., & Chrchill, E. (Eds.). (2000). *Embodied Conversational Agents.* Cambridge, MA: MIT Press.

Cassell, J., & Vilhjálmsson, H. (1999). Fully Embodied Conversational Avatars: Making Communicative Behaviors Autonomous. *Autonomous Agents and Multi-Agent Systems, 2*(1), 45–64. doi: 10.1023/a:1010027123541

Clark, A., & Chalmers, D. (1998). The Extended Mind. *Analysis, 58*(1), 7–19.

Clarke, R. (1994). The Digital Persona and its Application to Data Surveillance. *Int'l J. Information Soc. , 10*(2), 77–92.

De'Angeli, A. (2009). Ethical Implications of Verbal Disinhibition with Conversational Agents. *PsychNology, 7*(1), 49–57.

Friedman, D., Berkers, K., Salomon, O., & Tuchman, P. (2014). An architecure for a communication proxy for telepresence. *submitted.*

Friedman, D., Salomon, O., & Hasler, B. S. (2013). Virtual Substitute Teacher: Introducing the Concept of a Classroom Proxy. *London, 28–29 November 2013 King's College London, UK*, 186.

Friedman, D., & Tuchman, P. (2011, 15–17 September). *Virtual clones: Data-driven social navigation.* Paper presented at the 11th Int'l Conf. Intelligent Virtual Agents (IVA), Reykjavik, Iceland.

Gillies, M., Ballin, D., Pan, X., & Dodgson, N. (2008). Semi-Autonomous Avatars: A New Direction for Expressive User Embodiment. In L. Cañamero & R. Aylett (Eds.), *Animating Expressive Characters for Social Interaction* (pp. 235–255): John Benjamins Publishing Company.

Graesser, A. C., Chipman, P., Haynes, B. C., & Olney, A. (2005). AutoTutor: an intelligent tutoring system with mixed-initiative dialogue. *IEEE Transactions on Education, 48*(4), 612–618.

Guizzo, E. (2010). The man who made a copy of himself. *IEEE Spectrum, 47*(4), 44–56.

Hasler, B. S., Hirschberger, G., Shani-Sherman, T., & Friedman, D. (2014). Virtual peacemakers: Mimicry increases empathy in simulated contact with virtual outgroup members. *Cyberpsychology, Behavior, and Social Networking*, in press.

Hasler, B. S., Salomon, O., Tuchman, P., Lev-Tov, A., & Friedman, D. A. (2013). Real-time Gesture Translation in Intercultural Communication. *Artificial Intelligence & Society, in press.*

Hasler, B. S., Tuchman, P., & Friedman, D. (2013). Virtual research assistants: Replacing human interviewers by automated avatars in virtual worlds. *Computers in Human Behavior, 29*(4), 1608–1616.

Heeter, C. (1992). Being there: The subjective experience of presence. *Presence: Teleoperators and virtual environments, 1*(2), 262–271.

Isbister, K., & Nass, C. (2000). Consistency of personality in interactive characters: Verbal cues, non-verbal cues, and user characteristics. *Int. J. Human-Computer Studies, 53*, 251–267.

Lee, J. K., Toscano, R. L., Stiehl, W. D., & Breazeal, C. (2008). *The design of a semi-autonomous robot avatar for family communication and education.* Paper presented at the Robot and Human Interactive Communication, 2008. RO-MAN 2008. The 17th IEEE International Symposium on.

Looks, M., Goertzel, B., & Pennachin, C. (2004). *Novamente: An integrative architecture for general intelligence.* Paper presented at the AAAI Fall Symposium, Achieving Human-level intelligence.

Ma, J., Wen, J., Huang, R., & Huang, B. (2011). Cyber-Individual Meets Brain Informatics. *IEEE Intelligent Systems, 26*(5), 30–37.

Ong, K. W., Seet, G., & Sim, S. K. (2008). An implementation of seamless human-robot interaction for telerobotics. *International Journal of Advanced Robotic Systems, 5*(2), 167–176.

Paulos, E., & Canny, J. (2001). Social tele-embodiment: Understanding presence. *Autonomous Robots, 11*(1), 87–95.

Pelachaud, C. (2005). *Multimodal expressive embodied conversational agents.* Paper presented at the Proceedings of the 13th annual ACM international conference on Multimedia, Singapore.

Penny, S., Smith, J., Sengers, P., Bernhardt, A., & Schulte, J. (2001). Traces: Embodied Immersive Interaction with Semi-Autonomous Avatars. *Convergence, 7*(2), 47–65.

Prendinger, H., & Ishizuka, M. (2004). *Life-like characters: tools, affective functions, and applications*: Springer.

Purdy, R. (2011). Scoping Report on the Legal Impacts of BEAMING Presence Technologies. *Available at SSRN 2001418.*

Sheridan, T. B. (1992). *Telerobotics, Automation, and Supervisory Control.* Cambridge, MA: MIT Press.

Steed, A., Steptoe, W., Oyekoya, W., Pece, F., Weyrich, T., Kautz, J., . . . Tecchia, F. (2012). Beaming: An Asymmetric Telepresence System. *Computer Graphics and Applications, IEEE, 32*(6), 10–17.

Swartout, W. R., Gratch, J., Hill, R. W., Hovy, E., Marsella, S., Rickel, J., & Traum, D. (2006). Toward Virtual Humans. *AI Magazine, 27*(2), 96–108.

Turkle, S. (1984). *The Second Self*: MIT Press.

Turkle, S. (1997). *Life on the Screen: Identity in the Age of the Internet*: Touchstone Books.

Venolia, G., Tang, J., Cervantes, R., Bly, S., Robertson, G., Lee, B., & Inkpen, K. (2010). *Embodied social proxy: mediating interpersonal connection in hub-and-satellite teams.* Paper presented at the CHI '10 Proceedings of the 28th international conference on Human factors in computing systems

Vilhjlmsson, H. H., & Cassell, J. (1998). BodyChat: Autonomous Communicative Behaviors in Avatars *Int'l Conf. Autonomous Agents* (pp. 269–276). Minneapolis, Minnesota.

Vinayagamoorthy, V., Gillies, M., Steed, A., Tanguy, E., Pan, X., Loscos, C., & Slater, M. (2006). *Building Expression into Virtual Characters.* Paper presented at the Eurographics Conference State of the Art Reports.

Whitby, B. (2008). Sometimes it's hard to be a robot: A call for action on the ethics of abusing artificial agents. *Interacting with Computers, 20*(3), 326–333.

Robert Leeb, Ricardo Chavarriaga, and José d. R. Millán

10 Brain-Machine Symbiosis

Abstract: Imagine you want your computer or any computing device to perform an action. But before you have to get up and interact with it, the device is already doing it! Because directly from your intention, from your thoughts the control signal for the action is identified. Would such a novel interaction technique be of interest for us or would it be too scary? How far is the technology already towards the line of direct brain-controlled or brain-responsive devices? In this chapter we will introduce the field of brain-computer interfaces, which allows the direct control of devices without the generation of any active motor output. The control of brain-actuated robots, wheelchairs and neuroprosthesis will be presented and the concepts behind, like context awareness or hybrid systems are explained. Furthermore, also cognitive signals or mental states are possible sources of interaction. Whenever our brain identified an error performed by the system, we could automatically correct it, or based on our attention or other mental states the interaction system could adapt itself towards our current needs in speed, support or autonomy. Especially, since human computer confluence (HCC) refers to invisible, implicit, embodied or even implanted interaction between humans and system components. Brain-computer interfaces are just one possible option to achieve such a goal, but how would we or our brain embody such external devices into our body schema?

Keywords: Brain-computer Interface, Neuroprosthesis, Context Awareness, Hybrid System, Mental States

10.1 Introduction

A Brain-computer interface (BCI) establishes a direct communication channel between the human brain and a computer or an external device, which can be used to convey messages directly so that no motor activity is required (Wolpaw et al., 2002). The brain activity is acquired and in real-time analyzed to interpret the independent thought or action of the user, which can be transformed into a control signal. Particularly for people suffering from severe physical disabilities or those who are in a "locked-in" state, a BCI offers a possible new communication channel, but also augmenting or repairing human cognitive or sensory-motor functions.

Different types of BCIs exist and various methods can be used to acquire brain activity, but since the electroencephalogram (EEG) is the most practical modality (Mason et al., 2007) – if we want to bring BCI technology to a large population – this chapter will focus on EEG based BCIs only. Nevertheless we would like to say, that brain activity can be measured through non-electrical means as well, such as through magnetic and metabolic changes, which can be also measured non-invasively. Magnetic fields can be recorded with magnetoencephalography (MEG), while brain metabolic activity (reflected in changes in blood flow) can be observed with positron emission tomography (PET), functional magnetic resonance imaging (fMRI), and optical imaging (NIRS). Unfortunately, such alternative techniques require sophisticated devices that can be operated only in special facilities (except for NIRS). Moreover, techniques for measuring blood flow have long latencies compared to EEG systems and thus are less appropriate for interaction, although they may provide good spatial resolution. Besides EEG, electrical activity can also be measured through invasive means such as Electrocorticogram (ECoG) or intracranial recordings. Both methods require surgery to implant electrodes. The relative advantages and disadvantages of currently available noninvasive and implanted (i.e., invasive) methodologies are discussed in (Wolpaw et al., 2006).

Two different neurophysiological phenomena of the EEG can be used as input to a BCI. Either event-related potentials (ERPs) or event-related oscillatory changes in the ongoing EEG are analyzed. An ERP can be seen as an event- and time-locked response of a stationary system to an external/internal event, which is the response of the existing neural network. A significant number of reports are focused on the analysis of ERPs, including slow cortical potentials (Birbaumer et al., 1999), P300 component (a positive waveform occurring approximately 300 ms after an infrequent task-relevant stimulus) (Allison et al., 2007b, Donchin et al., 2000), steady-state visual evoked potentials (SSVEP) while looking at flickering lights (Gao et al., 2003). Event-related oscillatory changes on the other hand can be interpreted as result of changes in the functional connectivity within the neuronal network which are time- but not phase-locked. These internally triggered changes in the rhythmic components of the ongoing brain signal results in relative power increase or decrease, which can be associated with active information processing within these networks. For example, the imagination of different types of movements (MI) results in power changes over the motor cortex.

Most of the existing BCI applications are either software oriented, like mentally writing text via a virtual keyboard on a screen (Birbaumer et al., 1999), or hardware oriented, like controlling a small robot (Millán et al., 2004). These typical applications require a very good and precise control channel to achieve performances comparable to healthy users without a BCI. However, current day BCIs offer low information throughput and are insufficient for the full dexterous control of such complex applications, because of the inherent properties of the EEG. Therefore, the requirements and the skills don't match at all. Techniques like context awareness can enhance the interaction to a similar level, despite the fact that BCI is not such a perfect control channel (Tonin et al., 2011, Galán et al., 2008). In such a control scheme, the responsibilities are then shared between the user, who gives high-level commands, and the system, which executes fast and precise low-level interactions.

The classic user group in BCI research is severely disabled patients: persons who are unable to communicate through other means (Birbaumer et al., 1999). However, recent progress in the field of BCI technology shows that BCIs could also be helpful to less disabled users. New user groups are emerging as new devices and applications develop and improve. Rehabilitation of disorders has gained a lot of attention recently, especially for users with other disabilities such as stroke, addiction, autism, ADHD and emotional disorders (Allison et al., 2007b, Birbaumer & Cohen, 2007, Lim et al., 2010, Pineda et al., 2008). Furthermore, BCIs could also help healthy users in specific situations, such as when conventional interfaces are unavailable, cumbersome, or do not provide the needed information (Allison et al., 2007a).

Such passive monitoring offers potential benefits for both patients and healthy subjects. Furthermore, another area of research, interesting for healthy subjects, are BCI controlled or supported games; by augmentation of the operation capabilities or by allowing multi-task operations (Menon et al., 2009), or possible space applications (Millán et al., 2009). Another recent extension of BCI for healthy users is in the field of biometrics. Since the brainwave pattern of every person is unique, a person authentication based on BCI technology could use EEG measures to help authenticate a user's identity, either by mental tasks (Marcel & Millán, 2007) or reactive frequency components (Pfurtscheller & Neuper, 2006).

Many new BCI devices and applications have recently been validated mostly with healthy users, such as control of smart home or other virtual environment (Leeb et al., 2007b, Scherer et al., 2008), games (Lalor et al., 2005, Millán et al., 2008, Nijholt et al., 2008), orthosis or prosthesis (Müller-Putz & Pfurtscheller, 2008, Pfurtscheller et al., 2008), virtual or real wheelchairs (Leeb et al., 2007a, Cincotti et al., 2008, Galán et al., 2008), and other robotic devices (Bell et al., 2008, Graimann et al., 2008). We can even turn the BCI shortcomings into challenges (Nijholt et al., 2009, Lotte, 2011), by e.g. explicitly requiring a gamer to issue BCI commands to solve a task. Thereby far from perfect control 'solutions' are more interesting and challenging. These and other emerging applications adumbrate dramatic changes in user groups. Instead of being devices that only help severely disabled users and the occasional curious technophile, BCIs could benefit a wide variety of disabled and even healthy users.

Furthermore, when controlling complex devices via a BCI, the brain signals not only carry information about the mental task that is executed, but also about other cognitive processes that take place simultaneously. These processes reflect the way the user perceives the interaction and how much the device behavior truly reflects his/her intent. These cognitive processes can be exploited in a human-machine interaction, for allowing to recognize erroneous conditions during the interaction via the error potential (ErrP), or to detect the preparation or onset of motor actions, as well as identification of attentional and perceptual processes.

10.2 Applied Principles

We will first explain the underlying principles in this chapter, before moving towards examples of brain controlled devices and cognitive signals in the next chapters.

10.2.1 Brain-Computer Interface Principle

In the direct control examples presented later on (see section 10.3), a BCI based on motor imagery (MI) is used. MI is described as the mental rehearsal of a motor act without any overt motor output (Decety, 1996), which involves similar brain regions to those which are used in programming and preparing such real movements (Ehrsson et al., 2003, Jeannerod & Frak, 1999). The imagination of different types of movements (e. g. right hand, left hand or feet), results in an amplitude suppression (known as event-related desynchronization, ERD (Pfurtscheller & Lopes da Silva, 1999)) or in an amplitude enhancement (event-related synchronization, ERS) of Rolandic mu rhythm (7–13 Hz) and the central beta rhythm (13–30 Hz) recorded over the sensorimotor cortex of the participant (Pfurtscheller & Neuper, 2001).
Therefore, the brain activity is acquired via 16 active EEG channels over the sensorimotor cortex. From the Laplacian filtered EEG, the power spectral density was calculated. Canonical variate analysis was used to select subject-specific features, which were classified with a Gaussian classifier (Galán et al., 2008). Decisions with low confidence on the probability distribution were filtered out and evidence was accumulated over time (see the basic principle in Figure 10.1).

Before being able to use a BCI, participants have to go through a number of steps to learn to voluntarily modulate the EEG oscillatory rhythms by performing MI tasks. Furthermore, the BCI system has to learn what the participant-specific patterns are, that can be used for that particular user for online experiments. If participants achieve good online control they are allowed to test the application prototypes (see Section 10.3). More details about the experimental paradigm, signal processing and machine learning (feature extraction, feature selection, classification and evidence accumulation) and the feedback are given in (Leeb *et al.*, 2013).

10.2.2 The Context Awareness Principle

For example, let us consider driving a wheelchair in a home or indoor environment (scattered with obstacles like chairs, tables, doors ...) that requires precise control to navigate through rooms. A context aware and smart wheelchair will help the user to navigate through. The user issues via the BCI the high level commands such as left, right and forward, which are then interpreted by the wheelchair controller based on the contextual information from its sensors, also called shared control in robotics.

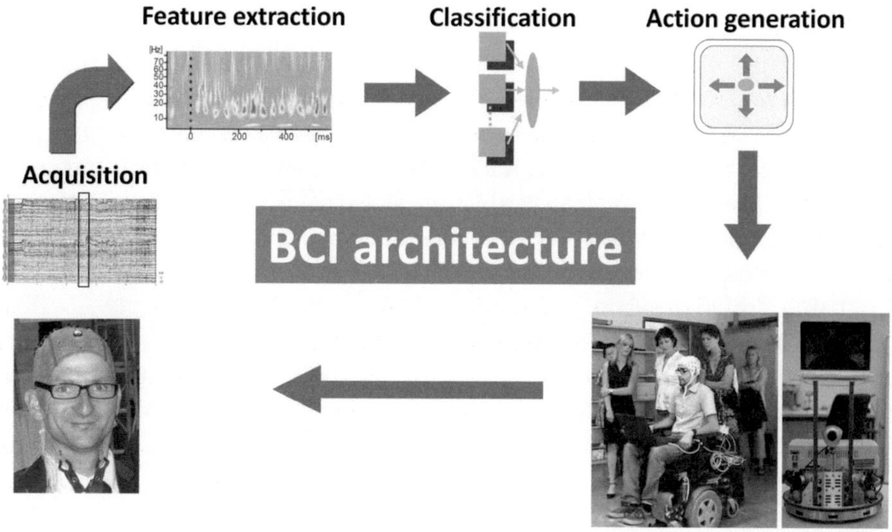

Figure 10.1: Basic principle of a BCI: The electrical signals from the brain are acquired, before feature –characteristic with the given task– are extracted. These are then classified to generate action, which are controlling the robotic devices. The participant immediately either sees the output of the BCI and/or the generated action

Based on these interpretations, the wheelchair can perform intelligent maneuvers (e.g. obstacle avoidance, guided turnings).

Despite the low information transfer rate of a BCI, researchers have demonstrated the feasibility of mentally controlling complex robotic devices from EEG (Flemisch et al., 2003, Vanhooydonck et al., 2003, Carlson & Demiris, 2008). In the case of neuroprosthetics, Millán's group has pioneered the use of shared control that takes the continuous estimation of the operator's mental intent and provides assistance to achieve tasks (Millán et al., 2004, Tonin et al., 2010, Galán et al., 2008). Generally, in a context awareness framework, the BCI's outputs are combined with information about the environment (obstacles perceived by the robotic sensors) and the robot itself (position and velocities) to better estimate the user's intent (see Figure 10.2). Some broader issues in human – machine interaction are discussed in (Flemisch et al., 2003), where the H-Metaphor ("horse" metaphor) is introduced, suggesting that interaction should be more like riding a horse or controlling a horse carriage, with notions of "loosening the reins", allowing the system more autonomy. Context awareness is a key component of any future BCI systems, as it will shape the closed-loop dynamics between the user and the brain-actuated device so tasks can be performed as easily as possible and effectively. As mentioned above, the idea is to integrate the user's mental commands with the contextual information gathered by the intelligent brain-actuated device, so as to help the user to reach the target or override the mental commands in critical situations. In other words, the actual commands sent to the device and the feedback to the user will adapt to the context and inferred goals. Therefore, context awareness can make target-oriented control easier, can inhibit pointless mental commands (e.g. driving zig-zag), and can help determine meaningful motion sequences (e.g., for a neuroprostheses). Context awareness is helping on a direct interaction with the environment but is conveying a different principle than autonomous control. In autonomous control high-level commands which are more abstract (e.g. drive to the kitchen or the living room) are issued and then executed autonomously by the robotic device without interaction of the user, till the selected target is reached (Carlson & Millán, 2013), which could be suboptimal in cases of interaction with other people.

A critical aspect of context awareness for BCI is coherent feedback —the behavior of the robotic device should be intuitive to the user and the robot should unambiguously understand the user's mental commands. Otherwise, people find it difficult to form mental models of the neuroprosthetic device.

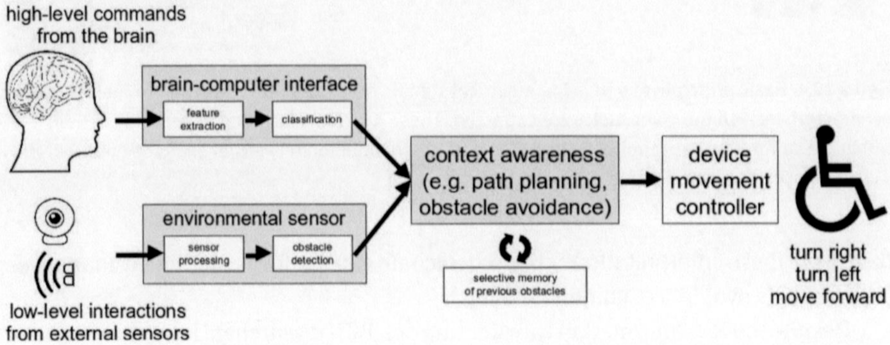

Figure 10.2: The context awareness principle: The user issues high-level commands via a brain-computer interface mostly on a lower pace. The system is acquiring fast and precise the environmental information (via sonars, webcams...). The context awareness system combines the two information to achieve a path planning and obstacle avoidance, so that a control of the robotic device is possible (shared control) and e.g. the wheelchair can move forward, turn left or right. Modified from Rupp et al. (2014)

10.2.3 Hybrid Principle

Despite the progress in BCI research, the level of control is still very limited compared to natural communication or existing assistive technology products. Practical brain-computer interfaces for disabled people should allow them to use all their remaining functionalities as control possibilities. Sometimes these people have residual activity of their muscles, most likely in the morning when they are not exhausted. In such a hybrid approach, where conventional assistive products (operated using some residual muscular functionality) are enhanced by BCI technology, leads to what is called a hybrid BCI (hBCI).

As a general definition, a hBCI is a combination of different input signals including at least one BCI channel (Millán et al., 2010, Pfurtscheller et al., 2010). Thus, it could be a combination of two BCI channels but, more importantly, also a combination of a BCI and other biosignals (such as EMG, etc.) or special AT input devices (e.g., joysticks, switches, etc.). There exist a few examples of hybrid BCIs. Some hBCIs are based on multiple brain signals: such as MI for control and ErrP detection for correction of false commands (Ferrez & Millán, 2008b), or an offline combination of MI and SSVEP (Allison et al., 2010, Brunner et al., 2010).

Other hBCIs combine brain and other biosignals: switching an standard SSVEP BCI on/off via an heart rate variation (Scherer et al., 2007), or fusing electromyographic (EMG) with EEG activity (Leeb et al., 2011) so that the subjects could achieve a good control of their hBCI independently of their level of muscular fatigue. Finally, EEG signals could be combined with eye gaze (Danoczy et al., 2008). Pfurtscheller et al. (2010) recently reviewed preliminary attempts, and feasibility studies, to develop hBCIs combining multiple brain signals alone or with other biosignals. Millán et al. (2010) reviewed the state of the art and challenges in combining BCI and assistive technologies and Müller-Putz et al. (2015) presented an hBCI framework, which was used in studies with non-impaired as well as end-users with motor impairments.

10.3 Direct Brain-Controlled Devices

In a traditional BCI fashion controlling complex devices such as brain-controlled wheelchair or mobile tele-presence platform in natural office environments would be a complex and frustrating task, especially since the timing and speed of interaction is limited by the BCI. Furthermore, the user has to share his attention between the BCI and the device, and also remember the place where he is and where he wants to go. In contrary, combing the above mentioned principles of BCI with context awareness and hybrid approaches allow subjects to control such complex devices easily.

10.3.1 Brain-Controlled Wheelchair

In case of brain-controlled robots and wheelchairs, Millán's group has pioneered the development of the shared autonomy approach to estimate the appropriate assistance which greatly improved BCI driving performance (Vanacker et al., 2007, Galán et al., 2008, Millán et al., 2009, Tonin et al., 2010). Although asynchronous spontaneous BCIs seem to be the most natural and suitable alternative, there are a few examples of synchronous evoked P300 BCIs for wheelchair control (Iturrate et al., 2009, Rebsamen et al., 2010), whereby the system flashes the possible predefined target destinations several times in a random order. The stimulus that elicits the largest P300 is chosen as the target. Then, the intelligent wheelchair reaches the selected target autonomously. Once there, it stops and the subject can select another destination – a process that takes around 10 seconds.

Here, we describe our recent work (Carlson & Millán, 2013), during which subjects controlled the movement of an electric wheelchair (InvaCare Europe) by thought. The wheelchair's turnings to the left and right are controlled via a 2-class BCI (see section 10.2.1). Whenever the BCI output exceeds the left or right threshold a command was delivered to the wheelchair. In addition, the participant can intentionally decide not to deliver any mental commands to maintain the default behavior of the wheelchair, which consists of moving forward and avoiding obstacles with the help of a shared control system using its on-board sensors. More details see (Carlson & Millán, 2013).

For controlling, the user asynchronously sent high-level commands for turning to the left or right (with the help of a motor-imagery based BCI) to achieve the desired goals, while short-term low-level interaction for obstacle avoidance was done by the context awareness (see Figure 10.3.a and section 10.2.2). In the applied context awareness paradigm, the wheelchair pro-actively slows down and turns to avoid obstacles as it approaches them. For that reason the wheelchair was equipped with proximity sensors and two webcams for obstacle detection. Using the computer vision algorithm described in (Carlson & Millán, 2013), we constructed a local 10 cm resolution occupancy grid (Borenstein & Koren, 1991), which was then used by the shared control module for local planning. Generally, the vision zone was divided into three zones. Obstacles detected in the left or right zone triggered rotation of the wheelchair, whereas obstacle in center (in front) slowed it down. We also implemented a docking mode, additionally to the obstacle avoidance. Therefore, we considered any obstacle to be a potential target, provided it was located directly in front of the wheelchair. Consequently, the user was able to dock to any "obstacle", be it a person, table, or even a wall. The choice of using cheap webcams and not using an expensive laser range-finder was taken to facilitate the development of affordable and useful assistive devices. If we want to bring the wheelchair to patients, the additional equipment should not cost more than the wheelchair itself.

In an experiment four healthy subjects (aged 23–28) participated successfully in driving the wheelchair (Carlson & Millán, 2013). The task was to enter an open – plan environment, through a narrow doorway, dock to two different desks, whilst navigating around natural obstacles and finally reach the corridor through a second doorway (see Figure 10.3.b). The experiment was performed twice, once with BCI control with the help of context awareness and once with the normal manual control, whereby the analog joystick was replaced by two discrete buttons. Across subjects, it took an average of 160.0 s longer to complete the task under the BCI condition. In terms of path efficiency, there was no significant difference among subjects between the distance traveled in the manual benchmark condition (43.1 ± 8.9 m) and that in the BCI condition (44.9 ± 4.1 m) (Carlson & Millán, 2013). The longer time is probably due to a combination of subjects issuing manual commands with a higher temporal accuracy and a slight increase in the number of turning commands that were issued when using the BCI, which yielded in a lower average translational velocity. Especially, inexperienced users had a bigger difference than experience ones. This is likely to be due to the fact that performing an MI task, while navigating and being seated on a moving wheelchair, is much more demanding than simply moving a cursor on the screen and when the timing of delivering commands becomes very important (Leeb et al., 2013).

We want to highlight that, in this study not only a complex task had to be performed, but also the potential stressfulness of the situation, since the user was co-located with the robotic device that he or she was controlling and was subject to many external factors. This means the user had to put trust in the context awareness system and expected that negative consequences (e.g. a crash) could result in the system failing (although an experimenter was always in control of a fail-safe emergency stop button).

In the future we are planning to add a start/stop or a pausing functionality for the movement of the robotic device, in parallel to the frequently-occurring commands of turning left or right. In the framework of a hybrid BCI, such rare start/stop commands could also be delivered through other channels such as residual muscular activity, which can be controlled reliably—but not very often, because of the quick fatigue.

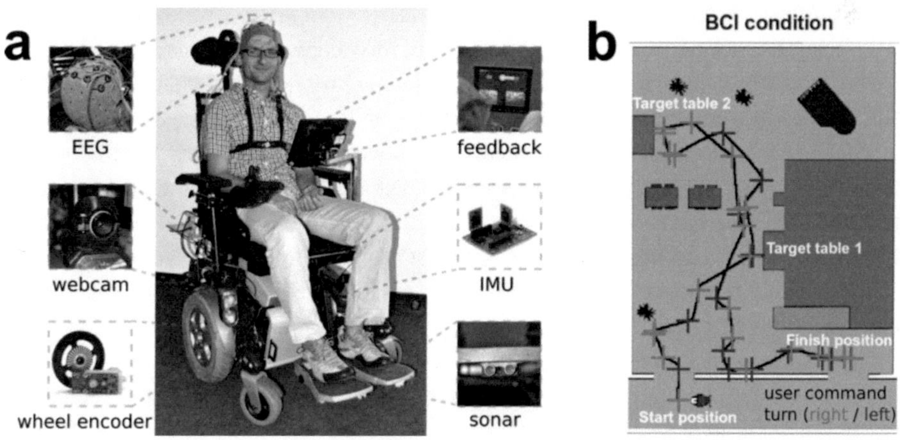

Figure 10.3: (a) Picture of a healthy subject sitting in the BCI controlled wheelchair. The main components on our brain-controlled robotic wheelchair are indicated with close-ups on the sides. The obstacles identified via the webcams are highlighted in red on the feedback screen and will be avoided by the context awareness system. (b) Trajectories of a subject during BCI control reconstructed from the odometry. The start, end and target positions as well as the BCI triggered turnings are indicated. Modified from Carlson & Millán (2013)

10.3.2 Tele-Presence Robot Controlled by Motor-Disable People

Moving on from healthy people to motor-disabled end users as BCI participants, we present a study in which a tele-presence robot was remotely navigated within a natural office environment. The space contains natural obstacles (i.e. desks, chairs, furniture, people) in the middle of the pathways and some predefined target positions. Importantly, participants have never been in such an environment. The robot's turnings to the left and right are controlled via a 2-class BCI similar to the aforementioned study with the wheelchair.

The implementation of context awareness used the dynamical system concept (Schöner et al., 1995), to control two independent motion parameters: the angular and translation velocities of the robot. The systems can be perturbed by adding attractors or repellors in order to generate the desired behaviors. The dynamical system implements the following navigation modality. The default device behavior is to move forward at a constant speed. If repellors or attractors are added to the system, the motion of the device changes in order to avoid the obstacles or reach the targets. At the same time, the velocity is determined according to the proximity of the repellors surrounding the robot. The robot is based on Robotino™ by FESTO (Esslingen, Germany) a small circular mobile platform (diameter 36 cm, height 65 cm), which is equipped with nine infrared sensors that can detect obstacles up to ~30 cm distance and a webcam that can also be used for obstacle detection. Furthermore, a notebook with a camera is added on top of the robot for tele-presence purposes (see Figure 10.4.a), so that the participant can interact with the remote environment via Skype™.

Nine severely motor-disabled end-users, who had never visited the laboratory in person, were able to use such a tele-presence robot to successfully navigate around the lab (see Figure 10.4.b), whilst they were located in their own homes or clinics at distances of up to 550 km away (Leeb et al., 2015). In some extreme tests, a healthy subject was attending a conference in South Korea, where he demonstrated that he could use our motor imagery based BCI to reliably control the tele-presence robot, which was located in our lab in Switzerland. As before, the same paths were followed with BCI control and with manual control (i.e. button presses). Furthermore, context awareness was either applied or not. The time and number of commands needed were previously reported for healthy users (Tonin et al., 2010) and recently for patients (Tonin et al., 2011, Leeb et al., 2015). Remarkably, the patients performed similar to the healthy users who were familiar with the environment (91.5 ± 17.5 versus 102.6 ± 26.3 seconds).

Context awareness also helped all subjects (including novel BCI subjects or users with disabilities) to complete a rather complex task in similar time and with similar number of commands to those required by manual commands without context awareness. More details are given in (Tonin et al., 2010, 2011, Leeb et al., 2013, 2015). Thus, we argue that context awareness reduces subjects' cognitive workload as it: (i) assists them in coping with low-level navigation issues (such as obstacle avoidance and allows the subject to focus the attention on his final destination) and thereby (ii) helps BCI users to maintain attention for longer periods of time (since the amount of BCI commands can be reduced and their precise timing is not so critical).

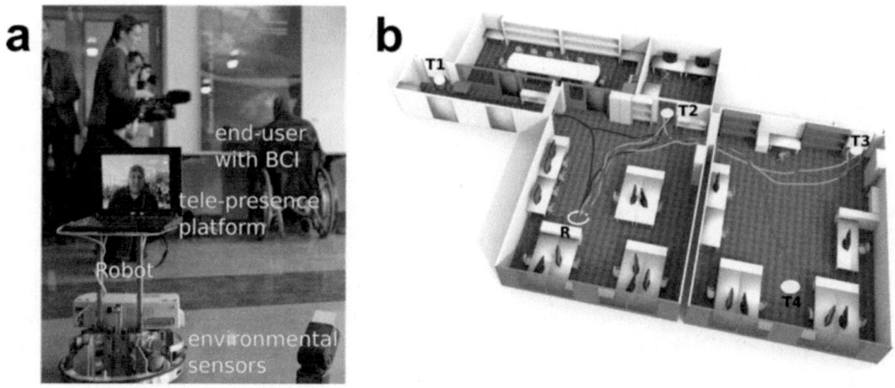

Figure 10.4: (a) A tetraplegic end-user (C6 complete) demonstrates his acquired motor imagery skills, manoeuring the brain-controlled tele-presence robot in front of participants and press at the "TOBI Workshop IV", Sion, Switzerland, 2013. (b) Layout of the experimental environment with the four target positions (T1, T2, T3, T4), start position (R)

10.3.3 Grasp Restoration for Spinal Cord Injured Patients

The restoration of grasp functions in spinal cord injured (SCI) patients or patients suffering from paralysis of upper extremities typically rely on Functional Electrical Stimulation (FES). In this context, the term neuroprosthesis is used for FES systems that seek to restore a weak or lost grasp function when controlled by physiological signals. Some of these neuroprostheses are based on surface electrodes for external stimulation of muscles of the hand and forearm (Ijzermann et al., 1996, Thorsen et al., 2001, Mangold et al., 2005). Others, like the Freehand system (NeuroControl, Cleveland, US), uses implantable neuroprostheses to overcome the limitations of surface stimulation electrodes concerning selectivity and reproducibility (Keith & Hoyen, 2002), but this system is no longer available on the market.

Pioneering work by the groups in Heidelberg and Graz showed that a BCI could be combined with an FES-system with surface electrodes (Pfurtscheller et al., 2003). In this study, the restoration of a lateral grasp was achieved in a spinal cord injured subject (see Figure 10.5.b). The subject suffered from a complete motor paralysis with missing hand and finger function. The patient could trigger sequential grasp phases by imagining foot movements. After many years of using the BCI, the patient can still control the system, even during conversation with other persons. The same procedure could be repeated with another tetraplegic patient who was provided with a Freehand system (Müller-Putz et al., 2005). All currently available FES systems for grasp restoration can only be used by patients with preserved voluntary shoulder and elbow function, which is the case in patients with an injury of the spinal cord below C5. So neuroprostheses for the restoration of forearm function (like hand, finger and elbow) require the use of residual movements not directly related to the grasping process. To overcome this restriction, a new method of controlling grasp and elbow function with a BCI was introduced recently via pulse-width coded brain patterns for controlling sequentially more degrees of freedom (Müller-Putz et al., 2010).

BCIs have been used to control not only grasping but also other complex tasks like writing. Millán's group used the motor imagery of hand movements to stimulate the same hand for a grasping and writing task (Tavella et al., 2010). Thereby the subjects had to split his/her attention to multitask between BCI control, reaching, and the primary handwriting task itself. In contrast with the current state of the art, an approach in which the subject was imagining a movement of the same hand he controls through FES was applied.

Moreover, the same group developed an adaptable passive hand orthosis (see Figure 10.5.a), which evenly synchronizes the grasping movements and applied forces on all fingers (Leeb et al., 2010). This is necessary due to the very complex hand anatomy and current limitations in FES-technology with surface electrodes, because of which these grasp patterns cannot be smoothly executed. The orthosis support and synchronize the movement of the fingers stimulated by FES for patients with upper extremity palsy to improve everyday grasping and to make grasping more ergonomic and natural compared to the existing solutions. Furthermore, this orthosis also avoids fatigue in long-term stimulation situations, by locking the position of the fingers and switching the stimulation off (Leeb et al., 2010).

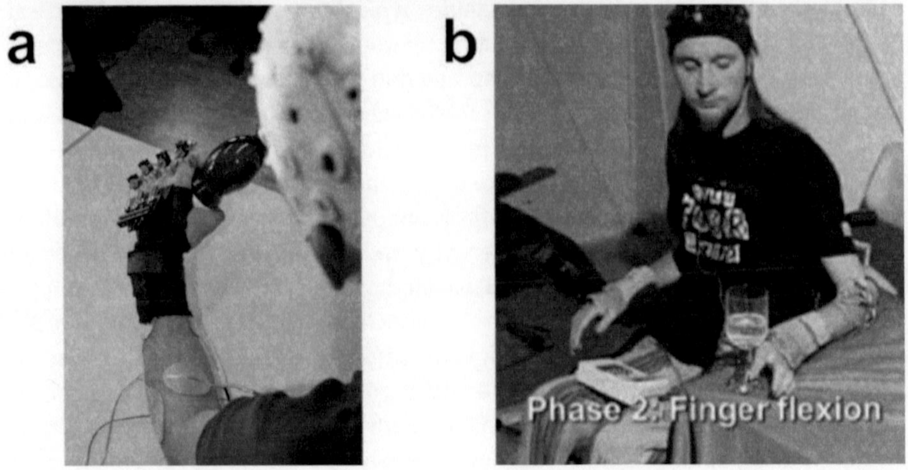

Figure 10.5: (a) Picture of BCI subject with an adaptable passive hand orthosis. The orthosis is capable of producing natural and smooth movements when coupled with FES. It evenly synchronizes (by bendable strips on the back) the grasping movements and applied forces on all fingers, allowing for naturalistic gestures and functional grasps of everyday objects. (b) Screen shot from the pioneering work showing the first BCI controlled grasp by a tetraplegic patient (Pfurtscheller et al., 2003)

10.4 Cognitive Signals and Mental States

Previous sections illustrate how it's possible to control complex devices by the decoding of user's intention from the execution of specific mental tasks (i.e. motor imagery – complemented by contextual information in order to increase the robustness of the system. However, when controlling a BCI, brain signals not only carry information about the mental task that is executed, but also about other cognitive processes that take place simultaneously. These processes reflect the way the user perceives the interaction and how much the device behavior truly reflects his/her intent. In this section we present several ways to exploit these cognitive processes to overall human-machine interaction.

In particular, we will review different potentials that convey useful information allowing to recognize erroneous conditions during the interaction, preparation of motor actions as well as attentional and perceptual processes.

10.4.1 Error-Related Potentials

Error recognition is crucial for efficient behavior in both animals and humans. Wealth of studies have identified brain activity patterns that are naturally elicited whenever a person commits an error in tasks requiring a rapid response (Falkenstein et al., 2000). Interestingly, similar potentials are also observed when the person perceives error committed by other person (van Schie et al., 2004) or even machines (Ferrez & Millán, 2008a). These error-related potentials (ErrPs) provide a mean to obtain information about the subject evaluation of the interaction. Allowing to synergistically incorporate detection of erroneous situations – decoded from the brain activity – into the control of the external device. Enabling us to correct these situations or even improve performance via error-driven adaptation.

Error-related potentials can be observed in the EEG signals over fronto-central areas. In the case of self-generated errors differences between the correct and error condition appear at about 120 ms after the action, while differential responses to external feedback appear at about 200–500 ms after the erroneous stimuli. Interestingly, these signals are naturally elicited during the interaction, therefore no user training is required. Moreover, they are rather stable across time (Chavarriaga & Millán, 2010) and similar waveforms appear across different tasks (Iturrate et al., 2014) and feedback modalities (Chavarriaga et al., 2012).

One of the first attempts to exploit these signals during human-computer interaction was proposed by Parra and colleagues (Parra et al., 2003). In their study the user performed a two-forced choice task and the EEG was decoded to detect the error-related pattern after incorrect presses. This automatic correction yielded to a performance improvement of around 20%. Later on, it was demonstrated that error-related potentials were also elicited in the frame of brain-computer interaction (Ferrez

& Millán, 2008a). Importantly, it is possible to decode these potentials at a single trial basis, i.e. inferring whether a given trial correspond to the erroneous or correct condition. This paved the way for automatic correction of BCI commands Ferrez and colleagues demonstrate this in a MI-based BCI by simultaneous decoding of the BCI control signal (e.g. motor imagery) and the ErrPs (Ferrez & Millán, 2008b). Similar approaches have also been implemented for P300-based BCIs both in healthy and motor disabled subjects (Dal Seno et al., 2010, Spüler et al., 2012).

These systems allow for instantaneous response of the previous command. However, this does not prevent the same errors to appear in the future. An alternative approach is to exploit the ErrPs to drive the adaptation of an intelligent controller so as to improve the likelihood of generating correct responses (Chavarriaga & Millán, 2010, Llera et al., 2011, Förster et al., 2010). Based on the reinforcement learning paradigm, the ErrPs provide information akin to (negative) rewards that make it possible to infer control strategies that the subject considers as correct. In this approach the human is placed within a cognitive monitoring loop with the agent, thus making possible to tune the agent's behavior to the user's needs and preferences.

10.4.2 Decoding Movement Intention

The counterpart of interpreting the outcome of a specific action is the possibility of detecting the intention to move prior to the execution. This can help in the control of neuroprosthetics as early detection can reduce the delay between the motor intention and the device activation.

There has been evidence of preparatory and anticipatory activity since several decades. This includes seminal works showing slow deflections of cortical activity between timely separated contingent stimuli (i.e. contingent negative variation) (Walter et al., 1964) and lateralized slow cortical potentials preceding movements up to 1.5 s (Libet et al., 1982). However, only recently this type of signal has been successfully decoded for Non-invasive BCI applications. A key factor for this decoding is the appropriate selection of spatio-spectral features used for the decoding, as low-frequency EEG oscillations exhibit a large inter-trial variability (Garipelli et al., 2013). Regarding arm movements, Lew et al. used a center-out reaching task (see Figure 10.6.a) to show that onset of self-paced movement intention could be detected more than 460 ms before the movement, based on SCP off-line analysis (Lew et al., 2012) (see Figure 10.6.b). A similar approach was also used to predict intention both in movement execution and imagination (Niazi et al., 2011). In turn, oscillatory activity in the alpha and beta bands (8–30 Hz) was also shown to carry information that could be used to detect self-paced wrist extension movement (Bai et al., 2011).

However, the previous studies were performed with simplified protocols. So the question remains on whether similar signals can be observed and decoded in realistic conditions. Experiments in virtual environments and during car driving tasks suggest that this is the case (Chavarriaga et al., 2012, Khaliliardali et al., 2012) (see Figure 10.6.c). We have analyzed the EEG activity while drivers (N=6) perform self-paced lane changes in a simulated highway. Using classifiers trained on segments corresponding to straight driving and steering actions, the onset of the steering actions was detected on average 811 ms before the action with a 74.6% true positive rate (Gheorghe et al., 2013) (see Figure 10.6.d).

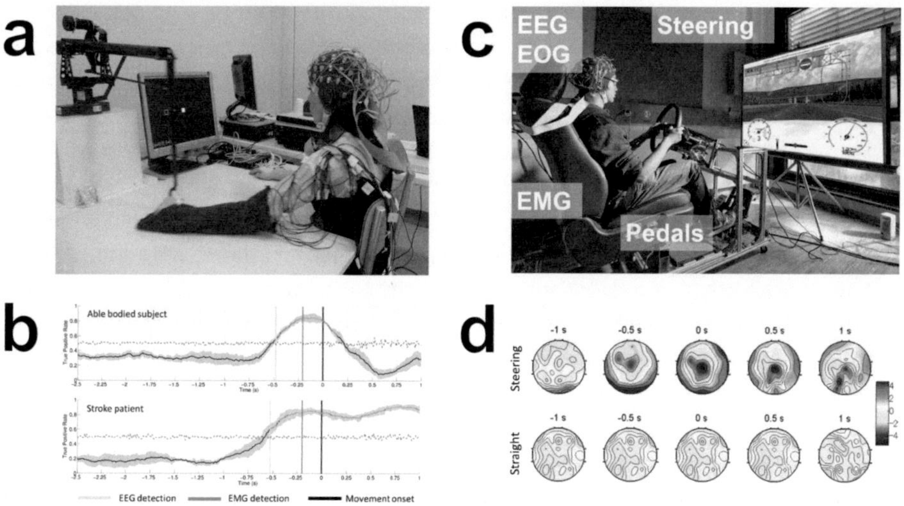

Figure 10.6: EEG correlates of movement intention: (a) Decoding of movement related potentials in both able-bodied and stroke subjects. (b) Single trial analysis of EEG signals in a center-out tasks yield recognition about chance level at about 500 ms before the movement onset (green line), earlier than any observable muscle activity (magenta line) (Lew et al., 2012). (c) Car driving scenario. Low-frequency oscillations (<1 Hz) reflect preparatory activity up to 1 s before steering actions in a car simulator. (d) As shown in the topographic representation this activity appears over central midline areas, consistent with movement-related potentials reported in simpler tasks (Gheorghe et al., 2013)

10.4.3 Correlates of Visual Recognition and Attention

Human machine interaction implies a closed-loop where information flows to, from and between the user and the device she/he is interacting with. For this reason there is an increased interest in identifying brain correlates of perceptual and attentional processes.

A clear example of combining human and machine capabilities can be found on applications of image retrieval. As of today, computer algorithms are quite efficient at processing large amounts of data based on their low-level features, but are less suitable to handle their semantic content. These applications decode the EEG responses to visual stimuli so as to identify those images that are interesting to the subject. They constitute labeled exemplars that can be exploited by computer vision algorithms to retrieve similar images from a larger database (Sajda et al., 2010, Bigdely-Shamlo et al., 2008, Uscumlic et al., 2013).

Interaction with complex system necessarily implies to attend to different stimuli. In the case of vision, attentional deployment can be produced with or without changes in the gaze direction (i.e. overt and covert attention). While the first one can be easily detected using eye-tracking techniques, the second one requires the analysis of the brain patterns, as no observable behavior is produced. Neurophysiological studies have shown that modulation of α rhythms signal voluntary changes of covert visual attention. Furthermore, there seems to be a specialized topographical representation of the attended locations (Rihs et al., 2007). Based on this, the use of covert shifts of attention – decoded from the EEG α activity – has been proposed as an alternative BCI paradigm (Treder et al., 2011, van Gerven & Jensen, 2009). Interestingly, a new approach allows for a more detailed spatio-temporal characterization of these processes by analyzing narrow sub-bands of the α rhythms, as well as the inherent temporal variability of such signals (Tonin et al., 2012). Experiments with able-bodied subjects over two days resulted in a mean on-line accuracy across the group of 70.6 ± 1.5% (N=8), and 88.8 ± 5.8% for the best subject (Tonin et al., 2013). Interestingly, these subjects that present a drop in performance also exhibited changes in the δ,θ, and α over frontal cortices. These changes have been previously reported as putative correlates of fatigue, increased workload or drowsiness (Borghini et al., 2012, Brouwer et al., 2012). This evidences the possibility of simultaneous monitoring of multiple cognitive signals.

10.5 Discussion and Conclusion

In this book chapter we gave a broad overview of the functionality of a brain-computer interface and showed possible scenarios and applications. We put emphasis on control of robotic devices (like wheelchair or tele-presence robots), motor substitution by functional electrical stimulation, decoding of erroneous decisions, intention of movements or actions, mental state monitoring of attention and visual recognition.

We presented examples of how healthy and disabled participants can use successfully the BCI to control robotic devices. Especially with the help of context awareness some of the BCI limitations can be overcome and the path in developing more practical BCIs is opened, especially towards the control of mobility (either a tele-presence robot or a wheelchair). We showed results from healthy users and end-users with disabilities, which were able to perform a rather complex navigation task. Remarkably, although the patients had never visited the remote location where the tele-presence robot was operating, their performances were similar to a group of healthy users who were familiar with the environment. Furthermore, the help of context awareness allowed all subjects to complete task in similar time and with similar number of commands to those required by manual commands without context awareness. Thus, we argue that context awareness reduces subjects' cognitive workload as it: (i) assists them in coping with low-level navigation issues (such as obstacle avoidance and allows the subject to focus the attention on his final destination) and (ii) helps BCI users to keep attention for longer periods of time (since the amount of BCI commands can be reduced and their precise timing is not so critical).

First steps are done in establishing the possibility to give the control back to patients, not only over robotic devices but directly of simple grasp patterns. Brain-controlled functional electrical stimulation of the muscles together with orthotic devices will allow a self-paced long term use. However, BCIs are not ready yet for an independent use at home (Leeb et al., 2013) and some gaps for usability and reliability have to be addressed.

The exploitation of cognitive signals, which carry valuable information in parallel to the mental task being performed, is pushing BCIs to the next level. Information like how the interaction is perceived or about erroneous decisions, or even about the attention to the task, will allow us to modulate the level of support which is needed for BCI control, or value the received signals. We can envision that a future car, could modify its behavior depending on the state of the user, it could help more or less, or even become more proactive in case the attention of a user is going down, or he is getting more and more distracted.

We expect even faster progress in the next years, since the BCI field is still gaining attention from funding agencies and companies. More practical and powerful tools for disabled people will develop. Furthermore, BCIs can benefit from other signals and human-computer interaction techniques, and vice-versa. BCIs can be used to extract cognitive-relevant information to improve standard interactions, which is becoming increasingly interesting for healthy users.

A further future key component for a successful application of BCI devices is the availability of dry and wireless electrodes systems with a sufficient data quality. First systems are appearing on the market, but long term studies are still missing. Furthermore, more translational studies involving end-users at their homes are needed to address the problems which are arising from application control outside laboratory environments. Adopting a user-centered iterative approach (for the end-users as well as for the healthy population) will allow addressing the specific needs and requirements of the different future user groups.

Acknowledgement: This work was supported by the European ICT programme projects TOBI: Tools for Brain-Computer Interaction (FP7-224631) and Opportunity: Activity and Context Recognition with Opportunistic Sensor Configuration (ICT-225938). This paper only reflects the authors' views and funding agencies are not liable for any use that may be made of the information contained herein.

References

Allison, B., Graimann, B., & Gräser, A. (2007a). Why use a BCI if you are healthy? In *Proceedings of BRAINPLAY 2007 "Playing with your brain"*, (pp. 7–11).

Allison, B. Z., Brunner, C., Kaiser, V., Müller-Putz, G. R., Neuper, C., & Pfurtscheller, G. (2010). Toward a hybrid brain-computer interface based on imagined movement and visual attention. *Journal of Neural Engineering*, *7*(2), 026007.

Allison, B. Z., Wolpaw, E. W., & Wolpaw, J. R. (2007b). Brain-computer interface systems: Progress and prospects. *Expert Review of Medical Devices*, *4*(4), 463–474.

Bai, O., Rathi, V., Lin, P., Huang, D., Battapady, H., Fei, D.-Y., Schneider, L., Houdayer, E., Chen, X., & Hallett, M. (2011). Prediction of human voluntary movement before it occurs. *Clinical Neurophysiology*, *122*(2), 364–372.

Bell, C. J., Shenoy, P., Chalodhorn, R., & Rao, R. P. N. (2008). Control of a humanoid robot by a noninvasive brain-computer interface in humans. *Journal of Neural Engineering*, *5*, 214–220.

Bigdely-Shamlo, N., Vankov, A., Ramirez, R. R., & Makeig, S. (2008). Brain activity-based image classification from rapid serial visual presentation. *IEEE Transactions on Neural Systems and Rehabilitation Engineering*, *16*(5), 432–441.

Birbaumer, N., & Cohen, L. G. (2007). Brain-computer interfaces: communication and restoration of movement in paralysis. *The Journal of Physiology*, *579*, 621–636.

Birbaumer, N., Ghanayim, N., Hinterberger, T., Iversen, I., Kotchoubey, B., Kübler, A., Perelmouter, J., Taub, E., & Flor, H. (1999). A spelling device for the paralysed. *Nature*, *398*(6725), 297–298.

Borenstein, J., & Koren, Y. (1991). The vector field histogram – fast obstacle avoidance for mobile robots. *IEEE Transactions on Robotics and Automation*, *7*(3), 278–288.

Borghini, G., Astolfi, L., Vecchiato, G., Mattia, D., & Babiloni, F. (2012). Measuring neurophysiological signals in aircraft pilots and car drivers for the assessment of mental workload, fatigue and drowsiness. *Neuroscience and Biobehavioral Reviews*, 44, 58–75.

Brouwer, A.-M., Hogervorst, M. A., van Erp, J. B. F., Heffelaar, T., Zimmerman, P. H., & Oostenveld, R. (2012). Estimating workload using EEG spectral power and ERPs in the n-back task. *Journal of Neural Engineering*, *9*(4), 045008.

Brunner, C., Allison, B. Z., Krusienski, D. J., Kaiser, V., Müller-Putz, G. R., Pfurtscheller, G., & Neuper, C. (2010). Improved signal processing approaches in an offline simulation of a hybrid brain-computer interface. *Journal of Neuroscience Methods*, *188*(1), 165–173.

Carlson, T., & Demiris, Y. (2008). Human-wheelchair collaboration through prediction of intention and adaptive assistance. In *Proceedings of the IEEE International Conference on Robotics and Automation*, (pp. 3926–3931). Pasadena, CA.

Carlson, T., & Millán, J. d. R. (2013). Brain-controlled wheelchairs: A robotic architecture. *IEEE Robotics and Automation Magazine*, *20*(1), 65–73.

Chavarriaga, R., & Millán, J. d. R. (2010). Learning from EEG error-related potentials in noninvasive brain-computer interfaces. *IEEE Transactions on Neural Systems and Rehabilitation Engineering*, *18*(4), 381–388.

Chavarriaga, R., Perrin, X., Siegwart, R., & Millán, J. d. R. (2012). Anticipation- and error-related EEG signals during realistic human-machine interaction: A study on visual and tactile feedback. In *Proceedings of International Conference of the IEEE Engineering in Medicine and Biology Society*. 6723–6726.

Cincotti, F., Mattia, D., Aloise, F., Bufalari, S., Schalk, G., Oriolo, G., Cherubini, A., Marciani, M. G., & Babiloni, F. (2008). Non-invasive brain-computer interface system: towards its application as assistive technology. *Brain Research Bulletin*, *75*, 796–803.

Dal Seno, B., Matteucci, M., & Mainardi, L. (2010). Online detection of P300 and error potentials in a BCI speller. *Computational Intelligence and Neuroscience*, *2010*, 307254.

Danoczy, M., Fazli, S., Grozea, C., Müller, K. R., & Popescu, F. (2008). Brain2robot: A grasping robot arm controlled by gaze and asynchronous EEG BCI. In *Proceedings of International BCI Workshop and Trainings Course*, 355–360.

Decety, J. (1996). The neurophysiological basis of motor imagery. *Behavioural Brain Research*, *77*(1–2), 45–52.

Donchin, E., Spencer, K. M., & Wijesinghe, R. (2000). The mental prosthesis: assessing the speed of a P300-based brain-computer interface. *IEEE Transactions on Neural Systems and Rehabilitation Engineering*, *8*, 174–179.

Ehrsson, H. H., Geyer, S., & Naito, E. (2003). Imagery of voluntary movement of fingers, toes, and tongue activates corresponding body-part-specific motor representations. *Journal of Neurophysiology*, *90*, 3304–3316.

Falkenstein, M., Hoormann, J., Christ, S., & Hohnsbein, J. (2000). ERP components on reaction errors and their functional significance: A tutorial. *Biological Psychology*, *51*(2–3), 87–107.

Ferrez, P. W., & Millán, J. d. R. (2008a). Error-related EEG potentials generated during simulated brain-computer interaction. *IEEE Transactions on Biomedical Engineering*, *55*, 923–929.

Ferrez, P. W., & Millán, J. d. R. (2008b). Simultaneous real-time detection of motor imagery and error-related potentials for improved BCI accuracy. In *Proceedings of International BCI Workshop and Trainings Course*. Graz, Austria, 197–202.

Flemisch, O., Adams, A., Conway, S. R., Goodrich, K. H., Palmer, M. T., & Schutte, P. C. (2003). The H-Metaphor as a guideline for vehicle automation and interaction. Tech. Rep. NASA/TM–2003-212672, NASA.

Förster, K., Biasiucci, A., Chavarriaga, R., Millán, J. d. R., Roggen, D., & Tröster, G. (2010). On the use of brain decoded signals for online user adaptive gesture recognition systems. In *Pervasive 2010 The Eighth International Conference on Pervasive Computing*. 427–444.

Galán, F., Nuttin, M., Lew, E., Ferrez, P. W., Vanacker, G., Philips, J., & Millán, J. d. R. (2008). A brain-actuated wheelchair: Asynchronous and non-invasive brain-computer interfaces for continuous control of robots. *Clinical Neurophysiology*, *119*(9), 2159–2169.

Gao, X., Xu, D., Cheng, M., & Gao, S. (2003). A BCI-based environmental controller for the motion-disabled. *IEEE Transactions on Neural Systems and Rehabilitation Engineering*, *11*, 137–140.

Garipelli, G., Chavarriaga, R., & Millán, J. d. R. (2013). Single trial analysis of slow cortical potentials: a study on anticipation related potentials. *Journal of Neural Engineering*, *10*(3), 036014.

Gheorghe, L. A., Chavarriaga, R., & Millán, J. d. R. (2013). Steering Timing Prediction in a Driving Simulator Task. In *Proceedings of International Conference of the IEEE Engineering in Medicine and Biology*. 6913–6916.

Graimann, B., Allison, B. Z., Mandel, C., Lüth, T., Valbuena, D., & Gräser, A. (2008). Non-invasive brain-computer interfaces for semi-autonomous assistive devices. In A. Schuster (Ed.) *Robust intelligent systems*, (pp. 113–137). London: Springer.

Ijzermann, M. J., Stoffers, T. S., Klatte, M. A., Snoeck, G., Vorsteveld, J. H., & Nathan, R. H. (1996). The NESS handmaster orthosis: Restoration of hand function in C5 and stroke patients by means of electrical stimulation. *Journal of Rehabilitation Sciences*, *9*, 86–89.

Iturrate, I., Antelis, J. M., Kübler, A., & Minguez, J. (2009). A noninvasive brain-actuated wheelchair based on a P300 neurophysiological protocol and automated navigation. *IEEE Transactions on Robotics*, *25*(3), 614–627.

Iturrate, I., Chavarriaga, R., Montesano, L., Minguez, J., & Millán, J. d. R. (2014). Latency correction of error potentials between different experiments reduces calibration time for single-trial classification. *Journal of Neural Engineering*, 11, 036005.

Jeannerod, M., & Frak, V. (1999). Mental imaging of motor activity in humans. *Current Opinion in Neurobiology*, *9*(6), 735–739. PMID: 10607647.

Keith, M. W., & Hoyen, H. (2002). Indications and future directions for upper limb neuroprostheses in tetraplegic patients: A review. *Hand Clinics*, *18*(3), 519–528, viii.

Khaliliardali, Z., Chavarriaga, R., Gheorghe, L. A., & Millán, J. d. R. (2012). Detection of anticipatory brain potentials during car driving. *Proceedings of International Conference of the IEEE Engineering in Medicine and Biology Society, 2012*, 3829–3832.

Lalor, E. C., Kelly, S. P., Finucane, C., Burke, R., Smith, R., Reilly, R. B., & McDarby, G. (2005). Steady-state VEP-based brain computer interface control in an immersive 3-d gaming environment. *EURASIP Journal on Applied Signal Processing, 19*, 3156–3164.

Leeb, R., Friedman, D., Müller-Putz, G. R., Scherer, R., Slater, M., & Pfurtscheller, G. (2007a). Self-paced (asynchronous) BCI control of a wheelchair in virtual environments: a case study with a tetraplegics. *Computational Intelligence and Neuroscience, 2007*(Article ID 79642), 1–8.

Leeb, R., Gubler, M., Tavella, M., Miller, H., & Millán, J. d. R. (2010). On the road to a neuroprosthetic hand: A novel hand grasp orthosis based on functional electrical stimulation. In *Proceedings of International Conference of the IEEE Engineering in Medicine and Biology Society*, (pp. 146–149).

Leeb, R., Lee, F., Keinrath, C., Scherer, R., Bischof, H., & Pfurtscheller, G. (2007b). Brain-computer communication: motivation, aim and impact of exploring a virtual apartment. *IEEE Transactions on Neural Systems and Rehabilitation Engineering, 15*, 473–482.

Leeb, R., Perdikis, S., Tonin, L., Biasiucci, A., Tavella, M., Molina, A., Al-Khodairy, A., Carlson, T., & Millán, J. d. R. (2013). Transferring brain-computer interfaces beyond the laboratory: Successful application control for motor-disabled users. *Artificial Intelligence In Medicine, 59*(2), 121–132.

Leeb, R., Sagha, H., Chavarriaga, R., & Millán, J. d. R. (2011). A hybrid brain-computer interface based on the fusion of electroencephalographic and electromyographic activities. *Journal of Neural Engineering, 8*(2), 025011.

Leeb, R., Tonin, L., Rohm, M., Desideri, L., Carlson, T., & Millán, J. d. R. (2015). Towards Independence: A BCI Telepresence Robot for People With Severe Motor Disabilities. *Proceedings of the IEEE*, 103(6), 969–982.

Lew, E., Chavarriaga, R., Silvoni, S., & Millán, J. d. R. (2012). Detection of self-paced reaching movement intention from EEG signal. *Frontiers in Neuroengineering, 5*(13).

Libet, B., Wright, E. W., & Gleason, C. A. (1982). Readiness-potentials preceding unrestricted 'spontaneous' vs. pre-planned voluntary acts. *Electroencephalogr Clinical Neurophysiology, 54*(3), 322–335.

Lim, C. G., Lee, T.-S., Guan, C., Sheng F., D. S., Cheung, Y. B., Teng, S. S. W., Zhang, H., & Krishnan, K. R. (2010). Effectiveness of a brain-computer interface based programme for the treatment of adhd: A pilot study. *Psychopharmacology Bulletin, 43*(1), 73–82.

Llera, A., van Gerven, M. A. J., Gómez, V., Jensen, O., & Kappen, H. J. (2011). On the use of interaction error potentials for adaptive brain computer interfaces. *Neural Networks, 24*(10), 1120–1127.

Lotte, F. (2011). Brain-computer interfaces for 3D games: Hype or hope? In *Proceedings of the 6th International Conference on Foundations of Digital Games*, (pp. 325–327). Bordeaux, France: ACM, New York, NY, USA.

Mangold, S., Keller, T., Curt, A., & Dietz, V. (2005). Transcutaneous functional electrical stimulation for grasping in subjects with cervical spinal cord injury. *Spinal Cord, 43*(1), 1–13.

Marcel, S., & Millán, J. d. R. (2007). Person authentication using brainwaves (EEG) and maximum a posteriori model adaptation. *IEEE Transactions on Pattern Analysis and Machine Intelligence, 29*, 743–748.

Mason, S. G., Bashashati, A., Fatourechi, M., Navarro, K. F., & Birch, G. E. (2007). A comprehensive survey of brain interface technology designs. *Annals of Biomedical Engineering, 35*(2), 137–169.

Menon, C., de Negueruela, C., Millán, J. d. R., Tonet, O., Carpi, F., Broschart, M., Ferrez, P., Buttfield, A., Tecchio, F., Sepulveda, F., Citi, L., Laschi, C., Tombini, M., Dario, P., Rossini, P. M., & de Rossi, D. (2009). Prospects of brain-machine interfaces for space system control. *Acta Astronautica, 64*, 448–456.

Millán, J. d. R., Ferrez, P. W., Galán, F., Lew, E., & Chavarriaga, R. (2008). Non-invasive brain-machine interaction. *International Journal of Pattern Recognition and Artificial Intelligence*, *22*(5), 959–972.

Millán, J. d. R., Ferrez, P. W., & Seidl, T. (2009). Validation of brain-machine interfaces during parabolic flight. *International Review of Neurobiology*, *86*, 189–197.

Millán, J. d. R., Galán, F., Vanhooydonck, D., Lew, E., Philips, J., & Nuttin, M. (2009). Asynchronous non-invasive brain-actuated control of an intelligent wheelchair. In *Proceedings of International Conference of the IEEE Engineering in Medicine and Biology Society*, (pp. 3361–3364).

Millán, J. d. R., Renkens, F., Mouriño, J., & Gerstner, W. (2004). Noninvasive brain-actuated control of a mobile robot by human EEG. *IEEE Transactions on Biomedical Engineering*, *51*(6), 1026–1033.

Millán, J. d. R., Rupp, R., Müller-Putz, G. R., Murray-Smith, R., Giugliemma, C., Tangermann, M., Vidaurre, C., Cincotti, F., Kübler, A., Leeb, R., Neuper, C., Müller, K., & Mattia, D. (2010). Combining brain-computer interfaces and assistive technologies: State-of-the-art and challenges. *Frontiers in Neuroscience*, *4*, 161.

Müller-Putz, G., Leeb, R., Tangermann, M., Höhne, J., Kübler, A., Cincotti, F., Mattia, D., Rupp, R., Müller, K.-R., & Millán, J. d. R. (2015). Towards Noninvasive Hybrid Brain-Computer Interfaces: Framework, Practice, Clinical Application, and Beyond. *Proceedings of the IEEE*, 103(6), 926–943.

Müller-Putz, G., Scherer, R., Pfurtscheller, G., & Neuper, C. (2010). Temporal coding of brain patterns for direct limb control in humans. *Frontiers in Neuroprosthetics*, *4*(34), 1–11.

Müller-Putz, G., Scherer, R., Pfurtscheller, G., & Rupp, R. (2005). EEG-based neuroprosthesis control: A step towards clinical practice. *Neuroscience Letters*, *382*, 169–174.

Müller-Putz, G. R., & Pfurtscheller, G. (2008). Control of an electrical prosthesis with an SSVEP-based BCI. *IEEE Transactions on Biomedical Engineering*, *55*, 361–364.

Niazi, I. K., Jiang, N., Tiberghien, O., Feldbæk Nielsen, J., Dremstrup, K., & Farina, D. (2011). Detection of movement intention from single-trial movement-related cortical potentials. *Journal of Neural Engineering*, *8*(6), 066009.

Nijholt, A., Plass-Oude Bos, D., & Reuderink, B. (2009). Turning shortcomings into challenges: Brain-computer interfaces for games. *Entertainment Computing*, *1*(2), 85–94.

Nijholt, A., Tan, D., Allison, B., Millán, J. d. R., Graimann, B., & Jackson, M. (2008). Brain-computer interfaces for HCI and games. In *Proceedings ACM CHI 2008*.

Parra, L. C., Spence, C. D., Gerson, A. D., & Sajda, P. (2003). Response error correction — A demonstration of improved human-machine performance using real-time EEG monitoring. *IEEE Transactions on Neural Systems and Rehabilitation Engineering*, *11*(2), 173–177.

Pfurtscheller, G., Allison, B., Bauernfeind, G., Brunner, C., Solis Escalante, T., Scherer, R., Zander, T., Müller-Putz, G., Neuper, C., & Birbaumer, N. (2010). The hybrid BCI. *Frontiers in Neuroscience*, *4*, 42.

Pfurtscheller, G., & Lopes da Silva, F. H. (1999). Event-related EEG/MEG synchronization and desynchronization: basic principles. *Clinical Neurophysiology*, *110*, 1842–1857.

Pfurtscheller, G., Müller, G. R., Pfurtscheller, J., Gerner, H. J., & Rupp, R. (2003). "Thought"-control of functional electrical stimulation to restore handgrasp in a patient with tetraplegia. *Neuroscience Letters*, *351*, 33–36.

Pfurtscheller, G., Müller-Putz, G., Scherer, R., & Neuper, C. (2008). Rehabilitation with brain-computer interface systems. *IEEE Computer Magazine*, *41*, 58–65.

Pfurtscheller, G., & Neuper, C. (2001). Motor imagery and direct brain-computer communication. *Proceedings of the IEEE*, *89*, 1123–1134.

Pfurtscheller, G., & Neuper, C. (2006). Future prospects of ERD/ERS in the context of brain-computer interface (BCI) developments. In C. Neuper, & W. Klimesch (Eds.) *Event-Related Dynamics of Brain Oscillations*, vol. 159 of *Progress in Brain Research*, (pp. 433–437). London: Elsevier.

Pineda, J. A., Brang, D., Hecht, E., Edwards, L., Carey, S., Bacon, M., Futagaki, C., Suk, D., Tom, J., Birnbaum, C., & Rork, A. (2008). Positive behavioral and electrophysiological changes following neurofeedback training in children with autism. *Research in Autism Spectrum Disorders, 2*(3), 557–581.

Rebsamen, B., Cuntai, G., Haihong, Z., Chuanchu, W., Cheeleong, T., Ang, M. H. & Burdet, E. (2010). A brain controlled wheelchair to navigate in familiar environments. *IEEE Transactions on Neural Systems and Rehabilitation Engineering, 18*(6), 590–598.

Rihs, T. A., Michel, C. M., & Thut, G. (2007). Mechanisms of selective inhibition in visual spatial attention are indexed by alpha-band eeg synchronization. *European Journal of Neuroscience, 25*(2), 603–610.

Rupp, R., Kleih, S. C., Leeb, R., Millán, J. d. R., Kübler, A., & Müller-Putz, G. R. (2014). Brain-Computer Interfaces and Assistive Technology. In G. Grübler, & E. Hildt (Eds.) *Brain-Computer-Interfaces in their ethical, social and cultural contexts, vol. 12 of the International Library of Ethics, Law and Technology,* (pp. 7–38). Netherlands: Springer.

Sajda, P., Pohlmeyer, E., Wang, J., Parra, L. C., Christoforou, C., Dmochowski, J., Hanna, B., Bahlmann, C., Singh, M. K., & Chang, S.-F. (2010). In a blink of an eye and a switch of a transistor: Cortically coupled computer vision. *Proceedings of the IEEE, 98*(3), 462–478.

Scherer, R., Lee, F., Schlögl, A., Leeb, R., Bischof, H., & Pfurtscheller, G. (2008). Toward self-paced brain-computer communication: navigation through virtual worlds. *IEEE Transactions on Biomedical Engineering, 55*, 675–682.

Scherer, R., Müller-Putz, G. R., & Pfurtscheller, G. (2007). Self-initiation of EEG-based brain-computer communication using the heart rate response. *Journal of Neural Engineering, 4*, L23-L29.

Schöner, G., Dose, M., & Engels, C. (1995). Dynamics of behavior: Theory and applications for autonomous robot architectures. *Robotics and Autonomous Systems, 16*, 213–245.

Spüler, M., Bensch, M., Kleih, S., Rosenstiel, W., Bogdan, M., & Kübler, A. (2012). Online use of error-related potentials in healthy users and people with severe motor impairment increases performance of a P300-BCI. *Clinical Neurophysiology, 123*(7), 1328–1337.

Tavella, M., Leeb, R., Rupp, R., & Millán, J. d. R. (2010). Towards natural non-invasive hand neuroprostheses for daily living. In *Proceedings of International Conference of the IEEE Engineering in Medicine and Biology Society*, (pp. 126–129).

Thorsen, R., Spadone, R., & Ferrarin, M. (2001). A pilot study of myoelectrically controlled FES of upper extremity. *IEEE Transactions on Neural Systems and Rehabilitation Engineering, 9*, 161–168.

Tonin, L., Carlson, T., Leeb, R., & Millán, J. d. R. (2011). Brain-controlled telepresence robot by motor-disabled people. In *Proceedings of International Conference of the IEEE Engineering in Medicine and Biology Society*, (pp. 4227–4230).

Tonin, L., Leeb, R., & Millán, J. d. R. (2012). Time-dependent approach for single trial classification of covert visuospatial attention. *Journal of Neural Engineering, 9*(4), 045011.

Tonin, L., Leeb, R., Sobolewski, A., & Millán, J. d. R. (2013). An online EEG BCI based on covert visuospatial attention in absence of exogenous stimulation. *Journal of Neural Engineering, 10*(5), 056007.

Tonin, L., Leeb, R., Tavella, M., Perdikis, S., & Millán, J. d. R. (2010). The role of shared-control in BCI-based telepresence. In *Proceedings of IEEE International Conference on Systems, Man and Cybernetics*, (pp. 1462–1466).

Treder, M. S., Schmidt, N. M., & Blankertz, B. (2011). Gaze-independent brain-computer interfaces based on covert attention and feature attention. *Journal of Neural Engineering, 8*(6), 066003.

Uscumlic, M., Chavarriaga, R., & Millán, J. d. R. (2013). An iterative framework for EEG-based image search: Robust retrieval with weak classifiers. *PLoS ONE, 8*, e72018.

van Gerven, M., & Jensen, O. (2009). Attention modulations of posterior alpha as a control signal for two-dimensional brain-computer interfaces. *Journal of Neuroscience Methods*, *179*(1), 78–84.

van Schie, H. T., Mars, R. B., Coles, M., & Bekkering, H. (2004). Modulation of activity in medial frontal and motor cortices during error observation. *Nature Neuroscience*, *7*(5), 549–554.

Vanacker, G., Millán, J. d. R., Lew, E., Ferrez, P., Galán Moles, F., Philips, J., Van Brussel, H., & Nuttin, M. (2007). Context-based filtering for assisted brain-actuated wheelchair driving. *Computational Intelligence and Neuroscience*, *2007*, ID 25130.

Vanhooydonck, D., Demeester, E., Nuttin, M., & Van Brussel, H. (2003). Shared control for intelligent wheelchairs: An implicit estimation of the user intention. In *Proceedings of International Workshop Advances in Service Robotics*, (pp. 176–182).

Walter, W. G., Cooper, R., Aldridge, V. J., McCallum, W. C., & Winter, A. L. (1964). Contingent negative variation: An electric sign of sensorimotor association and expectancy in the human brain. *Nature*, *203*, 380–384.

Wolpaw, J. R., Birbaumer, N., McFarland, D. J., Pfurtscheller, G., & Vaughan, T. M. (2002). Brain-computer interfaces for communication and control. *Clinical Neurophysiology*, *113*(6), 767–791.

Wolpaw, J. R., Loeb, G. E., Allison, B. Z., Donchin, E., do Nascimento, O. F., Heetderks, W. J., Nijboer, F., Shain, W. G., & Turner, J. N. (2006). BCI meeting 2005 – workshop on signals and recording methods. IEEE Transactions on Neural Systems and Rehabilitation Engineering, 14, 138–41.

Jonathan Freeman, Andrea Miotto, Jane Lessiter, Paul Verschure, Pedro Omedas, Anil K. Seth, Georgios Th. Papadopoulos, Andrea Caria, Elisabeth André, Marc Cavazza, Luciano Gamberini, Anna Spagnolli, Jürgen Jost, Sid Kouider, Barnabás Takács, Alberto Sanfeliu, Danilo De Rossi, Claudio Cenedese, John L. Bintliff, and Giulio Jacucci

11 The Human as the Mind in the Machine: Addressing Big Data

Abstract: A lot of what our brains process never enters our consciousness, even if it may be of potential value to us. So just what are we wasting by letting our brains process stimuli we don't even notice or attend to? This is one of the areas being explored in the 16-partner CEEDs project (ceeds-project.eu). Funded by the European Commission's Future and Emerging Technologies programme, CEEDs (the Collective Experience of Empathic Data systems) has developed new sensors and technologies to unobtrusively measure people's implicit reactions to multimodal presentations of very large data sets. The idea is that monitoring these reactions may reveal when you are surprised, satisfied, interested or engaged by a part of the data, even if you're not aware of being so. Applications of CEEDs technology are relevant to a broad range of disciplines – spanning science, education, design, and archaeology, all the way through to connected retail. This chapter provides a formalisation of the CEEDs approach and its applications and in so doing explains how the CEEDs project has broken new ground in the nascent domain of human computer confluence.

Keywords: Implicit Processing, Interaction, Big Data, Mixed Reality, Core Features

11.1 'Implicitly' Processing Complex and Rich Information

Over the past decades, researchers have become increasingly interested in how implicit cognitive processing works and how it influences our knowledge and behaviour. It has been claimed that a key element in the definition of implicit processing is the absence of conscious awareness of stimuli, or of patterns within stimuli. In contrast to explicit processing, which is related to those aspects of cognition and perception which are available to an individual's conscious awareness, "implicit processing refers to the acquisition of information expressed [...] in the absence of subjective awareness of the information acquired" (Morton & Barker, 2010, p. 1090; Faulkner, & Foster, 2002; Reber, 2013).

Much evidence supports the distinction between implicit and explicit processing on a number of distinct axes. In the cognitive domain, Zimmerman and Pretz

(2012) refer to explicit processing as rule-based, analytical and deliberate, and as dependent on awareness, attention, and effort, whilst describing implicit processing as associative, holistic, unaware, and effortless. According to this definition of implicit processing, these authors hypothesised that individuals can respond appropriately to complex relations without conscious effort and – more controversially – that the quality of scientific problem solving can sometimes benefit from operating in the absence of the goal to find a rule. Along these lines, Dijksterhuis et al. (2006) famously described such hypothesis as the 'deliberation-without-attention effect' (DWAE), which proposes that, under certain specific circumstances, as complexity of a decision increases, the quality of a decision made at the conscious level decreases. In contrast, decisions made at the unconscious level can be less affected by task, so that unconscious thought (i.e. deliberation without attention) may actually lead to better choices when encountering complex issues. Supporting this hypothesis, Dijksterhuis conducted four studies on consumer choice. In one study (Dijksterhuis, 2004), participants were asked to choose one of four apartments based on their attributes: one apartment was made to be attractive; another was made to be less appealing; the remaining two were average, with the same amount of positive and negative attributes. In the experiment, participants were either asked to choose their favourite immediately, or to think about the apartments for three minutes and then state their preferences. Participants in a third condition were asked for their preferences after being distracted for the same three minutes, thereby engaging in what is called unconscious thought. As predicted by DWAE, those who engaged in unconscious thought made better decisions than those who were given three minutes to think. Furthermore, those who were asked to choose immediately picked more poorly than did either of the thought groups. The results across the four studies were taken as support for the idea that conscious deliberation works very well for simple tasks involving a small amount of information, presumably because the limited capacity of conscious deliberation is able effectively to weigh a small number of attributes in a rational and efficient manner. However, when one is presented with large and complex information, unconscious deliberation can be more effective and more likely to lead to a more satisfying choice than mere conscious deliberation alone (Dijksterhuis & Van Olden, 2006).

The DWAE proposed by Dijksterhuis is only one of the empirically testable hypotheses that were used to describe a broader theory called *unconscious thought theory* (UTT), in an attempt to locate unconscious cognition within the broader decision-making literature. According to UTT, both conscious thought (CT) and unconscious thought (UT) have different characteristics and can be applied in different circumstances. The key difference between these two modes of thought is the presence (for CT) and absence (UT) of attention. During conscious thought, attention is directed toward the task at hand, and the problem is thoroughly considered before making a decision. In contrast, unconscious thought is characterized by attention that is directed away from the problem, and the problem is considered through processes outside of conscious awareness, resulting in deliberation-without-attention. The empirical support for UTT is still evolving, with some authors claiming that the early findings in support of DWAE can be explained by other mechanisms (e.g., Lassiter, Lindberg, González-Vallejo, Bellezza, Phillips, 2009). However, the basic idea remains powerful – there is simply no reason to suppose that explicit conscious processing should always be more effective than implicit unconscious processing.

According to the work of Gigerenzer and his group (1999), simple heuristics often perform better in complex decision situations than more elaborate strategies, perhaps because they can implicitly select the most relevant and robust aspects of the situations instead of explicitly taking all details into account.

The distinction between implicit and explicit processing is an important issue in consciousness research because it can provide for a better understanding of the processes underlying human behaviour. A fundamental question here concerns the extent to which brains can implicitly process information that is subliminally presented. Subliminal perception refers to a person's ability to perceive and respond to stimuli that are presented below the threshold for conscious perception.

Numerous studies and reviews of subliminal perception support the contention that some stimuli that are not consciously identified can influence the affective reactions of individuals, their brain activity and behavioural performance (Tsushima, Sasaki & Watanabe, 2006; Dupoux, De Gardelle & Kouider, 2008). Subliminal priming studies indicate that masked words can activate cognitive processes associated with the meanings of the words and thus have an influence at both perceptual and semantic levels (Allport, 1977, Kouider & Dehaene 2007). Masking experiments with Chinese characters demonstrate such effects already at the first stages of processing of visual information (Elze, Song, Stollhoff, Jost, 2011). Priming from masked stimuli has been shown not only with words, but also with auditory stimuli, pictures and videos. In a study on the effects of subliminal smiles on evaluative judgements (Tamir, Robinson, Clore, Martin & Whitaker, 2004), participants were led to believe that they were playing a competitive game in alternative runs and were then asked to passively watch the videos of their performances and those of their competitor. While watching the videos, subliminal smiles or frowns were flashed (for 32 milliseconds) and immediately masked. The results revealed that participants rated their performances as being better when they were exposed to smiling faces, whilst their opponent's performances were paired with frowning ones, creating the belief that they were doing well and their opponent were doing poorly.

There is also plentiful support for the notion that people's performance on *learning tasks* is affected by subliminal stimuli (Cleeremans & Sarrazin, 2007). This non-conscious acquisition of information allows for the development of procedural knowledge that may be important for a wide variety of cognitive functions (e.g., drawing inferences, and triggering emotional reactions) and evident in performance rather than in conscious recall. Lewicki, Hill and Czyzewska (1992) suggest that the procedural knowledge about complex information involves an advanced and structurally more complex organization that exceeds the one used in any consciously controlled inferences. These authors concluded that "our nonconscious information-processing system appears to be incomparably more able to process formally complex knowledge structures, faster, and 'smarter' overall than our ability to think and identify meanings of stimuli in a consciously controlled manner" [p. 801].

More recently, many other researchers have investigated the superiority of unconscious thought in processing, integrating, and searching through massive quantities of complex information (Payne, Samper, Bettman, & Luce, 2008; Smith, Dijksterhuis & Wigboldus, 2008). Apart from optimising complex decisions, implicit processing has also been found to facilitate divergent thinking, i.e. accessing a wide range of pre-stored information to produce more novel ideas, which improves the creative quality of unconscious thought (Zhong, Dijksterhuis & Galinsky, 2008).

Given the considerable evidence on the important role played by unconscious cognition and perception in the presence of rich information, it is not surprising that this concept is increasingly gaining interest in a broad range of domains where effective responses to large information and complex decision making is required. For example, in many professional occupations, such as air traffic control and stock market trading, a model of rapid decision making called 'recognition-primed decision' (RPD) is often employed to interpret and facilitate the flow of decision making. The RPD model stipulates that people integrate vast numbers of experiences within a given domain into patterns and recognise situational patterns within that domain. When faced with complex information or situations, the situational pattern recognition process should allow them to make fast decisions without invoking full awareness and conscious deliberation (Klein, 2008).

11.2 Exploiting Implicit Processing in the Era of Big Data: the CEEDs Project

Recent years have seen the physical environment becoming more and more saturated with sensing technologies that interact with users. More and more computing and communication entities are capable of sensing information from both the environment and users and responding to appropriate stimuli. A major problem raised by this technology-rich scenario is the rapid increase in the amount of information available and how to comprehend this information (i.e., the so called big data challenge). Experts in many specialist areas have to deal with large-scale, diverse and complex data sets which require efficient data-intensive decision-making, and they mostly rely on computational, statistical, data mining tools and techniques to find meaning in these large data sets. The big data phenomenon emphasises a need for research driving a new category of interfaces that considers the human implicit responses as an additional source of information to support human experience, understanding, and effective decision making in the context of large data sets.

Based on this accumulating evidence for influence of implicit forms of information processing in shaping explicit conscious experience, and in guiding our action and decision making, a European Commission Framework 7 funded project called Collective Experience of Empathic Data Systems (CEEDs) has, over the last four years, researched and developed new tools for interacting with rich and complex information that will assist our everyday decision making and information foraging (Betella et al. 2013; Wagner et al. 2013; Lessiter, Miotto, Freeman, Verschure, Bernardet, 2011; Verschure, 2011). To address this goal, the CEEDs technology monitors users' implicit responses when they are experiencing innovative visualisations of large data sets. Using this information, CEEDs technology automatically infers the extent to which users are surprised, satisfied, interested or engaged by a part of the data, even if they are not aware of being so. These implicit responses then guide users to discover patterns and meaning in the data sets.

The gearing mechanism that is at the core of this technology is called the CEEDs 'Sentient Agent' (CSA), a computational model of the implicit and explicit factors underlying consciousness, which derives indices of unconscious processing such as heart rate, skin conductance (arousal), pupil dilation and brain activity and defines how these feedback cues are presented to users to guide them through a complex data space. The CSA is modelled after the Distributed Adaptive Control theory of mind and brain (See Verschure 2012 for a review).

The overall user experience when interacting with large data sets is thus enhanced by CEEDs by merging the initial data representations with the changes made interactively due to user's implicit (and explicit, e.g., gesture, verbal responses/speech, motion) cues as well as the intentional actions of the CSA based on predictions about the user's behaviour. Additionally, the behaviour of multiple users can be combined to collectively control the data presentation.

Among the wide range of data-rich domains that could benefit from a more human experience centred solution to explore massive volumes of information, the CEEDs project identified a number of real world applications that are being used as test-beds for validating its approach and effectiveness at both scientific and technological levels. Below is a brief description on how implicit user reactions are combined with explicit reactions, and used to guide discovery of patterns and meaning in selected CEEDs-relevant domains.

- Archaeology: for archaeologists, the ability to sift automatically through pottery samples recovered from ancient cities is becoming a necessity. Their classification is manually done by pottery experts and archaeology students under their supervision, who methodically analyse piece by piece and classify these into the established type/variety classification system. Not surprisingly, a huge effort is put in this process, which can take from weeks to years to complete for a typical site. This also leads to the fundamental challenge of how to integrate these residues of ancient cultures into an understanding of their patterns of organization and interaction (such as functional zoning within ancient cities). Currently this remains intuitive and problematic and solutions beyond standard technological solutions are needed. In order to address these challenges, the CEEDs project proposes a two-step process based on sherd classification and statistical analysis of pottery dataset (Piccoli et al., 2013). Firstly, eye and gaze tracking are used to identify the parts of the sherd which gained most of the user's attention when attempting to classify it. These parts are matched by CEEDs with, for example, pots that share similar parts and shapes, and as a result, the most similar pots are retrieved and returned one by one to the user. CEEDs then assesses user satisfaction to the presented pots and filters out those with which the user is not satisfied, thus reducing the time of pottery classification. Secondly, collections of artifacts used to study cities from the whole of their surfaces can be data mined using statistical packages to reveal clusters of associations of artifact types with particular areas of the town. The clusters revealed scientifically can be compared with intuitive groupings based on experts' intuitive functional classes, and this could confirm or challenge the traditional expert system approach to mapping the infrastructure of the ancient site.

- Neuroscience: a goal for current neuroscience is to describe the "connectome" (Sporns, 2011), a comprehensive map of neural connections in the brain. Current versions of the connectome represent complex networks composed of hundreds of brain regions and their white-matter connection pathways, which are impossible to understand without the aid of models and data analysis techniques. The CEEDS neuroscience application supports the visualisation of large connectome data sets in virtual, synthetic reality environments. This allows scientists to virtually explore the intricate brain connectivity (both at the structural and functional level) and disclose different layers of complexity, test dynamical models and manipulate them in real time. These manipulations are displayed in an immersive real-time environment to support new discoveries, in particular, patterns of activation in the brain (see Figure 11.1).

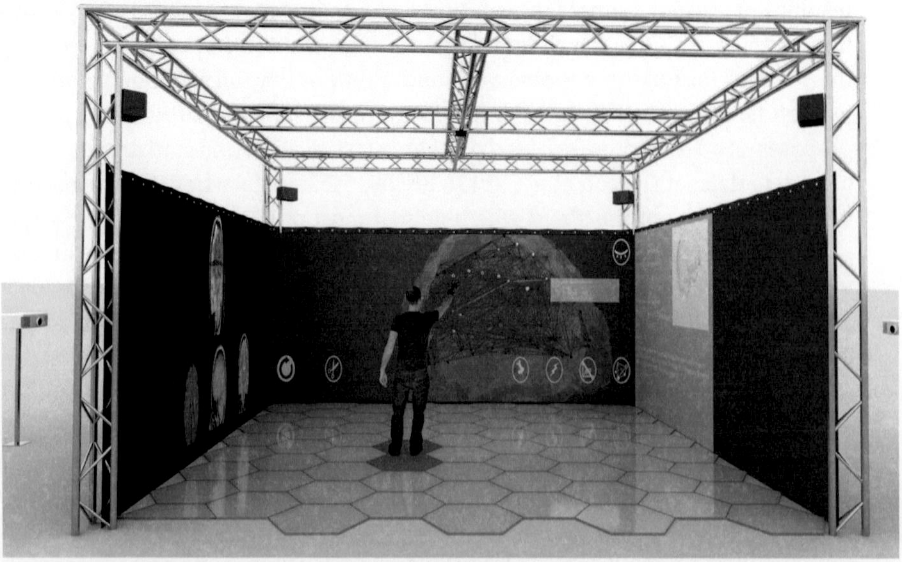

Figure 11.1: CEEDs eXperience Induction Machine, an immersive space equipped with a number of sensors and effectors (retrieved with permission from "BrainX³: embodied exploration of neural data" by Betella et al., 2014)

For example, immersed in the CEEDs eXperience Induction Machine (CXIM), a neuroscientist can explore the connectome to better understand brain structures and dynamics. She might do this by navigating in the CXIM to move her own body towards the desired point in the dataset representation. Her behaviour will be constantly analysed by the CSA, which interprets the user's implicit (e.g., galvanic skin response, hear rate, pupil dilation) and explicit (e.g., CXIM tracking data, gaze) signals obtained using special sensing technology worn by the user (e.g., sensing glove, shirt, eye tracking) or present in the CXIM environment (e.g., full body tracking system). The CSA uses these cues to build a model of arousal/cognitive load of the user and changes the data presentation accordingly. For example, when the user's arousal increases, the system records the position of the user in the dataset (location, gaze, options enabled, and path) and presents other sub-datasets with similar features. In another example, high levels of arousal or eye movement patterns signalling attentional overload would be used to 'dial down' the overall complexity of the dataset presentation, for example by thresholding the level at which connections are shown. First pilots have shown that naive users understand a connectome better in the CXIM than in the state of the art desktop tool.

- History: understanding the significance of the Holocaust remains of great importance today as it can help people engage in a critical reflection about the root causes of genocide, and in turn prevent the recurrence of such atrocities. However, the presentation of this event is problematic due to the vast and diverse amount of information available, but at the same time and in certain circumstances, to the lack of original structures remaining on memorial sites. For example, in concentration camps such as Bergen-Belsen in Germany, visitors have to rely upon their own imagination and interpretation of available information in order to picture the camp and events in their mind, as the site is now largely an empty field. This induces a dissonance which subverts the visitor's intention to re-imagine the events of the past. To address this problem, the CEEDS project developed a 'history' application that supports the acquisition and presentation of data that represents key aspects of both the Bergen-Belsen concentration camp and the holocaust. A virtual reconstruction of the space was developed to support public awareness and understanding of the significance of Bergen-Belsen. A mobile application (Figure 11.2) was also developed that allows visitors to navigate through a virtual reconstruction of the concentration camp displayed on a handheld device (iPad) while moving through the memorial site. Visitors can decide to follow different subject perspectives (e.g., survivors, victims, liberators of the camp, or guards) and discover factual information from these recollections. Implicit information regarding visitor locations can be used by CEEDs to provide visitors with relevant information when approaching locations significant to the selected subject perspective.

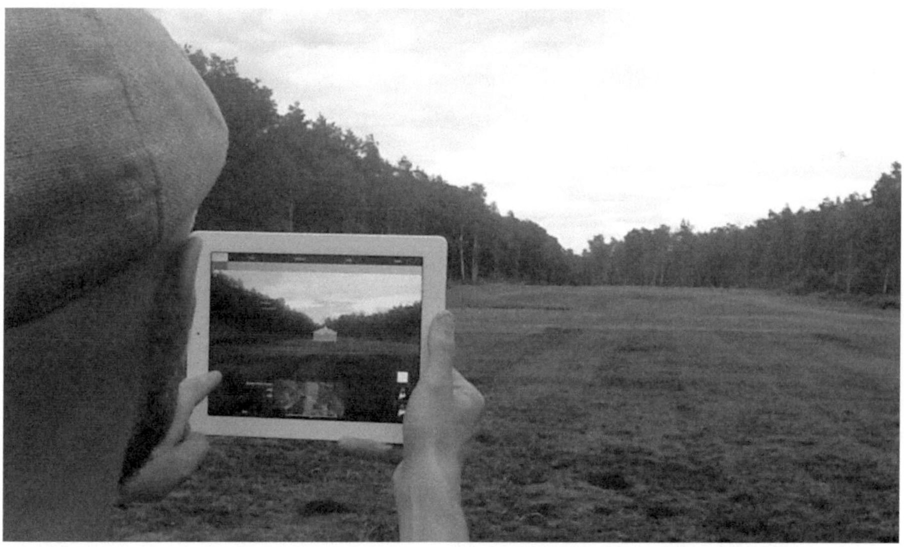

Figure 11.2: CEEDs 'history' application (retrieved with permission from "Spatializing experience: a framework for the geolocalization, visualization and exploration of historical data using VR/AR technologies" by Pacheco et al., 2014)

- Product design and commercial retail: the ongoing embrace of virtual, interactive media technology in product design and manufacturing opens new possibilities for testing ergonomic design by providing visual representations and exploration of products and prototypes. As part of this process, the CEEDs approach can be applied to support designers' understanding of their customers' preferences. In a hypothetical research session, potential customers can be located in front of an interactive large screen in one space within the design houses and interactively explore the range of virtual products, e.g., white goods. A design team in a second room is looking at the same display, and see what customers are looking at, how long they inspect areas, where they point, and where something looks odd or inconsistent with expectations. When appropriate, the design team vary the force required to turn the control (e.g., of what fridges or elements of fridges customers view) in real time and observes how this affects customers' implicit responses (e.g., interest, valence). The CEEDs system may use real-time information of customers to personalise the interactive experience and also induce the user to follow particular paths/journeys through the experience of the product, guided by subliminal stimuli. Indeed, our preliminary research suggests that subliminal priming is effective in guiding people through data in the CXIM (Cetnarski, Betella, Prins, Koudier & Verschure, 2014). This approach can be applied not only to design concept feedback, but to other scenarios including marketing and sales training, and end consumer information delivery. For example, an objective is to explore the use of CEEDS technologies to allow customers to develop CEEDS Universal Personal Preferences (CUPP) in retail environments. CUPPs will contain the explicit and implicit preferences of users with respect to their interests and behaviours. With the user's permission, CUPP files may be accessed by customers through their personal smartphones to receive services that are more tailored to their historical behaviours and interests.

11.3 A Unified High Level Conceptualisation of CEEDs

With such a diverse range of applications, a unified framework for CEEDs was needed to provide a better understanding of the commonalities across all real world applications, and to support the development of in-scope application scenarios, use cases and goals. The process, driven by open discussions with stakeholders and with CEEDs members, and critical and creative thinking, led to a unified high level conceptualisation of CEEDs uses and a more precise formalisation of what CEEDs *'is'*. The resulting framework consisted of two core use cases which specify how CEEDs may be used by potential users from different domains. These two core use cases are.

1. To communicate known meaning (e.g., transferring knowledge to students): with sensitivity to user's state, including to components of state of which user is not aware;
2. To enable discovery (e.g., supporting experts in the discovery of new patterns in datasets): exploiting recognition of user responses (implicit and explicit) according to the user model.

The CEEDs use cases are oriented towards, and may be implemented in, a wide range of domains that deal with complex and very large datasets, and that are in need of better analysis tools. Whether for archaeology, neuroscience, commercial or historical data, the datasets are also characterised as having structures which, without augmentation, are hard to conceptualise.

The use cases breaks down to five primary interdependent components of CEEDs experiences (identified as CEEDs 'core features') and two *associated databases*. The core features (CFs) are outlined below along with examples of how such features could be applied to the neuroscience scenario described above.

- *Associated Database 1: Raw Data Database (RDDB).* Exploring large datasets is fundamental to the primary objective of CEEDs. Any CEEDs experience requires an existing raw database from which data are represented (e.g., visualised) and displayed to the user.
- Core Feature 1: The display of a CSA-independent filtered view, perspective or flow of RDDB. CF1 defines the treatment of the raw data as it is displayed to users. It relates to the rules governing cue sequences including how the data is presented, the starting point and route taken. Importantly, CF1 is defined by its independence from the CSA, i.e., how the data is displayed does not require a user model derived from the CSA. Thus, passive sequences of data (akin to a 'fly-through') can be determined by outcomes of non-CSA variables such as 'sort' or 'match' (e.g., typologies), a directorial/producer preference, or a random sequence, and the data can be contextualised using a developer-designed virtual reconstruction. Active interactions between the user and the data displayed would be possible based on (reactive) rules specifying interaction paradigms (e.g., hand flick gesture to browse through object sequences). The way in which the data are presented provides the problem/data space.

  Example: a complex map of neural connections in the brain is visualised to a neuroscientist inside the CXIM; the neuroscientist can now interact naturally with the visualised data with gestures and body movements.
- Core Feature 2: The collection and storage of users' explicit and/or implicit responses to a dataset. In a CEEDs experience, users respond to datasets based on the output of CF1 or the output of CF4 (tagged dataset), and CF2 reflects the collection and storage of these responses. Raw user responses (e.g., GSR, ECG) are essential prerequisites for: (a) inferring how the user unconsciously interprets

the data (i.e., CF3); (b) the CSA to build a user model (defined in CF4) and (c) user response 'overlays' (review) (defined in CF5).

Example: while the neuroscientist actively engages with the data by changing the presentation properties (e.g., rotating the brain left and right, zooming in and out), his cognitive workload and arousal levels are collected and stored.

- Core Feature 3: The interpretation and storage of the output of CF2. Raw user responses require interpretation in order to establish whether the display has provoked in the user the desired response, which are variable across application scenarios/goals, and to understand what type of response the stimuli elicit (e.g., does the user's responses indicate implicit satisfaction?). In CF3, meaning is inferred through analysis of the pattern of user response data inputs from multiple sources (e.g., EEG, GSR). This information is used to drive CF4 and CF5.

  Example: the combination of the neuroscientist's physiological reactions to the abstract representation of data suggests that the student is not focused or overloaded with information.
- *Associated Database 2: User Response Database.* The CF-URDB stores outputs of CF2 and CF3, and in relation to the raw data (CF-RDDB input to CF1), this information is input to CF4.
- Core Feature 4: The display based on a user model of a CSA-dependent view, perspective or flow of a raw dataset. The autonomous CSA is a real-time goal driven agent which can control the data displayed and guide data exploration. The CSA coordinates the interaction between the user and the problem/data space. It does this by constructing a user model based on the outputs of CF2 and CF3 and, together with its own interests and intentions, modifies the display to guide users in their data exploration. CF4 defines the presentation of this real time CSA-influenced dynamic perspective of the raw dataset. As with CF1, cue sequences are rule based, but unlike CF1, in CF4 the rules are dependent on the CSA which may include subliminal and supraliminal influence to guide users through the data. This could be based on, for instance sort, match or typology functions (e.g., if the goal is to maintain a threshold level of interest or empathy). CF4 is analogous to car satnav systems by which a route is plotted and specified to the driver ("turn left") based on metadata of which the user is unaware (e.g., traffic congestion); that is, the metadata influences the presentation of raw data.

  Example: the system adapts the visualization and the interaction according to a predefined set of rules to avoid information overload (e.g., increasing the saliency of objects, reducing the field of view of the data, reducing the complexity of the dataset) and boost the exploration process.
- Core Feature 5: The display of users' responses and/or the data on which the CSA is making decisions as an overlay to the output of CF1 or CF4. CF5 defines an alternative representation of the raw data (CF1) or tagged data (CF4) by overlaying the outputs of CF2, CF3 to allow the user to access an overview perspective. This could be used in contexts where a user wishes to see which user data

(responses) have influenced the display, for instance, a professional examining the responses of a group of users, learning how experts classify stimuli, debugging, and general data exploration. In this sense, in contrast to CF4 in which metadata influences the display without the user being consciously aware of the relationships between their inputs and the output of the display, in CF5, the metadata is displayed. Analogous to a car satnav system, CF5 is where the driver can see the traffic congestion data in addition to, or instead of, being provided with instructions based on those data.

Example: both the information used by the system and the neuroscientist's implicit responses are made available to the user in order to provide transparency and insight in subconscious processing and decision making.

Across the implementation domains chosen by the project, the CEEDs research project has also uncovered evidence of consistency, for instance, among similar broad classes of users. These were identified and labelled as primary end users (or interactors) and beneficiaries. The former are those users who directly use and interact with the system. For instance, customers are supported in their product choices by CEEDs offering a personalised service based on their own (stored and/or real time) unconscious desires and preferences. As an alternative example, consider a team of neuroscientists attempting to validate/refute models to explain patterns of data. They are supported in this discovery process by CEEDs technology because it harnesses their unconscious responses to different visualisations of those models with the data. Primary CEEDs end users could be both expert/professional users as well as novices. On the other hand, other stakeholder goals suggested that some CEEDs users could be more correctly classified as CEEDs beneficiaries as they are (secondary) CEEDs users of others' data. These are characterised as CEEDs system/database owners who can analyse end user responses to data in all sorts of ways. Beneficiaries could use CEEDs user data to optimise displays for different goals (e.g., learning, empathy, sales); predicting and influencing a user's behaviour by understanding their states/plans/intentions in a given context. For instance, design teams may be beneficiaries if they explore their customers' implicit reactions to products to improve product design.

11.4 Conclusion

This chapter has provided an overview of the new scenarios enabled by the seamless integration between humans and intelligent technology. This synergistic interaction allows for novel solutions in the fields of data mining and knowledge discovery, and in particular to complex situations and environments requiring difficult decisions and rapid responses. Research has shown that unconscious cognition and perception to play an important role in human understanding of rich, complex information. The CEEDs project has adopted an innovative approach to this topic, which relies on two steps: a) monitoring signals of discovery or surprise in unconscious processes when people are experiencing visualisations of large data sets, and b) using such signals to direct users to areas of potential interest and guide meaning within the dataset, in real time. The CEEDs approach can be applied in a wide range of scenarios where performance and 'discovery' are hampered by a deluge of data. The data deluge is a source of increasing difficulty in analysis and sense making of data in fields as diverse as astronomy, neuroscience, archaeology, history and economics.

To support identification of use cases and scenarios that are not only possible but also in-scope for CEEDs, a framework of core features that apply across all applications was developed, which captures discrete components of any CEEDs experience. A shared understanding of the commonalities across all CEEDs applications is also important for identifying what can broadly be achieved with CEEDs-like technology independent of any implementation domain.

The broad consistency in the goals that CEEDs technology could support (i.e., supporting insight and adaptability to users' responses to data), in the core elements shaping the CEEDs experience, and in the characteristics of its users, makes CEEDs a unique system, and provides a high level framework that may be used as conceptual inspiration and the basis for future research and development in the new field of human computer confluence, and symbiotic interaction. CEEDS contributes to addressing the question of how people will interface with complex data and the systems that generate and analyse it, by placing human experience at the centre of the solution, thus breaking new ground in the shaping of a synergy between human and machine.

References

Allport, D. A. (1977). On knowing the meaning of words we are unable to report: The effects of visual masking. *Attention and performance VI*, 505–533.

Betella, A., Cetnarski, R., Zucca, R., Arsiwalla, X., Martínez, E., Omedas, P., Mura, A., & Verschure, P. F. M. J. (2014, April). BrainX 3: embodied exploration of neural data. In *Proceedings of the 2014 Virtual Reality International Conference* (p. 37). ACM.

Betella, A., Martínez, E., Zucca, R., Arsiwalla, X., Omedas, P., Wierenga, S., Mura, A., Wagner, J., Lingenfelser, F., André, E., Mazzei, D., Tognetti, A., Lanatà, A., De Rossi, D., Verschure, P. F. M. J. (2013, July). Advanced interfaces to stem the data deluge in mixed reality: placing human (un) consciousness in the loop. In *ACM SIGGRAPH 2013 Posters* (p. 68). ACM.

Cetnarski, R., Betella, A., Prins, H., Kouider, S., & Verschure, P. F. (2014). Subliminal Response Priming in mixed reality: The ecological validity of a classic paradigm of perception. *Presence: Teleoperators and Virtual Environments*, *23*(1), 1–17.

Cleeremans, A., & Sarrazin, J. C. (2007). Time, action, and consciousness. *Human Movement Science*, *26*(2), 180–202.

Dijksterhuis, A. (2004). Think different: the merits of unconscious thought in preference development and decision making. *Journal of personality and social psychology*, *87*(5), 586.

Dijksterhuis, A., & van Olden, Z. (2006). On the benefits of thinking unconsciously: Unconscious thought can increase post-choice satisfaction.*Journal of Experimental Social Psychology, 42*(5), 627–631.

Dijksterhuis, A., Bos, M. W., Nordgren, L. F., & Van Baaren, R. B. (2006). On making the right choice: The deliberation-without-attention effect. *Science, 311*(5763), 1005–1007.

Dupoux, E., De Gardelle, V., & Kouider, S. (2008). Subliminal speech perception and auditory streaming. *Cognition, 109*(2), 267–273.

Elze, T., Song, C., Stollhoff, R., & Jost, J. (2011). Chinese characters reveal impacts of prior experience on very early stages of perception. *BMC neuroscience, 12*(1), 14.

Faulkner, D., & Foster, J. K. (2002). The Decoupling of" Explicit" and" Implicit" Processing in Neuropsychological Disorders. *Psyche, 8*(02).

Gigerenzer, G., & Todd, P. M. (1999). *Simple heuristics that make us smart.* Oxford University Press, USA.

Klein, G. (2008). Naturalistic decision making. *Human Factors: The Journal of the Human Factors and Ergonomics Society, 50*(3), 456–460.

Kouider, S., & Dehaene, S. (2007). Levels of processing during non-conscious perception: a critical review of visual masking. *Philosophical Transactions of the Royal Society of London B: Biological Sciences, 362*(1481), 857–875.

Lassiter, G. D., Lindberg, M. J., González-Vallejo, C., Bellezza, F. S., & Phillips, N. D. (2009). The deliberation-without-attention effect evidence for an artifactual interpretation. *Psychological Science, 20*(6), 671–675.

Lessiter, J., Miotto, A., Freeman, J., Verschure, P., & Bernardet, U. (2011). CEEDs: unleashing the power of the subconscious. *Procedia Computer Science, 7,* 214–215.

Lewicki, P., Hill, T., & Czyzewska, M. (1992). Nonconscious acquisition of information. *American psychologist, 47*(6), 796.

Morton, N., & Barker, L. (2010). The contribution of injury severity, executive and implicit functions to awareness of deficits after traumatic brain injury (TBI).*Journal of the International Neuropsychological Society, 16*(06), 1089–1098.

Pacheco, D., Wierenga, S., Omedas, P., Wilbricht, S., Knoch, H., & Verschure, P. F. (2014, April). Spatializing experience: a framework for the geolocalization, visualization and exploration of historical data using VR/AR technologies. *Proceedings of the 2014 Virtual Reality International Conference* (p. 1). ACM.

Payne, J. W., Samper, A., Bettman, J. R., & Luce, M. F. (2008). Boundary conditions on unconscious thought in complex decision making. *Psychological Science, 19*(11), 1118–1123.

Piccoli, C., Aparajeya, P., Papadopoulos, G. T., Bintliff, J., Fol Leymarie, F., Bes, P., Van der Enden, M., Poblome, J., Daras, P. (2014). Towards the automatic classification of pottery sherds: two complementary approaches. In *Across Space and Time. Selected Papers from the 41st Computer Applications and Quantative Methods in Archaeology Conference.*

Reber, P. J. (2013). The neural basis of implicit learning and memory: a review of neuropsychological and neuroimaging research. *Neuropsychologia, 51*(10), 2026–2042.

Smith, P. K., Dijksterhuis, A., & Wigboldus, D. H. (2008). Powerful people make good decisions even when they consciously think. *Psychological Science, 19(12), 1258–1259*

Sporns, O. (2011). The human connectome: a complex network. *Annals of the New York Academy of Sciences, 1224*(1), 109–125.

Tamir, M., Robinson, M. D., Clore, G. L., Martin, L. L., & Whitaker, D. J. (2004). Are we puppets on a string? The contextual meaning of unconscious expressive cues. *Personality and Social Psychology Bulletin, 30*(2), 237–249.

Tsushima, Y., Sasaki, Y., & Watanabe, T. (2006). Greater disruption due to failure of inhibitory control on an ambiguous distractor. *Science, 314*(5806), 1786–1788.

Verschure, P. F. (2011, September). The complexity of reality and human computer confluence: stemming the data deluge by empowering human creativity. In *Proceedings of the 9th ACM SIGCHI Italian Chapter International Conference on Computer-Human Interaction: Facing Complexity* (pp. 3–6). ACM.

Verschure, P. F. (2012). Distributed adaptive control: a theory of the mind, brain, body nexus. *Biologically Inspired Cognitive Architectures*, *1*, 55–72.

Wagner, J., Lingenfelser F., André E., Mazzei D., Tognetti A., Lanatà A., De Rossi, D., Betella, A., Zucca, R., Omedas, P., Verschure, P. F. (2013, March). A sensing architecture for empathetic data systems. In *Proceedings of the 4th Augmented Human International Conference* (pp. 96–99). ACM.

Zhong, C. B., Dijksterhuis, A., & Galinsky, A. D. (2008). The merits of unconscious thought in creativity. *Psychological Science*, *19*(9), 912–918.

Zimmerman, C., & Pretz, J. E. (2012). The interaction of implicit versus explicit processing and problem difficulty in a scientific discovery task.

Alessandro D'Ausilio, Katrin Lohan, Leonardo Badino and Alessandra Sciutti

12 Studying Human-Human interaction to build the future of Human-Robot interaction

Abstract: Understanding human-to-human sensorimotor interaction, in a way that can be predicted and controlled, is probably one of the greatest challenges for the future of Human-Computer Confluence (HCC). This would allow, for example, the possibility of optimizing group decision-making or brain storming efficacy. On the other hand it would also offer the means to naturally introduce artificial embodied systems into our social landscape. This vision sees robots or software that smoothly interface with our social representations and adapt dynamically to social contexts. The path to such vision requires at least three components. The first, driven by cognitive neuroscience, has to develop methods to measure the real-time information flow between interacting participants – in ecological scenarios. The second, shaped by the Human-Robot Interaction (HRI) field, consists in building the proper information flow between robots and humans. Finally, the third will have to see the convergence of robotics, neuroscience and psychology in order to functionally evaluate the reality of a long-term HCC.

Keywords: HRI, Mirror Neurons, Sensorimotor Communication, Human-Human Interaction, Human-Robot Interaction, Behavioural Synchronization

12.1 Sensorimotor Communication

Understanding verbal and non-verbal communication in humans is a rather easy task we master in childhood. At the same time, it is true that communication is a rather vague concept, since there are too many unknown degrees of freedom or the same measurable configuration can change in a manner we cannot comprehend, predict nor control. However, the chemistry of group interaction e.g. the subjective feeling of being "in sync" with other people – is something we can perceive easily. We do that instinctively because we're innately social creatures that by definition send and receive (implicit) socially relevant messages in all our interactions (i.e. hand gestures, facial expressions, etc.). We do that in real time in an extremely adaptive manner, at no cost.

Such a capability may be supported by the complex sensory-motor properties present in the human motor system. In fact, in addition to the clear role in movement planning and execution, some premotor neurons have activity that could be interpreted as complex visual responses. For example, "mirror neurons" discharge both when the monkey executes an action and observes another individual making the same action in front of it (Gallese et al., 1996). This discovery has stimulated basic research on how, why and when we do send and receive explicit and implicit sensorimotor messages during social interaction. Along these lines, human research showed that hand muscles cortico-spinal excitability, tested via Transcranial Magnetic Stimulation (TMS), is modulated during the passive observation of hand actions (Fadiga, et al., 1995). Similarly, it was also shown that passive listening to speech, requiring tongue mobilization, modulated the tongue cortico-bulbar excitability (Fadiga et al., 2002). In both cases, the observer/listener shares similar motor programs with the actor/speaker. Therefore, the recognition of other's action/speech may exploit knowledge on how to produce that particular stimulus.

12.1.1 Computational Advantages of Sensorimotor Communication

This computational general principle has supported a major shift in cognitive systems research. In fact, the human motor system was once believed to be mainly an output system. However, the motor brain could also play a role in perceptual and cognitive functions. This challenges the classical sensory versus motor separation (Young, 1970) and opens the doors to embodied cognition and robotics research (Clark, Grush 1999). However, automated systems cannot reach human-like performance when dealing with real coding/decoding of these signals. This simple fact forces us to start exploiting human brain/body solutions. All attempts that do not take this fact into account are bound to be unreliable in variable environments, to fail in the generalization to new examples and to be unable to scale up to solve more complex problems.

These considerations in HCC are pivotal to humanoid robots, in which the explicit design of morphological and functional body features must be complemented with a human-like cognition in order to elicit a human-like interaction and communication (Ferscha, 2013). More importantly, such innate human "behavioural-coupling" capability has to interact with situational intervening factors, which can dramatically hinder a successful information flow. For example, in mediated communications, many relevant cues are often filtered-out because of particular constraints of the medium. As a consequence, things are even more complicated when designing the communication with artefacts (i.e. robots). Modelling and implementation of these automatic systems imposes the additional new challenge of adaptability to context.

Therefore, we suggest that the natural human-to-human coordination capability is the only guide in the development of the future human-to-robot and human-computer interaction in general. In the following sections we will describe the most updated efforts in measuring sensorimotor human-to-human interaction. Next we will overview the strategies to build robot-to-human interaction and finally we will stress the need to quantify the efficacy of the human-to-robot interaction.

12.2 Human-to-Human Interaction

Sensorimotor communication forms the basis of unmediated communication in animals and humans too (Rands et al., 2003; Couzin, et al., 2005; Nagy et al., 2010). Complex coordinated behaviour between multiple individuals can arise without the need for verbal communication to happen (Sebanz et al., 2010; Neda et al., 2000). One important aspect of this kind of communication is the absence of any symbolic component, making such information flow automatic and implicit in nature. Behavioural research has showed an implicit relationship between the stability of intrapersonal coordination and the emergence of spontaneous interpersonal coordination (Coey et al., 2011). Furthermore, individual differences on synchronization performance plays a significant role, suggesting that temporal prediction ability may potentially mediate the interaction of cognitive, motor, and social processes underlying joint action (Pecenka, Keller, 2011). In general, behavioural coordination results from establishing interpersonal synergies. Interpersonal synergies are higher-order control systems formed by coupling movement system degrees of freedom of two (or more) participants. Characteristic features of synergies identified in studies of intrapersonal coordination are revealed in studies of interpersonal coordination in interactive tasks (Riley et al., 2011).

Interestingly, a growing body of neuroscientific evidence indicates that such interpersonal coordination or "group mind" phenomena occurring during interactive tasks are mediated by synchronized cortical activity (Hasson et al., 2012; Loehr et al., 2013; Schippers et al., 2010; Lindenberger et al., 2009). However, classical approaches in social neuroscience, and the field of hyper-scanning, typically search for the significant changes in brain activities after specific training that is supposed to augment coordination (Yun et al., 2012) or during the engagement of a rather rigid/constrained social interaction in general (Hasson et al., 2012; Riley et al., 2011). Therefore, it is important to note that typical behavioural and neuroimaging experiments, rarely implement the ecological complexity of natural interaction. Rather, for control purposes, they devise forced turn taking or a constrained communication mode.

12.2.1 Ecological Measurement of Human-to-Human Information Flow

However, recent studies have approached the problem from a radically different perspective (D'Ausilio et al., 2012; Badino et al., 2014). These studies have indeed measured unobtrusive motion kinematics from "real" groups embedded in "real" social interaction and extracting continuous information flow from participants. This was made possible by recording the motion kinematics of ensemble musicians, and then the use of computational methods allowed the extraction of information flow between participants. Ensemble musicians are experts in non-verbal interaction and behave like processing units embedded within a complex system. Each unit possesses the capability to transmit sensory information non-verbally, and to decode other's movement potentially via the mirror matching system. As these two flows of information occur simultaneously, each unit, and the system as a whole, must rely heavily on predictive models. Thus, the musical ensemble behaves like a complex dynamical system having, however, important constraints that turn into benefits from an experimental perspective.

The quantification of inter-individual information transfer has rarely been attempted in the context of ecological and complex interaction scenarios. To this end, violinists' and conductors' movement kinematics was recorded during the execution of Mozart pieces, searching for causal relationships among musicians by using the Granger Causality method (GC). It was shown that the increase of conductor-to-musicians influence, together with the reduction of musician-to-musician coordination (an index of successful leadership) goes in parallel with quality of execution, as assessed by musical experts' judgments. This study shows that the analysis of motor behaviour provides a potentially interesting tool to approach the rather intangible concept of aesthetic quality of music and visual communication efficacy (D'Ausilio et al., 2012).

The subsequent work found a clear positive relationship between the amount of communication and complexity of the musical score segment. Furthermore, temporal and dynamical changes applied to the musical score were devised in order to force unidirectional communication between the leader of the quartet and the other participants. Results show that in these situations, unidirectional influence from the leader decreased, thus implying that effective leadership may require prior sharing of information between participants. In conclusion, it was possible to measure the amount of information flow and sensorimotor group dynamics suggesting that the fabric of leadership is not built upon exclusive information knowledge but rather on sharing it (Badino et al., 2014).

These studies suggest that, with minimal invasiveness and during real interaction, we can possibly measure the information flow between two (or more) human participants. The next step we suggest is to build robots that are capable of eliciting a realistic robot-to-human interaction. In this sense the goal is to foster a dynamical pattern of information flow between natural and artificial agents.

12.3 Robot-to-Human Interaction

It is usually predicted that the inclusion of robots in our society will progressively become more widespread. However, one of the biggest obstacles to a pervasive use of robots supporting and helping humans in their everyday chores relies on the absence of an intuitive communication between robotic devices and non-expert users. Several attempts have been made at achieving seamless human-robot interaction (e.g., Sisbot and Alami 2012; Dragan, Lee et al. 2013) even with positive outcomes in the context of the small manufacturing industries (e.g., the manufacturing robot Baxter). However the lack of a systematic understanding of what works and why, does not allow for a generalization of this success in different domains. Therefore, in order for robotics, and in particular humanoid robotics, to become a common and functional element of our society, a deeper comprehension of the principles of human-human interaction is needed. Only this knowledge will pave the way to the design of robotic platforms easily usable and understandable by everybody.

However, the investigation of social interaction is a very challenging task. The dynamics of two agents performing a joint action together is much more complex than just the sum of the behaviours of the two individuals. The actions, the movements and even the perceptual strategies each partner chooses are substantially modified and adapted to the cooperation. Traditional research on this topic has been conducted analysing a posteriori recordings of interactions, with the disadvantage of not being able to intervene or to selectively modulate the behaviour of the interacting partners. In more constrained scenarios, a human actor has been used as stimulus. Although this approach provides an increased level of control, not all aspects of human behaviour can be actually manipulated. In particular, the automatic behaviours that constitute a great part of natural coordination are very difficult to restrain. As a potential solution, the option of using video recordings as stimuli for an interaction has been often adopted, especially in the context of action observation and anticipation. This approach guarantees more control and a perfect repeatability, but on the other hand it eliminates some fundamental aspects of real collaborative scenarios, as the shared space of actions, the physical presence, the possibility to interact with the same objects and even the potential physical contact between the two partners.

A valuable, novel solution to these problems could be represented by robots and in particular by humanoid robots. These are embodied agents, moving in our physical world and therefore sharing the same physical space and being subject to the same physical laws that influence human behaviour. Robots with a humanoid shape have the additional advantage of being able to use the tools and objects that have been designed for human use, making them more adaptable to our common environments. Moreover, the human shape and the way humans move are encoded by the brain differently with respect to any other kind of shape and motion (Fabbri-Destro and Rizzolatti 2008). Consequently, humanoid platforms can probe some of the internal models already developed to interact with people and allow studying exactly those basic mechanisms that make human-human interaction fluid and efficient. Thus, humanoid robots represent an ideal stimulator, i.e. a “physical collaborator” whose behaviour could be controlled in a repeatable way. Not only do they share the partner’s action space and afford physical contact, but they can also monitor in real-time the performance of their partner through their on-board sensors and respond appropriately enabling the investigation of longer and more structured forms of interaction.

12.3.1 Two Examples on How to Build Robot-to-Human Information Flow

We suggest that this kind of technology is particularly suited to investigate the very basics mechanisms of interaction: how the motor and sensory models of action and perception change when an action is performed in collaboration rather than in solo, or which are the specific properties of motion that are most relevant in allowing an immediate comprehension between co-operators (Sciutti, Bisio et al. 2012). In this sense the focus is on implicit communication, one specific aspect of social interaction. A classic example of implicit communication is represented by gaze movements. We unconsciously move our eyes, fixating objects of interest or landmarks where our actions will be directed to (Flanagan and Johansson 2003). Human beings are extremely sensitive to the direction of others' gaze. For instance we follow someone else's gaze to recognize and share the focus of his attention and by looking at someone else's eyes we can infer if he is paying attention to what we are showing to him (Lohan, Griffiths et al. 2014). Moreover, we can often anticipate the intention of our partners by noticing what he is fixating, or even infer whether he is thinking or paying attention to us by observing the way he moves his eyes around.

To clarify the effect of this implicit signal on interaction, during a turn-taking game, a series of experiments manipulated the way in which the humanoid robot iCub moved its eyes. The robot either looked in the direction of the partner after its turn finished or kept its eyes fixed. We assessed whether the way participants played the game was influenced by this difference in gazing behaviour and by a different degree of robot autonomy. Interestingly, even if robot gazing was not relevant for the game play, participants modified their playing strategy, apparently attributing more relevance to robot actions when it exhibited an interactive gazing behaviour and more autonomy (Sciutti, Del Prete et al. 2013). Hence, a simple manipulation of robot's gaze motion has an actual impact on how humans behave in an interaction.

Not only eyes however, are carriers of unconscious communication. Indeed, even our common movements provide a quantity of information that it is implicitly read by human observers. When we are reaching to grasp a cup, someone looking at us can often anticipate which cup, among the ones on the table, we are going to take and whether we will drink from it or we will store it away. Moreover, when we transport the cup, our motion tells the observer whether it is full or empty or whether it is too hot to be handled. Understanding where all this information is encoded could potentially allow simplifying the design of robot shape and motion, by keeping at the same time the efficiency of a rich implicit communication.

To this aim the parameters of a lifting action were evaluated to verify whether they could convey enough information to the observer. This information might offer a cue not only to infer the weight that the agent is carrying, but also to be prepared to appropriately perform afterwards an action on the same object. On the humanoid robot iCub the velocity profile of the actions were changed to assess under which conditions robot observation was as communicative as human observation. Interestingly, even a simplified robotic movement, sharing with human actions only an approximation of the relationship between lifting velocity and object weight, was enough to guarantee both to adults (Sciutti, Patanè et al. 2014) and older children (10 years old, Sciutti, Patanè et al. 2014) a correct understanding of the load, with a performance comparable to that measured for the observation of human lifters.

Therefore, even a shape that is not exactly human-like and a motion which is a simplified version of that adopted by humans is enough to allow for a rich transfer of information through action observation. Hence, a very basic form of social intelligence, as the efficient transmission of implicit information through action execution (by gaze or by arm motion) can be achieved on humanoid robots, even with a strong simplification on the human-likeness of the robot shape and motion. We propose therefore that humanoid robots, before becoming companions or helpers, might play the fundamental role of interactive probes, i.e., of tools to derive in naturalistic contexts which human-like properties are actually relevant to foster a natural and seamless interaction. This process has two important consequences: on the one hand it allows shedding some light on the mechanisms of social interaction in humans, a complex topic which still requires the research of many neuroscientists and psychologists. On the other hand, it provides design indications, which could result in simpler and cheaper platforms, at the same time exhibiting a perfect and natural interface to their human users.

12.4 Evaluating Human-to-Robot Interaction

Humanoid robots are no humans, but their appearance and functionality sometime leans towards a human-like appearance and behaviour. In fact, here we suggest that replicating human-like features is useful only if these are central to the development of a natural interaction with humans. This functional stance on robotic design must be derived from basic research with the aim of removing superfluous computational and architectural costs, in a principled manner. The principle of replicating only the minimal human shape and motion features necessary to enable a natural interaction will have also the additional advantage of lowering the risk of entering in the Uncanny valley of eeriness (Mori 1970) in the attempt of mimicking the human being as a whole.

By following the principle of replicating only the minimal features needed, robots still have limitations. In fact, the ultimate minimalistic approach descends from a functional perspective and thus the human-likeness has to be judged by the users in a real/long term interaction and thus coping with the robots' limitations and potentialities.

12.4.1 Short term Human-to-Robot Interaction

Current research suggest that humans not only accept robots in social environments better when their behaviour and appearance is human-like but it also appreciates the fact that humans will be able to work with a natural interaction interface (like a humanoid robot) on a very efficient level (Sato, Yamaguchi, Harashima, 2007). To create such a natural interaction interface with a robot the appearance is supportive, but the promises given by the appearance must be kept by the robots' capabilities (Weiss, et al. 2008).

Keeping the balance between a human-like appearance and the functionality of the robot is a key point to keep in mind. In fact, the primary goal of social robotics should be that of building functionally effective and coherent implementations of behaviours on any given robotic platform. Thus, it is important to not only base a behaviour strategy for a robot on a human-based model, but also to understand the limitations of the robots capabilities and the discrepancies that have to be taken into account. Therefore, it is like saying that we need to be in the robot's shoes or look from the robots perspective.

By looking from the robots perspective, the implementation of models based on human behaviour need to take a second thought. In this second step we are not only evaluating the model implemented on the robot, but also the resulting behaviour of the robot and effects on humans. A method to evaluate the functional results of the implemented interaction is to evaluate the loop between human and robot. Hence, the idea is to evaluate the interplay presented in the interaction of human and robot (Lohan et al. 2012).

Therefore, evaluating human-to-robot interactions should be seen as a two-step process from the very beginning. First, the model based on human social behaviour is implemented on an appropriate robotic platform. This model has to be validated based on its given benchmarks and the given hypothesis to tested. Secondly, the resulting interface between human and robot in interaction may give a higher-level of insight into the capacity to establish a social connection, presented by the robot. However, even in a constrained scenario, the quantification of the effective establishment of the modelled interaction is not trivial. In this critical second step, measurements of human-human interaction could potentially be used as the ground truth to compare with the human-to-robot one.

At the same time, also methods derived from behavioural research have been recently employed. Among them, the methodology of conversation analysis is one possibility, which has been used in human-human interaction to evaluate this interplay (Hutchby and Wooffitt, 2008). Furthermore, there are other useful concepts like the measurement of contingency (Csibra and Gergely, 2009; Lohan et al., 2011) or synchronization (Kose-Bagci, et al. 2010), between interaction partners that can potentially hint towards the interaction quality. These methods are taking both interaction partners and therefore both sides into account. At the same time, it is also true that different social contextual conditions can change the meaning of interaction, not only based on the interaction partner's characteristics (i.e. when greeting someone close to you in a public place different social rules apply than when greeting the same person in a private space).

12.4.2 Long Term Human-to-Robot Interaction

When moving towards the direction of social interaction and long term or even life-long relationships with a robot we also need to understand the long-term dynamics behind these interactions. Hence, the robot needs to be able to adapt and act within its capability on the side of the human partner. In human-human interaction small changes in the sensorimotor communication can have a drastic impact on their behaviour, therefore the sensitivity and understanding of these small cues must be important for a robot. At the same, human behaviour has a broad and hierarchical variation in the communication complexity. For such a reason, those subtle cues sent by humans are not always central to the communicative interaction, and thus the robot needs to learn all the possible variations in a given context. Therefore, the robot will have to select the saliency of very different kinds of features in order to respond appropriately in accordance to the given social situation.

As a matter of fact, the embodiment of a system like a robot in social situations is defined as not only being dependent on its own sensory-motor experiences and capabilities but also dependent on the environmental changes, caused by social constraints (Dautenhahn, 1999). Thus, when moving robots into social environments they need to be able to take their surroundings and the rules given by these surroundings into account. This is why looking from a robots perspective, the interplay between its behaviour and the behaviour of its interaction partner, needs to be considered carefully.

When concentrating on a long-term perspective of social interaction, the evaluation of a robot that can create a relation with a human is a very complex problem, still requiring a credible solution. When looking towards methodologies used in developmental psychology we can see that it is difficult to create a quantitative strategy to evaluate the long-term evolution of the interactions. Current state of the art robotics is facing exactly these problems with the evaluation of long-term interaction. Therefore, models like social symbioses or emotional states are explored in creating strategies to give a robot the capability of dynamic adaptation (Rosenthal et al., 2010).

Overall, evaluating human-robot interaction has different levels of complexity. When evaluating human-to-robot interaction, we need to take also the robots perspective and therefore its capabilities into account to take a look at the loop created in the interaction. Furthermore, social rules created by environmental constraints and therefore the full embodiment of a social interaction, needs to be taken into account to functionally evaluate the success of the robotic design appropriately.

12.5 Conclusion

In conclusion here we are proposing the need for the field of HRI, to move from a "rigid" social contact between (social) bodies towards a "soft" interaction. By "soft" interaction we mean the dynamical compliance and long-term adaptability to human sensorimotor, cognitive, affective non-physical communication and interaction. Speaking in terms of control/planning, robotics is already moving from avoiding contacts with the environment to exploiting them, i.e., using them in motion control, thanks to the new compliant actuations and the sensors (Tsagarakis et al., 2010; Ferscha, 2013).

Along these lines, the field of HRI may be stimulated by current attempts to measure the real-time implicit information flow between human agents, embedded in a complex and ecological scenario. In fact, basic research in cognitive neuroscience we outlined earlier, may serve two critical functions. The first regards the principled building of a functionally effective human-robot interaction. The second technical advantage is that the same methods and models used to measure human-human flow can be applied to the future HRI implementations, as a benchmark to evaluate successful interaction with robots.

This means that the robot is not anymore studied in separation from its physical human-centred environment. Conversely, robot and environment (or other agents) are blended together to plan a new optimal and collaborative way to move. Similarly, in social cognition, both for human-human and human-robot interaction, we feel the need for a change: from the study of individual in isolation, to the study of complex systems of two or more people interacting together. Most importantly, these latter needs not to be treated as a linear sum of single individualities, but require again a "blending" which is manifested by the subtle mechanisms of implicit communication and which is modulated by the context and the long term interaction.

In general, we propose an integrated approach (as sketched in Figure 12.1) that starts with methods to quantify human-human interaction. The knowledge derived for this basic research is then translated into basic principles to build better robots. Finally, and by closing the conceptual loop, it uses those very same methods to functionally evaluate the efficacy of human-robot interaction.

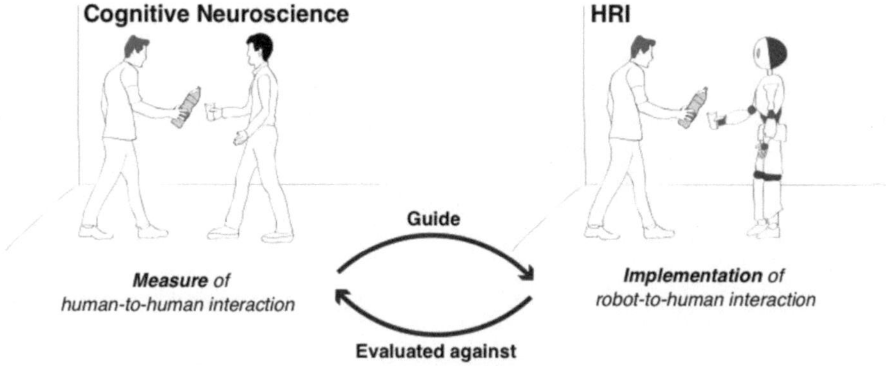

Figure 12.1: This graphical depiction represents the need to rigorously quantify human-to-human interaction for two main purposes. The first is to derive useful principles to guide the implementation of robot-to-human interaction. The second is that such artificially built interaction needs to be evaluated against its natural benchmark. Closing this conceptual loop, in our opinion, is the only way to establish an effective HCC with an embodied artefact.

References

Badino L, D'Ausilio A, Glowinski D, Camurri A, Fadiga L. (2014). Sensorimotor communication in professional quartets. *Neuropsychologia* 55(1), 98–104.

Clark, A., Grush, R. (1999). Towards a cognitive robotics. *Adaptive Behavior*, 7, 5–16.

Coey, C., Varlet, M., Schmidt, R. C., Richardson, M. J. (2011). Effects of movement stability and congruency on the emergence of spontaneous interpersonal coordination. *Experimental Brain Research*, 211, 483–493.

Couzin, I. D., Krause, J., Franks, N. R., Levin, S. A. (2005). Effective leadership and decision-making in animal groups on the move. *Nature*, 433, 147–150.

Csibra, G., & Gergely, G. (2009). Natural pedagogy. *Trends in cognitive sciences*, 13(4), 148–153.

D'Ausilio A., Badino L., Tokay S., Aloimonos Y., Li Y., Craighero L., Canto R., Fadiga L. (2012). Leadership in Orchestra Emerges from the Causal Relationships of Movement Kinematics. *PLoS ONE* 7(5): e35757.

Dautenhahn, K. (1999). Embodiment and interaction in socially intelligent life-like agents. In *Computation for metaphors, analogy, and agents* (pp. 102–141). Springer Berlin Heidelberg.

Dragan, A. D., Lee, K. C., Srinivasa, S. S. (2013). Legibility and predictability of robot motion. *8th ACM/IEEE International Conference on Human-Robot Interaction* (HRI), Tokyo, Japan.

Fabbri-Destro, M., Rizzolatti, G. (2008). Mirror neurons and mirror systems in monkeys and humans. *Physiology*, 23, 171–179.

Fadiga, L., Fogassi, L., Pavesi, G., Rizzolatti, G. (1995). Motor facilitation during action observation: a magnetic stimulation study. *Journal of Neurophysiology*, 73, 2608–2611.

Fadiga, L., Craighero, L., Buccino, G., Rizzolatti, G. (2002). Speech listening specifically modulates the excitability of tongue muscles: a TMS study. *European Journal of Neuroscience*, 15, 399–402.

Ferscha, A. (Ed.). (2013). *Human Computer Confluence: The Next Generation Humans and Computers Research Agenda*. Linz: Institute for Pervasive Computing, Johannes Kepler University Linz.

ISBN: 978-3-200-03344-3. Retrieved from http://smart.inf.ed.ac.uk/human_computer_confluence/

Flanagan, J. R., Johansson, R. S. (2003). Action plans used in action observation. *Nature*, 424(6950), 769–771.

Hasson, U., Ghazanfar, A. A., Galantucci, B., Garrod, S., Keysers, C. (2012). Brain-to-brain coupling: a mechanism for creating and sharing a social world. *Trends in Cognitive Sciences*, 16, 114–121.

Hutchby, I., & Wooffitt, R. (2008). Conversation analysis. Polity.

Kose-Bagci, H., Dautenhahn, K., Syrdal, D. S., Nehaniv, C. L. (2010). Drum-mate: interaction dynamics and gestures in human – humanoid drumming experiments. *Connection Science*, 22(2), 103–134.

Lindenberger. U., Li, S. C., Gruber, W., Muller, V. (2009). Brains swinging in concert: cortical phase synchronization while playing guitar. *BMC Neuroscience*, 10, 22.

Loehr, J. D., Kourtis, D., Vesper, C., Sebanz, N., Knoblich, G. (2013). Monitoring individual and joint action outcomes in duet music performance. *Journal of Cognitive Neuroscience*, 25(7), 1049–1061.

Lohan, K., Griffiths, S. S., Sciutti, A., Partmann, T. C., Rohlfing, K. (2014). Co-development of manner and path concepts in language, action and eye-gaze behavior. *Topics in Cognitive Science*. In Press.

Lohan, K. S., Rohlfing, K., Pitsch, K., Saunders, J., Lehmann, H., Nehaniv, C., Fischer, K., Wrede, B. (2012). Tutor spotter: Proposing a feature set and evaluating it in a robotic system. *International Journal of Social Robotics*, 4, 131–146.

Lohan, K. S., Pitsch, K., Rohlfing, K. J., Fischer, K., Saunders, J., Lehmann, H., Nehaniv, C., Wrede, B. (2011). Contingency allows the robot to spot the tutor and to learn from interaction. *2011 IEEE International Conference on Development and Learning* (ICDL).

Mori, M. (1970). Bukimi no tani The uncanny valley. *Energy*, 7(4), 33–35.

Nagy, M., Akos, Z., Biro, D., Vicsek, T. (2010). Hierarchical group dynamics in pigeon flocks. *Nature*, 464, 890–893.

Neda, Z., Ravasz, E., Brechet, Y., Vicsek, T., Barabasi, A. L. (2000). The sound of many hands clapping. *Nature*, 403, 849–850.

Pecenka, N., Keller, P.E. (2011). The role of temporal prediction abilities in interpersonal sensorimotor synchronization. *Experimental Brain Research*, 211(3–4), 505–15.

Rands, S. A., Cowlishaw, G., Pettifor, R. A., Rowcliffe, J. M., Johnstone, R. A. (2003). Spontaneous emergence of leaders and followers in foraging pairs. *Nature*, 423, 432–434.

Riley, M. A., Richardson, M. J., Shockley, K., Ramenzoni, V. C. (2011). Interpersonal synergies. *Frontiers in Psychology*, 2, 38.

Rosenthal, S., Biswas, J., Veloso, M. (2010). An effective personal mobile robot agent through symbiotic human-robot interaction. *9th International Conference on Autonomous Agents and Multiagent Systems*.

Sato, E., Yamaguchi, T., Harashima, F., (2007). Natural Interface Using Pointing Behavior for Human – Robot Gestural Interaction. *IEEE Transactions on Industrial Electronics*, 54(2), 1105–1112.

Schippers, M. B., Roebroeck, A., Renken, R., Nanetti, L., Keysers, C. (2010). Mapping the information flow from one brain to another during gestural communication. *Proceedings of the National Academy of Sciences U S A*, 107(20), 9388–9393.

Sciutti, A., Bisio, A., Nori, F., Metta, G., Fadiga, L., Pozzo, T., Sandini, G. (2012). Measuring human-robot interaction through motor resonance. *International Journal of Social Robotics*, 4(3), 223–234.

Sciutti, A., Del Prete, A., Natale, L., Burr, D., Sandini, G., Gori, M., (2013). Perception during interaction is not based on statistical context. *8th ACM/IEEE International Conference on Human-Robot Interaction (HRI)*, Tokyo, Japan.

Sciutti, A., Patanè, L., Nori, F., Sandini, G., (2014). Development of perception of weight from human or robot lifting observation. *9th ACM/IEEE International Conference on Human-Robot Interaction (HRI)*, Bielefeld, Germany.

Sciutti, A. Patane, L., Nori, F., Sandini, G. (2014). Understanding object weight from human and humanoid lifting actions. *IEEE Transactions on Autonomous Mental Development*, 6(2), 80–92.

Sebanz, N., Bekkering, H., Knoblich, G. (2010). Joint action: bodies and minds moving together. *Trends in Cognitive Sciences*, 10, 70–76.

Sisbot, E. A., Alami, R. (2012). A Human-Aware Manipulation Planner. *IEEE Transactions on Robotics*, 28(5), 1045–1057.

Tsagarakis, N. G., Laffranchi, M., Vanderborght, B. and Caldwell, D. G. (2010). Compliant Actuation: Enhancing the Interaction Ability of Cognitive Robotics Systems. *Advances in Cognitive Systems*, Eds.: Nefti, S. and Gray, J.O., pp. 37–56.

Weiss, A., Bernhaupt, R., Tscheligi, M., Wollherr, D., Kuhnlenz, K., Buss, M., (2008). A methodological variation for acceptance evaluation of Human-Robot Interaction in public places. The *17th IEEE International Symposium on Robot and Human Interactive Communication*, RO-MAN, pp. 713–718.

Young, R. M. (1970). Mind, brain and adaptation in the nineteenth century. *Cerebral localization and its biological context from Gall to Ferrier*, Clarendon Press, Oxford.

Yun, K., Watanabe, K., Shimojo, S. (2012). Interpersonal body and neural synchronization as a marker of implicit social interaction. *Scientific Reports*, 2, 959.

Section III: **Applications**

Joris Favié, Vanessa Vakili, Willem-Paul Brinkman, Nexhmedin Morina and Mark A. Neerincx

13 State of the Art in Technology-Supported Resilience Training For Military Professionals

Abstract: Certain professions carry a risk of experiencing traumatic events and sometimes developing Posttraumatic Stress Disorder (PTSD). Researchers have been working on strategies to prevent professionals in those fields from developing PTSD. Recently, there has been a focus on applying technology that supports these preventive strategies, especially in a military context. This chapter provides an overview of the state of the art in technology-supported resilience training for military professionals, which has considerable common ground with the interdisciplinary field of human computer confluence (HCC). The effectiveness of these technologies and the resilience strategies they support are reviewed through the literature.

Keywords: Resilience, Training Systems, Posttraumatic Stress Disorder

13.1 Introduction

Soldiers, police officers, fire fighters, and ambulance staff are significantly more likely to experience traumatic events and other forms of intense stress at work. They might witness situations in which people are seriously injured or killed. They themselves might also be exposed to threatened or actual injury as well as threatened or actual death. Exposure to these and similar traumatic events can lead to posttraumatic stress disorder (PTSD). Individuals with PTSD re-experience the traumatic event via intrusive memories or nightmares, have increased physiological reactions upon exposure to reminders of the traumatic event, avoid distressing reminders of traumatic events, and have negative alterations in cognitions about themselves and the world as well as negative alterations in arousal and reactivity (American Psychiatric Association, 2013). Significant functional impairment has been shown in the daily lives of those meeting criteria for PTSD (Nemeroff et al., 2006). Extensive work has been done on the treatment of PTSD (Ehlers et al., 2010). Recently, research has also focused on ways to prevent PTSD by enhancing resilience before a trauma occurs with computer assisted training programs.

This work has considerable common ground with the HCC research agenda, which focuses on the science and technologies required to ensure an effective, transparent coexistence between humans and computers, and studies how to enable radically new forms of sensing, perception, interaction, and understanding. The HCC paradigm brings together fields such as bio-signals processing, neuroscience, electronics, robotics, pervasive computing, virtual & augmented reality (Ferscha, 2013).

Various resilience training environments employ pervasive technologies to collect biosignals to give professionals real time insight into their response to stressful events simulated, for example, in a virtual reality environment (Bouchard, Bernier, Boivin, Morin, & Robillard, 2012). To be effective, these technologies should not hinder the experience, but fade into the background of users' awareness. This can only be done with extensive understanding of the mental processes set in motion when an individual is confronted with traumatic events, and the psychology behind resilience training as well as resilience measurement. This chapter gives a coherent overview of these issues before discussing various resilience training-systems that have been developed recently across the world.

13.2 Psychology

PTSD symptoms have been explained as the result of an inability to inhibit learned fear in a safe environment. During a traumatic event, certain neutral stimuli become associated with fearful stimuli. After the event, the neutral stimuli continue to elicit the negative or fearful responses they have now been associated with. Social-cognitive theories like Horowitz's (1986) stress response theory explain how trauma breaks existing mental structures, and how incompatible information is reconciled with previous beliefs. Horowitz argued that when faced with trauma, two responses occur: (1) outcry at the realization of the trauma, and (2) an attempt to integrate the new trauma information with prior knowledge. Horowitz proposed that failure to process the trauma information in the second response leads to PTSD as the information remains in active memory and continues to intrude and be avoided. While social-cognitive theories focus on the wider personal and social context, cognitive information processing theories center mainly on the traumatic events itself (Creamer, Burgess, & Pattison, 1992; Foa, Steketee, & Rothbaum, 1989), or to be more precise on the encoding, storage, and recall of the traumatic events and their related stimuli and responses (Brewin & Holmes, 2003). The core idea is that traumatic events are represented in memory in a special way, and if they are not processed and integrated within the broader memory system appropriately, psychopathology may result.

13.2.1 Resilience

Although many individuals develop PTSD after experiencing a traumatic event, most individuals exposed to a traumatic event show psychological resilience in the sense that they do not fall victim to a long term debilitating disorder, but manage to recover from the initial blow after some time (Mancini & Bonanno, 2006). This has sparked research into the concept of resilience, which on the most basic level has been defined as the ability to adapt and cope successfully despite threatening or challenging situations (Bonanno, 2004). The empirical construct of resilience is however not that consistent, well defined and scientifically grounded yet. Resilience also is being perceived differently, as a set of characteristics, a trait, an outcome, a process or all of the above. Southwick and Charney (2012) describe resilience as the complex outcome of genetic, biological, psychological, social and spiritual factors. Resilience is often defined in terms of the presence of protective factors, which enables individuals to resist life stress (Kaplan et al., 1996). Rutter (1990) defined three general variables as protective factors: personality coherence, family cohesion, and social support. For personality factors he included level of autonomy, self-esteem and self-efficacy, good temperament, and positive social outlook.

13.2.2 Hardiness

Hardiness is a personality style introduced by Kobasa (1981), which is closely related to resilience. The construct of hardiness is posited as mediating stress and illness, potentially reducing the negative effects of stress. Theoretically, hardiness develops in early childhood and emerges as the result of rich, varied, and rewarding life experiences. Hardiness comprises three sub-constructs: (1) commitment as opposed to alienation, (2) control as opposed to powerlessness, and (3) challenge as opposed to threat. Individuals who are under stress will stay healthier if they feel committed to the various areas of their lives. Commitment is the valuing of one's life, one's self, one's relationships, and the investment of oneself in these valued dimensions of life. Commitment results in a sense of purpose that can carry a person through difficult times. Having a sense of control over what takes place in their lives helps individuals to understand stress and stay healthier than those who feel helpless in the face of external powers. People with control can integrate various kinds of events into a continuing life plan, and transform these events into something consistent with meaning, which makes them less destructive to their wellbeing. Persons with this view believe that change, rather than stability, is the norm in their life (Kobasa, 1982).

13.3 Measuring Resilience

Instead of trying to measure resilience directly, it is often measured indirectly as a function of other constructs (e.g. hardiness), clinical outcomes (e.g., absence of depression or PTSD), or behavioral measures (e.g. academic performance). Self-report instruments are used widely in studies related to resilience training. There are a number of self-report measurement scales and instruments related with resilience to support research and clinical practice:

- Baruth protective factors inventory (Baruth & Carroll, 2002)
- Youth risk and resilience inventory (Brady, 2006)
- Connor-Davidson resilience scale (Connor & Davidson, 2003)
- Resilience Scale for Adults (Friborg, et al., 2006)
- Resilience scale (Wagnild & Young, 1993)

In addition, the Deployment Risk and Resilience Inventory (King, King & Vogt et al., 2006) has been specially developed for military personnel.

13.3.1 Biomarkers

To improve objectivity, psychosocial instruments could be expanded to integrate biomarkers with demonstrated relevance to resilience. A biomarker is an objectively measured indicator of a biological state. Examples of biomarkers are hormones, genetic data and neurological factors. Biomarker research related to psychological performance and dysfunction is currently in the early stages. Rather than attempting to measure resilience itself, it is often measured using biomarkers that are associated with better-defined constructs such as stress or arousal, e.g. skin conductivity, heart rate, heart rate variability (HRV), and salivary cortisol.

Cortisol is a hormone released in response to stress. Skin conductance, also known as galvanic skin response (GSR), is a measure of the electric conductance of the skin, which varies with the level of sweat released in response to arousal. GSR has been found to be associated with self-reported sadness (Kreibig, Wilhelm, Roth, & Gross, 2007) and writing about traumatic experiences (Hughes, Uhlmann, & Pennebaker, 1994). HRV reflects the fluctuations in time between two consecutive heartbeats, which is considered to be an indication of the constant interaction of the sympathetic and parasympathetic circuits of the autonomous nervous system (ANS) innervating the heart (Taelman & Vandeput, 2009). HRV therefore provides a means to quantify the activity of the ANS, and may thus provide a measure for stress. Although the causes of HRV are still under debate, it can be considered a general measure of adaptability as HRV reduces as people become more vulnerable to stress (Lehrer, 2007).

Preliminary genetic studies have identified some loci for resilience, but which specific genes confer resilience via specific mechanisms is still an active area of research. Epigenetic factors have also emerged as candidates for gene-environment interactions that influence stress responsiveness (Franklin, Saab & Mansuy, 2012). Epigenetics is the study of heritable changes in gene expression without altering the DNA sequence itself, e.g. through DNA methylation: transcription of genes has found to be inhibited when methyl groups are attached to them. This process of DNA methylation may apparently be brought on by environmental factors: Meaney & Szyf (2005) found that in the pups of inattentive mother rats, genes regulating the production of glucocorticoid receptors, which regulate sensitivity to stress hormones, were highly methylated. Furthermore, this methylated DNA was passed on to the next generation. As epigenetic measures are thought to reflect enduring effects of environmental exposures, they may be useful in distinguishing e.g. combat-exposed veterans who do or do not develop PTSD (Yehuda, Daskalakis, Desarnaud, et. al, 2013).

The construct of allostatic load is based on multiple biomarkers. Allostatic load is a measure of cumulative wear and tear on physiological symptoms due to chronic stress (McEwen & Stellar, 1993) and is based on a response called allostasis.

13.3.2 Emotional Stroop Test

The Stroop effect demonstrates the presence of interference in the reaction time of a task (Stroop, 1935). When the name of a color is printed in a font color other than its name (e.g., the word red printed in blue instead of red), naming the color of the word takes longer than when the color of the font matches the name of the color. The emotional Stroop test (EST) is an adaptation of the original Stroop test, and measures an individual's ability to ignore irrelevant emotional content by examining the response time of the individual to name the colors of words that are emotionally charged for him or her. Instead of relying on mere lexical representations, images have also been used in a so-called Pictorial Emotional Stroop Task (PEST). In a PEST, images are either surrounded by a colored border, or they have been color-filtered so that they appear tinted in a single color. People are slower to name the color of a word or image that is emotionally charged for them, which is interpreted as a selective allocation of attentional processes to emotionally charged information (Williams, Mathews, MacLeod, 1996). This process takes a few milliseconds, and competes with other cognitive processes such as recognizing the color. The latter processes will thus be performed slower as compared to a situation lacking stimuli that are perceived as threatening. Research (MacLeod & Hagan, 1992) using the EST indicates that preexisting differences in attention control can predict adjustment to stress. Furthermore, in a meta-analysis of 26 studies Cisler et al. (2011) conclude that EST performance of PTSD groups was affected by PTSD-relevant words and generally threatening words relative to neutral words, and the performance of trauma exposed control groups was impaired only by PTSD-relevant words. These effects were not present in the non-trauma exposed control groups.

13.3.3 Startle Reflex

The startle reflex is a natural physiological response to unexpected, intense stimuli such as a loud noise or a bright flash of light. It manifests itself by muscle responses such as contraction of the neck muscles, jumping up and blinking of the eyes, and serves to protect the back of the neck (whole-body startle) or the eye (eye blink). The reflex is influenced by emotional states. For normal individuals the amplitude of the reflex is larger when presented together with unpleasant stimuli (e.g. pictures of a mutilated body), smaller with neutral stimuli (e.g. a picture of a closet), and still smaller when presented with pleasant stimuli (e.g. a picture of a smiling baby). (Vrana, Spence, & Lang, 1988). The amplitude is also larger when fear is elicited beforehand, which is referred to as the fear potentiated startle (FPS) (Brown, Kalish, & Farber, 1951). A conditioned fear response can be generated by e.g. repeatedly shining a light or showing a colored object on a screen followed by an aversive stimulus such as an air-blast to the larynx or an electric shock. If a loud noise that triggers the startle response is now presented shortly after (or together with) the shining light, the startle response will be significantly larger. The FPS response also occurs after seeing videos or slides with unpleasant or anxiety-provoking scenes (Vrana et al., 1988). An increased FPS response is present in individuals with PTSD, and several studies found that the FPS becomes even bigger when they experience stress (Lissek et al., 2005). Furthermore, people diagnosed with PTSD display a similar FPS response to threatening and neutral stimuli, indicating that they cannot distinguish between a stimulus as a genuine threat or being harmless (Pole, Neylan, Best, Orr & Marmar, 2003). Moreover, war veterans with severe, chronic PTSD have a significantly reduced ability for the extinction of conditioned fear responses (Milad et al., 2008).

13.3.4 Content Analysis of Narratives

There have been numerous studies on the beneficial effects of emotional writing. In a meta-analysis of 13 experimental writing studies, Smyth (1998) reported that personally disclosive writing was linked with improved physical and mental health. These positive effects have been explained by the idea that constructing a narrative helps individuals to better integrate the experience. Support for this idea is provided by studies showing that health improvements can be predicted by automated linguistic analysis, e.g. the number of emotion words people use may be indications about their emotional states, thought processes, motivations, and intentions (Tausczik & Pennebaker, 2009). Examples of other predicting word patterns are (1) an increasing use of cognitive or insight words over the days of writing (Pennebaker, Mayne, & Francis, 1997), (2) shifts in the use of pronouns from day to day (Campbell & Pennebaker, 2003), (3) higher use of positive relative to negative emotion words (Pennebaker et al., 1997).

13.4 Resilience Training

Concepts of cognitive behavior therapy (CBT) are used in applied training settings as discussed later on in this chapter. CBT is based on the assumption that cognitively distorted views of experiences and events may cause psychological problems. Furthermore, CBT theories presume that psychological problems are maintained by faulty thinking and behavior patterns. The basic cognitive behavior model in CBT states there is a two-way link between cognition, emotion and behavior in which cognitive processes can influence emotions and behavior, and behavioral change can influence cognitions and emotions (Mowrer & Orville, 1950). Here, fear is seen as a response resulting from classical conditioning, and it is maintained and negatively reinforced by avoidance. A core idea is also that there is no direct link between an event and how people feel, but it is the way they perceive situations, i.e. cognitive appraisal, that influences their emotions. The core tenet of CBT is that psychological problems arise when there is a mismatch between the perception of events and the available evidence of reality gets exaggerated beyond the available facts. CBT techniques are used to help people challenge their automatic thoughts and schemas, and replace maladaptive thoughts with more sound and healthy thoughts, in order to decrease emotional distress and dysfunctional behavior (Hassett & Gevirtz, 2009).

13.4.1 Stress Inoculation Training (SIT)

SIT (Meichenbaum & Deffenbacher, 1988) is a form of CBT aimed at the reduction and prevention of stress. The idea is that arousal levels of individuals in response to powerful stressors may be reduced by inoculating them to potentially traumatizing stressors. It is based on models that posit that stress arises when the perceived demands of a situation exceed an individual's (perceived) capability to cope. SIT is designed to enable individuals to manage minor stressors in order to increase their ability to manage major stressors, and to boost their confidence in use of their coping skills. Meichenbaum proposes three stages to SIT: (1) psycho-education (learning about stress responses and the need to control them), (2) training (learning a skill, such as arousal control, in order to tone down the harmful effects of stress), and (3) implementation (utilizing these skills in the stressful context).

13.4.2 Biofeedback Training

Biofeedback is a method used for teaching voluntary control of various physiological functions in order to improve health or performance by providing perceptible, real-time feedback for variations in physiological activity (Schwartz & Andrasik, 2003). Feedback is usually given in the form of visual and/or auditory signals derived from physiological recording devices. This provides both the trainee and the trainer with a continuous image of what is going on inside the body. The effect of a frightening thought, the way of breathing etc. is directly visible. There are three stages of biofeedback training: (1) acquiring awareness of the maladaptive response, here individuals learn the effect of certain thoughts and bodily events on a response, (2) learning to control the response, and (3) transfer these control skills into everyday life (Calderon & Thompson, 2004). In treatment of stress-related disorders, biofeedback is often combined with relaxation training, which is referred to as biofeedback-assisted relaxation training.

13.4.3 Cognitive Reappraisal

According to appraisal theories of emotion, emotion is determined by an individual's subjective appraisal of an event – the meaning and significance that the individual attaches to the event – rather than the event itself (Lazarus & Folkman, 1984). Therefore, learning to change one's own appraisal process is believed to be a key factor in many psychological interventions such as CBT (Samoilov & Goldfield, 2000). A cognitive-linguistic emotion regulation strategy known as cognitive reappraisal aims to achieve exactly this (Gross, 1998). Cognitive reappraisal refers to the implementation of cognitive strategies to assist individuals in changing the intensity of their response to an event (Ochsner & Gross, 2005). In reappraisal tasks, trainees may be asked to systematically apply certain appraisal themes so as to reduce the negative affect they experienced. Schartau, Dalgleish, & Dunn (2009) found that many of the dysfunctional appraisal themes mentioned in the CBT literature reflect a difficulty to see the bigger picture. They selected four functional appraisal themes focused on perspective broadening, e.g. a theme that stresses that bad events do not happen often and good things occur all the time. In their study, they asked participants to watch a film and employ these appraisal themes to reduce their emotional reaction. Participants who practiced appraisal displayed reduced levels of self-reported negative emotional responses to a final distressing test film. Furthermore, appraisal practice resulted in reduced intrusion and avoidance of the target memories in the week after the study.

Several other laboratory studies (e.g. Dandoy & Goldstein, 1990) also found that people instructed to use reappraisal reported less negative emotion after watching an emotional film clip compared to those in a just watch condition. Moreover, Gross & John (2003) reported that individuals who frequently use reappraisal, experience less negative emotions in emotionally charged events and exhibit positive outcomes over time.

13.5 Review of Resilience Training Systems

The focus on HCC in the mental healthcare domain is not new as applications such as brain interfacing, mobile devices, body computing, and virtual reality have been studied in this context (Viaud-Delmon, Gaggioli, Ferscha, et al., 2012). The same seems to apply for the current resilience training systems as described below.

13.5.1 Predeployment Stress Inoculation Training (Presit) & Multimedia Stressor Environment (Mse)

Hourani, Kizakevech, et al. (2011) developed a SIT based intervention as a preventative effort against combat related stress disorders in armed forces personnel. The main goal of this approach is to train personnel to lower their physiologic arousal in response to a stressor. A group-administered program was chosen because it was cost-effective, and because marines are used to working in groups where they can also support each other. The skills acquisition phase of the training is a presentation of two types of breathing and focus-retraining techniques. The eyes-open technique focuses on in-combat situations, while the eyes-closed technique focuses on post-combat situations. Trainees are also trained in stress reduction using a biofeedback training software package that provides paced breathing exercises via a graphical user interface, including display of HRV and a stress index. The training is practiced in a combat relevant MSE. Up to 20 individuals are seated in front of a large screen, and they are taken on a virtual journey through an Iraqi village from a first person perspective, as if they are all in the same multi-passenger vehicle. Trainees are instructed to perform a reaction time task by pressing specific buttons upon noticing specific events. A controlled pilot study was carried out to compare the efficacy of PRESIT with current best practices of the Navy's and Marine's Combat and Operational Stress Control programs by examining HRV and reaction time in response to events in the MSE. Participants with deployment experience, especially those with PTSD, showed greater relaxation during the MSE of a follow-up session relative to that of a baseline session. There was no significant effect for individuals without combat experience.

13.5.2 Stress Resilience in Virtual Environments (Strive)

In contrast to the narrow focus of the PRESIT study on lowering physiologic arousal in response to a stressor through breathing and focus re-training, STRIVE aims for a broader CBT based approach. STRIVE is a set of combat simulations that are part of a multi-episode free-agency narrative experience, forming an experiential learning approach for delivering psycho-educational material, stress management techniques and cognitive-behavioral emotional coping strategies prior to deployment

(Rizzo et al., 2011). This approach draws input from CBT and teaches soldiers the distinction between factual events and emotion caused by their appraisal that can be taught. STRIVE is designed as a virtual emotional obstacle course, including various cinematic VR episodes that are narrated in the first-person as if by the individual experiencing the training. At the end of each episode an emotionally challenging event occurs, and a virtual mentor appears, who guides the soldiers through rational restructuring exercises relevant to the event. This facilitates state-dependent learning as skills are taught in a similar state in which they have to be applied later on. STRIVE uses cinematic techniques, such as a storyline and character development, so that soldiers can become engaged on an emotional level.

13.5.3 Immersion and Practice of Arousal Control Training (Impact)

Bouchard et al (2012) developed a stress management training (SMT) program to test whether practicing stress management skills would benefit the usual training offered to military personnel. A stressful 3D horror/first person shooting game was modified by making it more stressful and including biofeedback components, so that it could be used as an SIT based training tool for biofeedback-assisted SMT. Visual biofeedback was provided by reducing the visual field of the player more and more as arousal (as measured by skin conductivity and heart rate variability) of the participant increased. Auditory feedback was provided by the sound of a thumping heart that grew progressively louder and faster. Trainees play the game during three 30-minute training sessions, and a human coach is present to personally help train participants in tactical breathing during these sessions. The program was evaluated by measuring salivary cortisol and heart rate during a live first-aid training simulation after soldiers participated in the ImPACT program. A significant reduction in stress level was found for the soldiers that followed the program as compared with training as usual.

13.5.4 Personal Health Intervention Tool (PHIT) for Duty

Kizakevich, Hubal and Brown (2012) developed a personal health assessment and self-help intervention application for smartphones and tablets to help build resilience in healthy military personnel and support prevention in high-risk personnel. The application collects a host of health assessments using self-report forms and questionnaires. In addition data are acquired via interactive exercises and optional non-intrusive physiological and behavioral sensors measuring e.g. HRV and body motion. An intelligent advisor analyzes these assessments using a personal health status model to recommend, tailor and present self-help advisories to reduce symptoms and prevent disease, such as stress relaxation, mindfulness meditation, progressive muscle relaxation, behavior therapy, and links to professional care.

13.5.5 Stress Resilience Training System

Cohn, Weltman, Ratwani et al (2010) developed an application that combines cognitive learning methodologies grounded in learning theory and biofeedback techniques. It is based on the idea that fighters adapt to combat stress after the first few experiences by learning self-awareness of their stress state and self-regulation of stress effects, and the idea that training can help duplicate this process. The application consists of three parts: (1) know-how, (2) coherence training, and (3) HRV-controlled games, which roughly correspond to the three stages of SIT. The know-how part consists of brief audiovisual presentations. The main goal is to provide the trainee with techniques to inoculate against negative stress effects and use positive effects of stress. The coherence training includes two elements. A HRV-controlled game allows trainees to practice and master a coherence breathing technique. To practice their technique the trainees are presented with games with ascending levels of difficulty. A virtual coach advises the trainees during the training.

13.5.6 Physiology-Driven Adaptive Virtual Reality Stimulation for Prevention and Treatment of Stress Related Disorders

Cosic, Popovic, Kukolja et al. (2010) describe a concept for an adaptive control of virtual reality affect stimulation. Exposure levels are automatically controlled according to physiological input levels, which would alleviate trainers from performing this task. The three main components are: (1) stimulus generator that contains various rated and categorized multimedia stimuli, (2) emotional state estimator, which collects physiological samples from trainees in order to estimate their valence/arousal, and (3) adaptive controller, which applies a strategy for the control of the stimulus generator based on this estimation. A stimulus-delivery algorithm is also described that automatically adjusts for the participants' habituation, by choosing for stimuli that are either more or less intense.

13.6 Conclusions

Concepts from CBT are found to be widely used, and both SIT and biofeedback training have been implemented within technology-supported resilience trainings. Cognitive reappraisal has also been implemented in one existing training system. The preferred approach to measure resilience currently seems to combine subjective self-report with objective measures such as biomarkers, of which GSR and HRV are often used. Most of the current systems involve breathing and relaxation techniques as a means to reduce stress or arousal during stressful activities. Unfortunately, limited empirical evidence is currently available regarding the efficacy of these systems in helping individuals staying more relaxed during stressful exercises, which often made it only possible for this chapter to describe the systems and the psychology behind them, and not their efficacy. A major limitation of the current programs is also the lack of longitudinal evaluation. At this point no conclusion can be made on the long-term efficacy of these training systems. Existing systems still need further empirical evaluation and new technology-supported training paradigms need to be explored. Although some elements of HCC are already being employed, integrating a more full set of interdisciplinary HCC components into an effective resilience training tool remains both a challenge and an opportunity.

Acknowledgement: This study was supported by the Dutch Economic Structure Enhancement Fund (FES) "Brain and Cognition: Societal Innovation" program (NWO project no 056-25-012).

References

American Psychiatric Association (2013). Diagnostic and statistical manual of mental disorders, 5th edition. Arlington: American Psychiatric Association.

Baruth, K. E., & Caroll, J. J. (2002). A formal assessment of resilience: The Baruth Protective Factors Inventory. *The Journal of Individual Psychology; The Journal of Individual Psychology*.

Bonanno, G. A. (2004). Loss, trauma, and human resilience: have we underestimated the human capacity to thrive after extremely aversive events? *The American psychologist*, *59*(1), 20–28.

Bouchard, S., Bernier, F., Boivin, E., Morin, B., & Robillard, G. (2012). Using biofeedback while immersed in a stressful videogame increases the effectiveness of stress management skills in soldiers. *PloS one*, *7*(4), e36169.

Brady, R. P. (2006). *Youth Risk and Resilience Inventory*. JIST Publishing.

Brewin, C. R., & Holmes, E. A. (2003). Psychological theories of posttraumatic stress disorder. *Clinical Psychology Review*, *23*(3), 339–376.

Brown, J. S., Kalish, H. I., & Farber, I. E. (1951). Conditioned fear as revealed by magnitude of startle response to an auditory stimulus. *Journal of Experimental Psychology*, *41*(5), 317.

Calderon, K. S., & Thompson, W. W. (2004). Biofeedback relaxation training: A rediscovered mind-body tool in public health. *American Journal of Health Studies*, *19*(4), 185.

Campbell, R. S., & Pennebaker, J. W. (2003). Research Article The Secret Life Of Pronouns : Flexibility in Writing Style and Physical Health. *Psychological Science*, *14*(1), 60–65.

Cisler, J. M., Wolitzky-Taylor, K. B., Adams, T. G., Babson, K. A., Badour, C. L., & Willems, J. L. (2011). The emotional Stroop task and posttraumatic stress disorder: a meta-analysis. *Clinical psychology review*, *31*(5), 817–828.

Cohn, J., Weltman, G., Ratwani, R., Chartrand, D., & McCraty, R. (2010). Stress Inoculation through Cognitive and Biofeedback Training. *The Interservice/Industry Training, Simulation & Education Conference (I/ITSEC)* (Vol. 2010, pp. 1–11).

Connor, K. M., & Davidson, J. R. T. (2003). Development of a new resilience scale: The Connor-Davidson resilience scale (CD-RISC). *Depression and anxiety*, *18*(2), 76–82.

Cosić, K., Popović, S., Kukolja, D., Horvat, M., & Dropuljić, B. (2010). Physiology-driven adaptive virtual reality stimulation for prevention and treatment of stress related disorders. *Cyberpsychology, behavior and social networking*, *13*(1), 73–78.

Creamer, M., Burgess, P., & Pattison, P. (1992). Reaction to trauma: a cognitive processing model. *Journal of Abnormal Psychology*, *101*(3), 452–459.

Dandoy, A. C., & Goldstein, A. G. (1990). The use of cognitive appraisal to reduce stress reactions: A replication. *Journal of Social Behavior & Personality; Journal of Social Behavior & Personality*.

Driskell, J. E., & Johnston, J. H. (1998). Stress exposure training. *Making decisions under stress: Implications for individual and team training*, 191–217.

Ehlers, A., Bisson, J., Clark, D. M., Creamer, M., Pilling, S., Richards, D., Yule, W. (2010). Do all psychological treatments really work the same in posttraumatic stress disorder? *Clinical psychology review*, *30*(2), 269–276.

Ferscha, A. (Ed.). (2013). Human computer confluence, The Next Generation Humans and Computers Research Agenda: Institute for Pervasive Computing, Johannes Kepler University Linz.

Foa, E. B., Steketee, G., & Rothbaum, B. O. (1989). Behavioral/cognitive conceptualizations of post-traumatic stress disorder. *Behavior Therapy*, *20*(2), 155–176.

Franklin, T. B., Saab, B. J., & Mansuy, I. M. (2012). Neural mechanisms of stress resilience and vulnerability. *Neuron*, *75*(5), 747–761

Friborg, O., Hjemdal, O., Rosenvinge, J. H., & Martinussen, M. (2006). A new rating scale for adult resilience: What are the central protective resources behind healthy adjustment? *International journal of methods in psychiatric research*, *12*(2), 65–76.

Gross, J. J. (1998). The emerging field of emotion regulation: An integrative review. *Review of general psychology*, *2*(3), 271.

Gross, J. J., & John, O. P. (2003). Individual differences in two emotion regulation processes: implications for affect, relationships, and well-being. *Journal of personality and social psychology*, *85*(2), 348–362.

Hassett, A. L., & Gevirtz, R. N. (2009). Nonpharmacologic treatment for fibromyalgia: patient education, cognitive-behavioral therapy, relaxation techniques, and complementary and alternative medicine. *Rheumatic diseases clinics of North America*, *35*(2), 393.

Horowitz, M. J. (1986). Stress-response syndromes: A review of posttraumatic and adjustment disorders. *Hospital & Community Psychiatry*, *37(3)*, 241–249.

Hourani, L., Kizakevich, P., & Hubal, R. (2011). Predeployment stress inoculation training for primary prevention of combat-related stress disorders. *Journal of cybertherapy & rehabilitation*, *4*(1).

Hughes, C. F., Uhlmann, C., & Pennebaker, J. W. (1994). The Body's Response to Processing Emotional Trauma: Linking Verbal Text with Autonomic Activity. *Journal of Personality*, *62*(4), 565–585.

Ilnicki, S., Wiederhold, B. K., Maciolek, J., & Kosinska, L. (2012). Effectiveness Evaluation for Short-Term Group Pre-Deployment VR Computer- Assisted Stress Inoculation Training Provided to Polish ISAF Soldiers. In B. K. Wiederhold & G. Riva (Eds.), *Annual Review of Cybertherapy and Telemedicine* (pp. 113–117). IOS Press.

Kaplan, C. P., Turner, S., Norman, E., & Stillson, K. (1996). Promoting resilience strategies: A modified consultation model. *Children & Schools*, *18*(3), 158–168.

King, L. A., King, D. W., Vogt, D. S., Knight, J., & Samper, R. E. (2006). Deployment Risk and Resilience Inventory: A collection of measures for studying deployment-related experiences of military personnel and veterans. *Military Psychology*, *18*(2), 89–120.

Kizakevich, P., Hubal, R., & Brown, J. (2012). PHIT for Duty, a Mobile Approach for Psychological Health Intervention. *Studies in health technology and informatics*, 268–272.

Kobasa, Suzanne C, Maddi, S. R., & Courington, S. (1981). Personality and Constitution as Mediators in the Stress-Illness Relationship. *Journal of Health and Social Behavior*, *22*(4), pp. 368–378.

Kobasa, Suzanne C, & others. (1982). The hardy personality: Toward a social psychology of stress and health. *Social psychology of health and illness*, *4*, 3–32.

Kreibig, S. D., Wilhelm, F. H., Roth, W. T., & Gross, J. J. (2007). Cardiovascular, electrodermal, and respiratory response patterns to fear- and sadness-inducing films. *Psychophysiology*, *44*(5), 787–806.

Lazarus, R. S., & Folkman, S. (1984). *Stress, appraisal, and coping*. Springer Publishing Company.

Lehrer, P. M. (2007). Biofeedback training to increase heart rate variability. *Principles and practice of stress management*, 227–248.

Lissek, S., Powers, A. S., McClure, E. B., Phelps, E. A., Woldehawariat, G., Grillon, C., & Pine, D. S. (2005). Classical fear conditioning in the anxiety disorders: a meta-analysis. *Behaviour research and therapy*, *43*(11), 1391–1424.

MacLeod, C., & Hagan, R. (1992). Individual difference in the selective processing of threatening information, and emotional responses to a stressful life event. *Behaviour Research and Therapy*, *30*(2), 151–161.

Mancini, A. D., & Bonanno, G. A. (2006). Resilience in the face of potential trauma: clinical practices and illustrations. *Journal of clinical psychology*, *62*(8), 971–985.

McEwen, B. S., & Stellar, E. (1993). Stress and the individual: mechanisms leading to disease. *Archives of internal medicine*, *153*(18), 2093.

Meaney, M., & Szyf, M. (2005). Environmental programming of stress responses through DNA methylation: life at the interface between a dynamic environment and a fixed genome. *Dialogues in Clinical Neuroscience*, *3*, 103–123.

Meichenbaum, D. H., & Deffenbacher, J. L. (1988). Stress inoculation training. *The Counseling Psychologist*, *16*(1), 69–90.

Milad, M. R., Orr, S. P., Lasko, N. B., Chang, Y., Rauch, S. L., & Pitman, R. K. (2008). Presence and acquired origin of reduced recall for fear extinction in PTSD: results of a twin study. *Journal of psychiatric research*, *42*(7), 515–520.

Mowrer, O. (1950). Learning theory and personality dynamics: selected papers. New York: Ronald Press.

Nemeroff, C. B., Bremner, J. D., Foa, E. B., Mayberg, H. S., North, C. S., & Stein, M. B. (2006). Posttraumatic stress disorder: a state-of-the-science review. *Journal of psychiatric research*, *40*(1), 1–21.

Ochsner, K. N., & Gross, J. J. (2005). The cognitive control of emotion. *Trends in cognitive sciences*, *9*(5), 242–249.

Pennebaker, J., Mayne, T. J., & Francis, M. E. (1997). Linguistic predictors of adaptive bereavement. *Journal of personality and social psychology*, *72*(4), 863–871.

Pole, N., Neylan, T. C., Best, S. R., Orr, S. P., & Marmar, C. R. (2003). Fear-potentiated startle and posttraumatic stress symptoms in urban police officers. *Journal of Traumatic Stress*, *16*(5), 471–479.

Rizzo, A., Parsons, T. D., Lange, B., Kenny, P., Buckwalter, J. G., Rothbaum, B., Difede, J., et al. (2011). Virtual reality goes to war: a brief review of the future of military behavioral healthcare. *Journal of clinical psychology in medical settings*, *18*(2), 176–187.

Rutter, M. (1990). Psychosocial resilience and protective mechanisms. In J. Rolf, A. S. Masten, D. Cicchetti, K. H. Neuchterlein, & S. Weintraub (Eds.), *Risk and protective factors in the development of psychopathology* (pp. 181–214). New York: Cambridge University Press.

Samoilov, A., & Goldfried, M. R. (2000). Role of Emotion in Cognitive-Behavior Therapy. *Clinical Psychology: Science and Practice*, *7*(4), 373–385.

Schartau, P. E. S., Dalgleish, T., & Dunn, B. D. (2009). Seeing the bigger picture: training in perspective broadening reduces self-reported affect and psychophysiological response to distressing films and autobiographical memories. *Journal of abnormal psychology*, *118*(1), 15.

Schwartz, M. S., & Andrasik, F. (2003). *Biofeedback: A practitioner's guide*. Guilford Press.

Smyth, J. M. (1998). Written emotional expression: effect sizes, outcome types, and moderating variables. *Journal of consulting and clinical psychology*, *66*(1), 174–184.

Southwick, S. M., & Charney, D. S. (2012). *Resilience: The Science of Mastering Life's Greatest Challenges* (p. 204). Cambridge University Press.

Stroop, J. R. (1935). Studies of interference in serial verbal reactions. *Journal of experimental psychology*, *18*(6), 643.

Taelman, J., & Vandeput, S. (2009). Influence of mental stress on heart rate and heart rate variability. *IFMBE Proceedings*, *22*, 1366–1369.

Tausczik, Y. R., & Pennebaker, J. W. (2009). The Psychological Meaning of Words: LIWC and Computerized Text Analysis Methods. *Journal of Language and Social Psychology*, *29*(1), 24–54.

Viaud-Delmon, I., Gaggioli, A., Ferscha, A., & Dunne, S. (2012). Human Computer Confluence Applied in Healthcare and Rehabilitation. *Studies in health technology and informatics*, *181*(Annual Review of Cybertherapy and Telemedicine), 42–45.

Vrana, S. R., Spence, E. L., & Lang, P. J. (1988). The startle probe response: A new measure of emotion? *Journal of abnormal psychology*, *97*(4), 487.

Wagnild, G. M., & Young, H. M. (1993). Development and psychometric evaluation of the Resilience Scale. *Journal of Nursing Measurement*, 1(2), 165–178

Williams, J. M. G., Mathews, A., & MacLeod, C. (1996). The emotional Stroop task and psychopathology. *Psychological bulletin*, *120*(1), 3–24.

Yehuda, R., Daskalakis, N. P., Desarnaud, F., Makotkine, I., Lehrner, A. L., Koch, E., ... Bierer, L. M. (2013). Epigenetic Biomarkers as Predictors and Correlates of Symptom Improvement Following Psychotherapy in Combat Veterans with PTSD. *Frontiers in Psychiatry*, *4*(September), 118.

Mónica S. Cameirão and Sergi Bermúdez i Badia

14 An Integrative Framework for Tailoring Virtual Reality Based Motor Rehabilitation After Stroke

Abstract: Stroke is a leading cause of life-lasting motor impairments, undermining the quality of life of stroke survivors and their families, and representing a major challenge for a world population that is ageing at a dramatic rate. Important technological developments and neuroscientific discoveries have contributed to a better understanding of stroke recovery. Virtual Reality (VR) arises as a powerful tool because it allows merging contributions from engineering, human computer interaction, rehabilitation medicine and neuroscience to propose novel and more effective paradigms for motor rehabilitation. However, despite evidence of the benefits of these novel training paradigms, most of them still rely on the choice of particular technological solutions tailored to specific subsets of patients. Here we present an integrative framework that utilizes concepts of human computer confluence to 1) enable VR neurorehabilitation through interface technologies, making VR rehabilitation paradigms accessible to wide populations of patients, and 2) create VR training environments that allow the personalization of training to address the individual needs of stroke patients. The use of these features is demonstrated in pilot studies using VR training environments in different configurations: as an online low-cost version, with a myoelectric robotic orthosis, and in a neurofeedback paradigm. Finally, we argue about the need of coupling VR approaches and neurocomputational modelling to further study stroke and its recovery process, aiding on the design of optimal rehabilitation programs tailored to the requirements of each user.

Keywords: Stroke Rehabilitation, Virtual Reality, Accessibility, Personalization, Computational Neuroscience

14.1 Introduction

Stroke remains one of the main causes of adult disability, with about one third of survivors experiencing permanent motor impairments that severely affect their quality of life (Feigin et al., 2008). This represents a challenge for modern societies, which have to handle the resulting social and economical burden that already accounts for 2–4% of total healthcare costs worldwide (Donnan et al., 2008). In the last years, important neuroscientific findings have contributed to the understanding of functional recovery after stroke, and it is nowadays widely accepted that recovery relies to a large extent on neuronal plasticity mechanisms, such as synapse strengthening and activity-dependent rewiring that can lead to the formation of new neural connections and/or altered pathways to regain function (Dimyan et al., 2011; Murphy et al., 2009).

Motor rehabilitation focused on physical and occupational therapy is still considered a critical driver for restoration, but the challenge remains identifying the optimal way to mobilize plasticity (Bowden et al., 2013; Dimyan et al., 2011).

Information and communication technologies are leading to new breakthroughs in this area, with Virtual Reality (VR) systems receiving special attention (Fluet et al., 2013; Laver et al., 2012). VR is a powerful tool because it enables personalizing artificial environments to particular users and manipulating feedback in such a way that users with disabilities can interact with the virtual environment in a way that would not be possible in the real world (Bohil et al., 2011). Because of its properties, VR technology has been incorporated in several systems aimed for stroke rehabilitation. Particularly, it has been widely used in conjunction with devices for robotic assistance for providing support to patients with limited motor function (Frisoli et al., 2012, Tyryshkin et al., 2014), devices that provide haptic feedback to increase the validity of the virtual interaction (Turolla et al., 2013b, Cameirao et al., 2012, Boos et al., 2011), and also in combination with EEG to study brain activation during virtual training (Steinisch et al., 2013, Bermúdez i Badia et al., 2013). A more recent trend focuses on using virtual reality based serious games that use sophisticated tracking and/or commercial games and movement controllers to increase challenge, enjoyment and adherence to training (Shin et al., 2014, Cameirao et al., 2010, Cho et al., 2012). Rehabilitation paradigms that combine VR with well-defined clinical and neuroscientific guidelines have been shown to moderately improve motor function in stroke patients when compared to traditional physical and occupational therapy (Cameirao et al., 2011, Lohse et al., 2014, Turolla et al., 2013a). While the potential of these technologies for supporting recovery is large, the amount of evidence on the benefit of such paradigms is still limited, and consequently a consensus has not yet been reached concerning the best way of personalizing rehabilitation protocols in terms of system type, method and dose (Laver et al., 2012). This is largely because patients display mismatched outcomes depending on the neural areas and networks affected by stroke (Carey et al., 2005; Stinear et al., 2012). Further, most VR based rehabilitation paradigms usually focus on a specific subset of patients, mainly those with a mild to intermediate impairment level, who allow exploring more inexpensive solutions.

In this chapter, we present strategies that rely on the use of multi-interface and customizable VR solutions for addressing the interindividual variability of stroke survivors and providing training protocols tailored to the specific requirements of each individual.

14.2 Human Computer Confluence (HCC) in neurorehabilitation

The scientific and technological advancements in the rehabilitation area have reached a point in which the mere application of technology leads to unsatisfactory solutions. The use of VR and associated technologies in rehabilitation post-stroke was initially popularized by its surface properties, such as the affinity with gaming elements, capacity of objectively assessing performance, monitoring over time by clinicians, active involvement of the patient, or ease of transferring the technology to home environments (Iosa et al., 2012, Laver et al., 2012). Although these are very useful and necessary features, they describe features of the implementation of VR based neurorehabilitation but not necessarily operational principles that are able to boost rehabilitation's efficacy. However, taking also into consideration neuroscientific principles of brain functioning it is possible to utilize VR in a more effective way to tackle specific mechanisms that support recovery after stroke. We are therefore not dealing anymore with the application of technology to rehabilitation but instead working towards its confluence with the patient's specificities.

The pressing need to find novel and more effective solutions require us to work at the confluence of computer science, human computer interaction, engineering, rehabilitation medicine and neuroscience. It is by exploiting the synergies among those disciplines that a deeper understanding about the brain and the underlying processes of stroke recovery may arise, and consequently, also novel rehabilitation approaches. In this respect, two core aspects of HCC are particularly well suited to enhance the motor rehabilitation process by enabling a more targeted intervention at the level of the brain: 1) the use of (physical and/or mental) invisible interfaces; and 2) the augmentation of the patient's abilities, not only through training but also through technology.

– Invisible interfaces: The capacity of patients to perform meaningful goal oriented motor actions depends on the existence and extent of residual movement after stroke. This is an important limiting factor because motor rehabilitation requires the active involvement of error correction and planning processes (Beets *et al.*, 2012). Because interfaces carry the responsibility of mediating between the patient's intentions and the motor training tasks, interfaces have to support the correct physical and/or mental execution of actions to ensure that the motor training experience engages those planning and error correction processes. Hence, the role of interfaces for post-stroke motor rehabilitation is of major importance and goes beyond a mere selection of actions to be performed in VR. Interfaces need to be invisible (physically or mentally) in the mediation between the intents of patients and their perceived actions. This is, however, very challenging because of the heterogeneity of motor deficits we find in stroke patients, which result in a yet greater diversity of training paradigms. A VR training paradigm that is adapted to the deficits of a particular patient may require a very specific use of interface technology. Patients' interactions with VR training tools can be based on body kinematics (movement and electromyography), but also on autonomic nervous system responses (such as galvanic skin response, respiration, and heart rate among other) or even brain activity (such as electroencephalography, near-infrared spectroscopy or functional magnetic resonance imaging), extending motor rehabilitation paradigms beyond physical execution. As a result, there is the need to work towards a unified and coherent framework for interfaces for motor rehabilitation that is able to accommodate a large variety of motor deficits and map motor intent to VR training paradigms in a transparent way.

- Augmenting patient's abilities: Similar to what happens with the interfaces, VR training paradigms need to go beyond the mere computerization or "gamification" of motor training, which has already been shown effective to contribute to recovery (Takeuchi and Izumi, 2013). It has already been shown that the use of controlled multimodal (visual, auditory and/or tactile) cues for reward and error correction is important for motor learning (Levin, 2010). Thus, VR motor training tools need to be designed, together with its interfaces, to maximally exploit the remaining neural mechanisms of stroke survivors in order to mobilize brain plasticity (Tunik *et al.*, 2013). By means of the possibility of altering the feedback provided in VR training, we propose to use VR to create an alternative reality to allow for a more direct intervention at the level of the central nervous system. VR allows us to augment the motor abilities of the patient in order to be able to restore compromised sensorimotor contingencies, closing the sense-act loop in a very controlled manner. Consequently, VR will enable patients to generate meaningful goal oriented motor actions despite their physical limitations. Hence, personalizing the parameters of motor training to each patient as well as maximizing the recruitment of the Mirror Neurons (MN) system – responsible for action recognition (Rizzolatti *et al.*, 2009) – and the engagement of motor adaptation, error feedback and sensorimotor integration networks (Shadmehr *et al.*, 2010) (Figure 14.1).

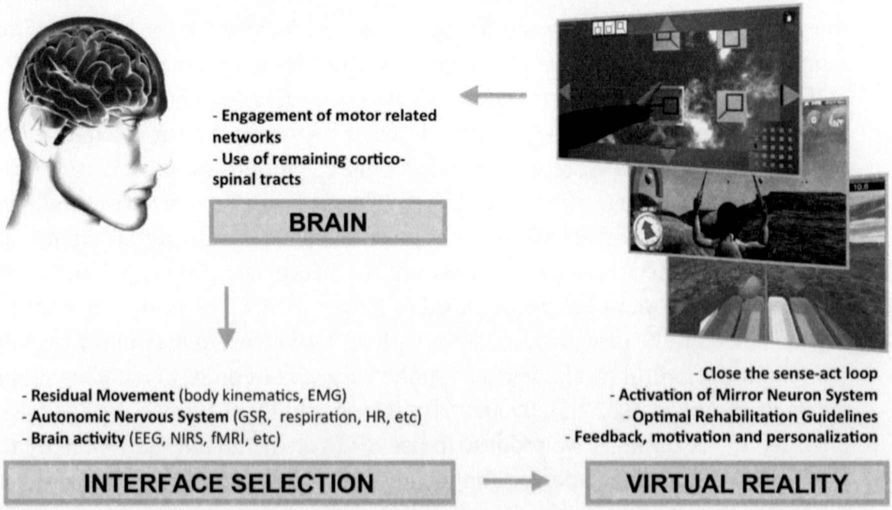

Figure 14.1: Framework for tailoring VR based motor rehabilitation after stroke. The goal is to utilize HCC concepts to achieve a maximal engagement of motor control brain related networks, to mobilize cortical plasticity for maximizing the use of remaining cortico-spinal tracts, and to generate meaningful functional movement. There is therefore a confluence of technology with the patient in which interface technology captures the available voluntary and involuntary control signals, and VR closes the act-sense loop to generate meaningful actions. This approach is designed to recruit motor related networks, to support optimal rehabilitation guidelines and to provide appropriate feedback, motivation and personalization in training

In the following sections we will introduce RehabNet, a technological framework that has been implemented to support the proposed neurorehabilitation approach. We will show in several pilot experiments how the RehabNet framework supports the confluence of technology and patient, allowing interfaces and VR to work in a symbiotic relation with the patient. In previous research we showed that the interface technology of a VR based intervention can have an impact and modulates motor improvements as well as the retention of gains in follow up measures (Cameirao et al., 2012). In RehabNet, interfaces are used to enable patient's access to novel training paradigms unavailable when motor control is seriously compromised, at the same time that VR offers a more direct intervention at the central nervous system level that is not possible by traditional therapy. Thus, interfaces are both enablers and determinant factors of VR based rehabilitation. Nevertheless, there is still limited knowledge available on how to best utilize interfaces and VR to mobilize the remaining motor related networks after stroke. For this reason, in the last section of this chapter we discuss the need of studying the effect of these approaches with brain imaging as well as combining it with a complementary computational modelling effort. A combined effort, bringing together neurocomputational modelling and clinical research, can give rise to very specific testable model-driven hypothesis on how to improve current neurorehabilitation practices, and enable us to further elucidate the brain mechanisms of recovery after stroke.

14.3 The RehabNet Framework

RehabNet's primary goal is to enable patient's access to novel training paradigms unavailable when motor control is seriously compromised. The existing variability in motor deficits in stroke patients, ranging from mild impairment to no movement, require a broad spectrum of training paradigms based on sensibly different principles, such as for instance training of active movement, robotic assisted movement or neurofeedback (see (Takeuchi et al., 2013) for a review). Thus, technological solutions need to be flexible enough to accommodate numerous interfaces and training paradigms. However, access to therapy does depend exclusively on the availability or use of appropriate interfaces. There are many other factors that influence the access of patients to VR based therapies, among them location, versatility and cost. VR technologies installed at health centres have a great potential of reaching many users but they also require shared usage, transportation from the patient's place, and support by trained professionals. Additionally, the cost of these systems is still prohibitive for the large majority of patients. Either of these factors may result in impossibility of access or in a lack of compliance with the desired frequency of use of VR therapy. Hence, there is the need to develop technological solutions that enable patient's access to VR therapy, but that also consider the economical and social aspects. That is, they should be designed for home usage, be scalable and compatible with low cost mass consumption devices.

To face the above problems we have developed RehabNet, a low cost and accessible system architecture for VR based rehabilitation that provides VR based training directly from the web, supporting several interface technologies and enabling more accessible training paradigms (Figure 14.2) (Vourvopoulos et al., 2013). VR training content is accessible via any standard web browser and is compatible with all major operating systems and android based smart TVs. The control panel, a client application that runs on the home computer, acts as a bridge between the hardware and the online VR training content. The control panel supports multiple low cost and medical grade interface technologies, ranging from a mouse to Brain Computer Interfaces (BCIs). In addition, it translates and maps the information provided by the different interfaces (currently openVibe compatible (Renard et al.) and EPOC (Emotiv Systems, Australia) BCIs), myo-electric robotic orthosis (mpower 1000, Myomo Inc, USA), MS kinect tracking, webcam tracking (Bermúdez i Badia, 2004–2013), android phones as pointing devices, and any VRPN (Taylor Ii et al., 2001) and OSC (Wright, 2005) compatible hardware) onto meaningful control commands for the VR training tasks. While keeping the VR training tasks consistent and interface independent, the control panel enables adapting the VR training paradigms to a broader range of patients and disabilities, ranging from an active movement based upper limb training to a neurofeedback paradigm based on Sensory Motor Rhythms (SMR) detection using BCIs (Pfurtscheller et al., 1997).

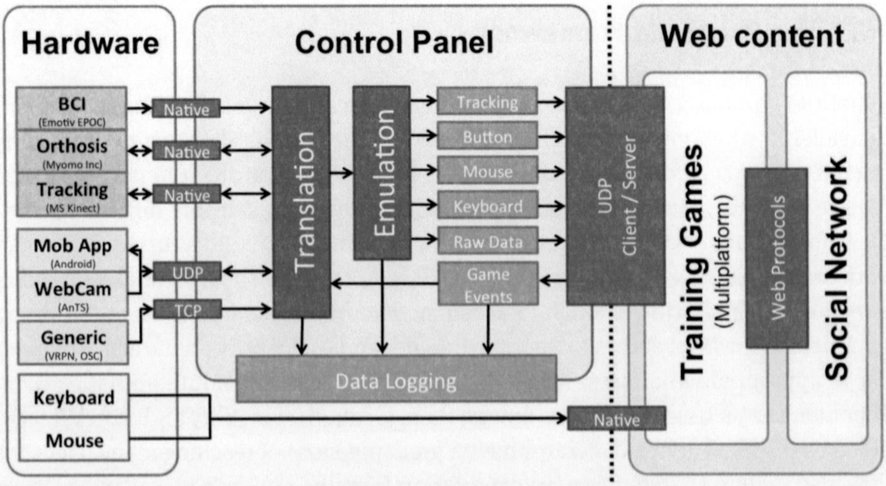

Figure 14.2: The RehabNet system architecture. It consists of three main building blocks: Hardware for device support, Control Panel for data translation and emulation, and Web content for accessing the rehabilitation content. All blocks are interconnected in a client-server (open) architecture. Adapted from (Vourvopoulos et al., 2013)

14.4 Enabling VR Neurorehabilitation Through its Interfaces

14.4.1 Low Cost at Home VR Neurorehabilitation

The Neurorehabilitation Training Toolkit (NTT) is a rehabilitation system implemented with the RehabNet architecture (Bermúdez i Badia & Cameirao, 2012). This rehabilitation system was designed with the primary focus of enabling upper limb VR training anywhere at the lowest possible cost. Therefore, it is a free and worldwide accessible tool for at home rehabilitation with minimal technical requirements[18]. The VR training system is operated using only two computer mice and is accessible through a web browser. Because the NTT is designed for home use, it has a strong emphasis on intelligent and automated personalization of training (see section 14.5

18 Available at http://neurorehabilitation.m-iti.org/NTT

for details on personalization). It trains bimanual coordinated movements on a table-top in a simulated glider control task, allowing support of the paretic arm by the non paretic arm (Figure 14.3a). Despite the simplicity and limitations of the use of two computer mice as interface technology, we have shown that this configuration allows extracting relevant movement kinematic data such as movement smoothness, range of motion and arm coordination, and can successfully adapt the training to each user accordingly (Figure 14.3b).

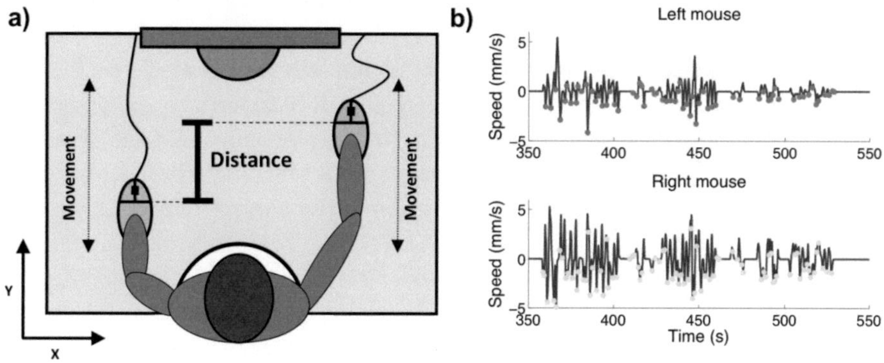

Figure 14.3: The Neurorehabilitation Training Toolkit (NTT). a) The NTT trains bimanual coordination and requires the use of a personal computer and 2 computer mice. b) Mice data provide accurate information on movement speed and acceleration that is used to adapt the rehabilitation training parameters. Adapted from (Bermúdez i Badia & Cameirao, 2012)

14.4.2 Enabling VR Neurorehabilitation Through Assistive Robotic Interfaces

Despite the clear benefits that a system such as the NTT provides, they come at a cost. In its simplest configuration, the NTT can only be used by patients that have sufficient control of active movements and can grasp a computer mouse. Although the adaptation of the physical aspects of interfaces for patients suffering spasticity or flaccidity is feasible, the training does not hold for patients without or with minimal active movement capabilities. For those patients we propose the use of adaptive assistive interfaces for the restoration of active movement. Previous myo-electric driven robotic interventions have been shown to lead to improved motor function and reduced spasticity of the upper extremities (Hu et al., 2009). Consequently, we augmented the NTT with a portable myo-electric limb orthosis equipped with 2 electromyography (EMG) channels and 1 actuated joint (mpower, Myomo Inc., USA) to restore active movement. The orthosis can detect residual muscle activity and provide an adaptive robotic assistance to facilitate movement. The mpower assists in the completion of arm movement based on the detection of biceps and/or triceps EMG activity.

In this new configuration, the NTT integrates the myo-electric robotic system, a camera based hand position tracking and a VR training task for granting access to active movement training to patients with minimal or no active movement capabilities but with residual EMG activation (Figure 14.4a). In order to assess how the provided assistance affects movement quality, task performance and training outcome we evaluated the system in a pilot study with stroke survivors with very low level of control of their paretic arm but still able to generate voluntary EMG activation (Bermúdez i Badia, Lewis et al., 2012). Results showed that the level of myo-electric assistance provided a linear increase of bíceps flexion/extension (Figure 14.4b). An analysis of biceps movement assisted by the robotic orthosis revealed a positive but low correlation coefficient with that of the end effector (Pearson's $r = .37$), indicating that most of the arm movement was supported by the glenohumeral joint (shoulder) (Figure 14.4c). When compared to the movement of the non paretic arm, we observed that with myo-electric assistance we could restore active movement up to about 60% of the non paretic arm capabilities (Figure 14.4d). Thus, this robotic interface enables a match between motor intent and performed action transparent to the patient, what is consistent with the recruitment of both the motor control networks and the MN system. In addition, this system allows objectively assessing and monitoring the active contribution of the elbow joint to overall arm movement, and detecting and quantifying the presence of compensatory strategies.

14.4.3 Closing the Act-Sense Loop Through Brain Computer Interfaces

In some cases active movement therapies are not possible even with the aid of assistive interfaces. Without the existence of a physical action, the patient's capability to recruit the brain mechanisms necessary for re-learning – such as motor planning, motor adaptation, or sensorimotor integration – may be disrupted. In these cases there is the need to provide an alternative channel to associate motor intent and perceived action. One solution is to use BCIs in electroencephalography (EEG) based neurofeedback paradigms to promote cortical plasticity (Bundy et al., 2012; Grosse-Wentrup et al., 2011). Mental imagery or simulation training has been shown to be able to engage neuronal systems consistent with those activated during motor training (Miller et al., 2010). VR is very well suited for providing multisensory feedback on mentally simulated motor actions, allowing closing the act-sense loop even in absence of physical movement. We have shown in a study with healthy participants that (1) mental simulation and (2) combined mental simulation and physical motor training are more effective at engaging cortical motor related networks than motor actions alone (Figure 14.5). This effect is most visible in β and γ EEG frequency bands, generally associated to SMRs, active concentration, busyness, alertness, and cross-modal processing and binding (see (Bermúdez i Badia et al., 2013) for details). Consequently, the potential of VR based neurofeedback paradigms based on SMRs

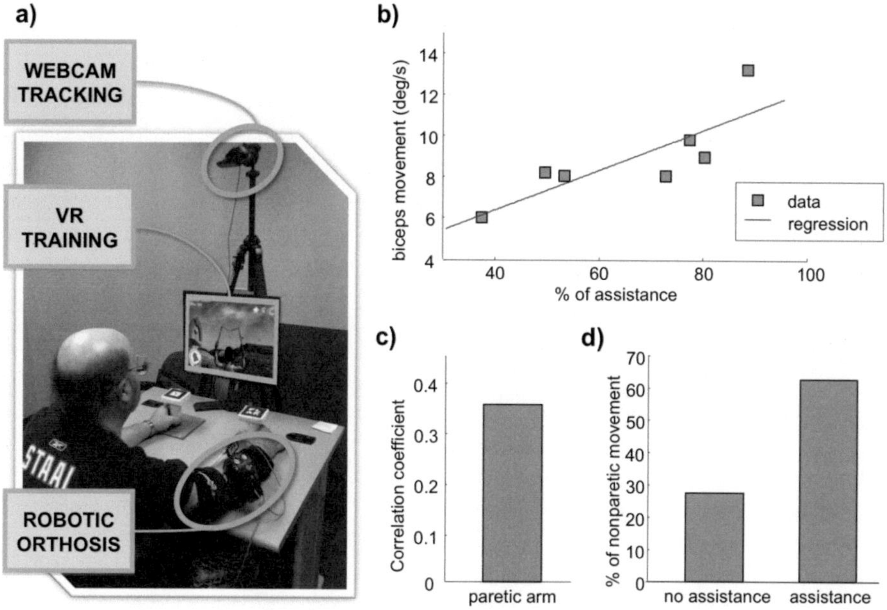

Figure 14.4: NTT with a myo-electric robotic system. a) Components of the system (robotic orthosis, tracking setup, and training game task) while being used by a stroke patient. b) Effect of the level of assistance of the limb orthosis on the amount of biceps movement. c) Quantification of the correlation of biceps movement and overall arm movement. d) Restoration of paretic arm movement as % of non-paretic arm in presence and absence of robotic assistance. Adapted from (Bermúdez i Badia, Lewis et al., 2012)

generated by motor imagery is enormous considering that they can enable access to VR based therapies to most stroke patients, regardless of their level of motor impairment.

14.5 Creating Virtual Reality Environments For Neurorehabilitation

Two critical aspects have to be considered when creating virtual rehabilitation environments for neurorehabilitation: 1) how to adjust automatically the task, assessing patient's skills and matching them with task difficulty; and 2) how to keep the user engaged by controlling the levels of stress and challenge. An efficient way of combining task personalization with challenge within VR rehabilitation scenarios is creating training tasks presented in the form of games. Serious games for stroke rehabilitation have received increased attention during the last few years mainly because of their potential to increase engagement with the rehabilitation task and keep patients working during longer periods of time (Deutsch et al., 2011; Peters et al., 2013). Compliance with training is in fact one critical aspect, particularly when considering the deployment of home based solutions for enduring rehabilitation. The main obstacle

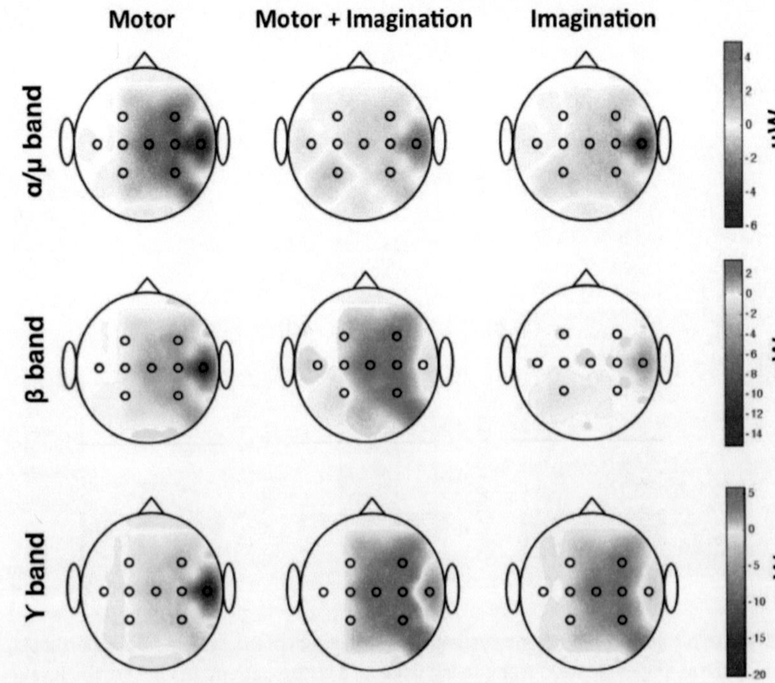

Figure 14.5: Analysis of brain activity for different motor training conditions: motor only, motor and mental imagination, and mental imagination only. Blue indicates de-synchronization of neural responses and red enhanced synchronization of neural responses as compared to baseline. EEG mapping realized with electrodes at F3, C3, P3, T3, F4, C4, P4, T4 and Cz of the international 10–20 system. Adapted from (Bermúdez i Badia et al., 2013)

is to get patients to use these solutions in a systematic way (Jurkiewicz et al., 2011). Here, games have the potential to motivate users and increase adherence to training. From the rehabilitation point of view there are however some aspects that have to be considered when developing serious VR games that aim at promoting recovery following stroke. First, games should be specifically designed for the stroke population and incorporate therapy approaches. Hence, games should target the training of specific movements (for example, reaching and grasping) with realistic short- and long-term goals. Most commercial of-the-shelf games are not appropriate because they lack the specificity of the movements to be executed, and because the tasks are often too demanding. Second, games should be related to functional movements, preferably related to activities of daily living, within a meaningful context (Hochstenbach-Waelen et al., 2012). For example, if the goal is to learn how to reach and grasp and object, performing the movement sequence without an object to be grasped is meaningless and may not contribute to motor learning (Arya et al., 2011; Wu et al., 2000).

Finally, ideally games should be varied and aesthetically pleasant to sustain interest and long-term use.

One of the main advantages of VR rehabilitation when compared to traditional treatment is that it allows implementing artificial environments for task-specific training that determine in real-time the most appropriate task parameters for each user based on his/her specific requirements. This enables bringing to patients tailored rehabilitation tasks fully adjusted to their individual capabilities and with goals that patients are able to accomplish within the range of their motor limitations. Goal oriented task-specific training is common practice in stroke rehabilitation and there is a large body of evidence that suggests its relevance for promoting cortical reorganization, hence recovery after stroke (Buma et al., 2013; Takeuchi et al., 2013). VR has potential to reinforce this effect by allowing users to interact and accomplish goals in a way that would not be possible in the real world, effectively augmenting their capabilities through VR. However, this requires identifying the capabilities of patients and tailoring training exercises depending on their specific motor deficits. In most cases, this is done by having experienced therapists allocating tasks and adjusting the parameters (Duff et al., 2013; Turolla et al., 2013a). While we believe that the involvement of rehabilitation practitioners is crucial for the development of novel VR approaches, we also think that these systems should be somehow autonomous in allocating personalized rehabilitation exercises. We have two main reasons for defending this view. First, it allows having unified frameworks for personalization, i.e., the same set of rules is applied to all users, which will ease assessing the impact of VR based rehabilitation approaches as a function of the profile of stroke patients. Second, one of the main advantages of low-cost VR rehabilitation systems is that patients have the possibility of using them at home after hospital discharge. Hence, these systems should be independent in the decision process and require only minimum intervention of the therapist.

Adjusting the task to the user requires assessing his/her current performance and setting the difficulty level with the task parameters accordingly. Matching appropriate difficulty levels in multi-parameter virtual tasks requires the development of patient based performance models. These models need to be trained with sufficient performance data to provide a thorough assessment of the specific contribution of each VR feature to the overall task difficulty. Hence, these models provide an objective way of tuning task parameters to specific difficulty levels. One specific example of the implementation of this methodology is the Rehabilitation Gaming System (Cameirao et al., 2010). The detailed psychometrics of a sphere catching game were assessed by exposing stroke patients to random combinations of the game parameters, and this information was used to build an adaptation module for adjusting the game difficulty to users. Moreover, it is yet more valuable when these models are able to capture not only task difficulty but also clinically relevant performance metrics (for example, interjoint coordination, velocity of movement, movement smoothness or range of movement) and provide a more clinically relevant adaptation (Figure 14.6) (Bermúdez i Badia & Cameirao, 2012).

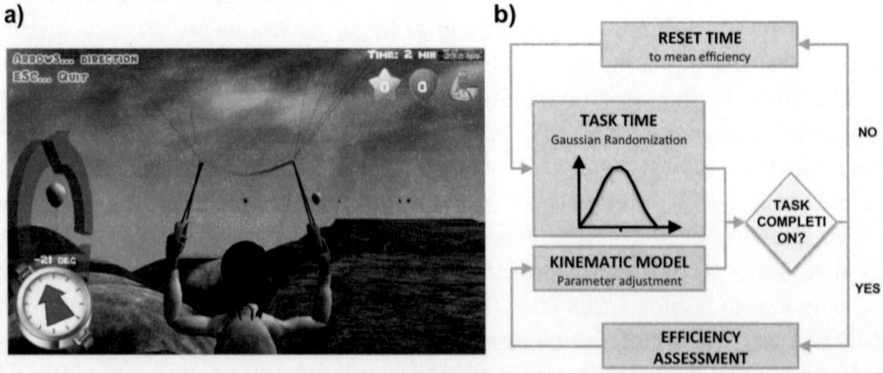

Figure 14.6: Personalization in the Neurorehabilitation Training Toolkit (NTT). a) The user controls the movements of an avatar that flies a glider to collect a number of objects in a VR environment. The target direction is achieved by balancing left and right arm movements. b) The training task is adjusted to the performance of the user through an algorithm that captures the efficiency of actions and adapts the parameters of the task accordingly. Adapted from (Bermúdez i Badia & Cameirao, 2012)

Another critical aspect in personalization is engagement. It has been acknowledged that optimum levels of performance and engagement are obtained at intermediate levels of stress, i.e., when the task is neither too easy nor too hard (Csikszentmihalyi 2002). This means that a degree of failure is necessary for keeping the user challenged and interested. In the context of rehabilitation, strategies based on incremental task complexity have been shown to correlate with cortical reorganization after stroke (Page et al., 2009; You et al., 2005). One way to sustain challenge is by increasing gradually the difficulty of the task while keeping the user in a level that he/she can perform, thus avoiding high levels of stress and frustration. For example, one possible rule can be: for a specific difficulty level, if the user performs without errors the difficulty level is increased; if the failure rate is higher than the success rate, the difficulty is decreased; otherwise, the difficulty level stays the same. In the case of the NTT the user has to collect items in a virtual environment within a limited time window, the time-to-collect of new items being derived from the time used when collecting previous items (Figure 14.6) (Bermúdez i Badia & Cameirao, 2012). Based on the efficiency of motor performance in a race against time task, the personalization algorithm provides an adaptive training that is neither too easy nor too hard to avoid boredom and frustration. This means that the more efficient the user the more demanding and challenging the task. An interesting feature of the NTT's race against time model is that it enables to control stress levels (time-to-perform) independently from motor skills (kinematic training parameters) (Figure 14.6b). In previous studies, we have shown that VR tasks that personalize training and adjust difficulty based on failure rates have a positive impact in both acute and chronic stroke patients (Cameirao et al., 2012; Cameirao et al., 2011). Although further evidence is needed to assess and understand the particular benefits of personalized VR gaming in stroke rehabilitation, we believe that these tools have all the ingredients to become common practice in rehabilitation in the near future.

14.6 Looking Forward: Tailoring Rehabilitation Through Neuro-Computational Modelling

With the aging of the population and the unsustainable cost of current rehabilitation, new solutions must come from novel scientific approaches that bring further insights on how to improve the effectiveness of rehabilitation. Although the field of stroke rehabilitation has advanced enormously during the last years and VR is a very promising tool for stroke recovery, we are likely to be reaching the boundaries of what can be achieved without a solid and integrated theoretical framework on stroke and its recovery. Rehabilitation approaches need to take into account how neuroanatomical determinants, such as lesion size and location, affect motor execution; how the corresponding brain mechanisms underlie recovery; and need to be able to provide optimal rehabilitation strategies for each individual case. Unfortunately we are still far from such a holistic understanding of stroke, and as consequence we cannot take full advantage of the technological advantages brought by VR training tools.

We believe that one way to address this challenge systematically is by using a neurocomputational modelling approach that considers the neural areas and circuits involved in movement planning and execution; replicates the effect of focal brain lesions in specific brain areas; and simulates recovery mechanisms. By simulating lesions to the model and integrating plasticity mechanisms following stroke, such an approach could be used to simulate stroke and study the effect of different rehabilitation approaches. Here VR is the key piece because the coupling of a computational model of motor control and a virtual body allows closing the act-sense control loop and having a cohesive framework to systematically study healthy and impaired motor control. There has been some work on computational modelling for stroke (Goodall et al., 1997; Han et al., 2008; Reinkensmeyer et al., 2012) but to our knowledge there is no work that couples a neurocomputational model with a VR rehabilitation environment. If the VR environments used for simulations of the neurocomputational models were consistent with those used for motor rehabilitation training, the generalization of results would be straightforward. In fact, the use of a common VR environment for both model simulation and patient training enables direct transfer of results from the clinical praxis to the computational modelling approach, enabling model training to fit available performance, kinematic and clinical patient data.

Although being a very ambitious and laborious research goal, this is a path that will increase our knowledge on stroke, its recovery and will enable us to design personalized VR rehabilitation programs that take into account the neuroanatomical constrains of each patient to maximize functional recovery, bringing personalization of VR training to the next level. This modelling effort enables investigating how recovery patterns are modulated by lesion location and training routines, in a unique manner not yet explored. The potential impact of such an approach is multifold. At the scientific level, it would provide a comprehensive and integrative platform for neuroscientists, engineers and clinicians to further understand the mechanisms underlying stroke recovery and the impact of different rehabilitation strategies. For rehabilitation medicine, it would represent an important step towards model based tailoring of rehabilitation protocols for maximizing recovery. Finally, in the long-term such a strategy would contribute to further increase the quality of life of stroke survivors; improve the management of healthcare services and resources; and reduce the overall socio-economic burden of stroke.

Acknowledgements: This work is supported by the European Commission through the RehabNet project – Neuroscience Based Interactive Systems for Motor Rehabilitation – EC (303891 RehabNet FP7-PEOPLE-2011-CIG) and the Fundação para a Ciência e Tecnologia (Portuguese Foundation for Science and Technology) through CMU-Pt/0004/2007, SFRH/BPD/84313/2012, and Projeto Estratégico – LA 9 – 2013–2014.

References

Arya, K. N., Pandian, S., Verma, R., et al. (2011). Movement therapy induced neural reorganization and motor recovery in stroke: a review. *J Bodyw Mov Ther, 15*(4), 528–537.

Beets, I. A., Mace, M., Meesen, R. L., et al. (2012). Active versus passive training of a complex bimanual task: is prescriptive proprioceptive information sufficient for inducing motor learning? *PLoS One, 7*(5), e37687.

Bermúdez i Badia, S. (2004–2013). Analysis and Tracking System [version 2]. Retrieved 28/10/2013, from http://sergibermudez.blogspot.com

Bermúdez i Badia, S., & Cameirao, M. S. (2012). The Neurorehabilitation Training Toolkit (NTT): A Novel Worldwide Accessible Motor Training Approach for At-Home Rehabilitation after Stroke. *Stroke Res Treat, 2012*, 802157.

Bermudez i Badia, S., Garcia Morgade, A., Samaha, H., et al. (2013). Using a hybrid brain computer interface and virtual reality system to monitor and promote cortical reorganization through motor activity and motor imagery training. *IEEE Trans Neural Syst Rehabil Eng, 21*(2), 174–181.

Bermúdez i Badia, S., Lewis, E., & Bleakley, S. (2012, September). *Combining virtual reality and a myo-electric limb orthosis to restore active movement after stroke: a pilot study.* Paper presented at the 9th Intl Conf. Disability, Virtual Reality & Associated Technologies, Laval, France.

Bohil, C. J., Alicea, B., & Biocca, F. A. (2011). Virtual reality in neuroscience research and therapy. *Nat Rev Neurosci, 12*(12), 752–762.

Boos, A., Qiu, Q., Fluet, G. G., & Adamovich, S. V. (2011). Haptically facilitated bimanual training combined with augmented visual feedback in moderate to severe hemiplegia. *Conf Proc IEEE Eng Med Biol Soc, 2011*, 3111–3114.

Bowden, M. G., Woodbury, M. L., & Duncan, P. W. (2013). Promoting neuroplasticity and recovery after stroke: future directions for rehabilitation clinical trials. *Curr Opin Neurol, 26*(1), 37–42.

Buma, F., Kwakkel, G., & Ramsey, N. (2013). Understanding upper limb recovery after stroke. *Restor Neurol Neurosci.* 31(6):707–722.

Bundy, D. T., Wronkiewicz, M., Sharma, M., et al. (2012). Using ipsilateral motor signals in the unaffected cerebral hemisphere as a signal platform for brain-computer interfaces in hemiplegic stroke survivors. *Journal of neural engineering, 9*(3), 036011.

Cameirao, M. S., Badia, S. B., Duarte, E., et al. (2012). The combined impact of virtual reality neurorehabilitation and its interfaces on upper extremity functional recovery in patients with chronic stroke. *Stroke, 43*(10), 2720–2728.

Cameirao, M. S., Badia, S. B., Oller, E. D., et al. (2010). Neurorehabilitation using the virtual reality based Rehabilitation Gaming System: methodology, design, psychometrics, usability and validation. *J Neuroeng Rehabil, 7*, 48.

Cameirao, M. S., Bermudez, I. B. S., Duarte, E., et al. (2011). Virtual reality based rehabilitation speeds up functional recovery of the upper extremities after stroke: a randomized controlled pilot study in the acute phase of stroke using the rehabilitation gaming system. *Restor Neurol Neurosci, 29*(5), 287–298.

Carey, L. M., Abbott, D. F., Egan, G. F., et al. (2005). Motor impairment and recovery in the upper limb after stroke: behavioral and neuroanatomical correlates. *Stroke, 36*(3), 625–629.

Cho, K. H., Lee, K. J., & Song, C. H. (2012). Virtual-reality balance training with a video-game system improves dynamic balance in chronic stroke patients. *Tohoku J Exp Med, 228*(1), 69–74.

Csikszentmihalyi , M. (2002). *Flow: The Classic Work on How to Achieve Happiness.* London: Rider & Co

Deutsch, J. E., Brettler, A., Smith, C., et al. (2011). Nintendo wii sports and wii fit game analysis, validation, and application to stroke rehabilitation. *Top Stroke Rehabil, 18*(6), 701–719.

Dimyan, M. A., & Cohen, L. G. (2011). Neuroplasticity in the context of motor rehabilitation after stroke. *Nat Rev Neurol, 7*(2), 76–85.

Donnan, G. A., Fisher, M., Macleod, M., et al. (2008). Stroke. *Lancet, 371*(9624), 1612–1623.

Duff, M., Chen, Y., Cheng, L., et al. (2013). Adaptive mixed reality rehabilitation improves quality of reaching movements more than traditional reaching therapy following stroke. *Neurorehabil Neural Repair, 27*(4), 306–315.

Feigin, V. L., Barker-Collo, S., McNaughton, H., et al. (2008). Long-term neuropsychological and functional outcomes in stroke survivors: current evidence and perspectives for new research. *Int J Stroke, 3*(1), 33–40.

Fluet, G., & Deutsch, J. (2013). Virtual Reality for Sensorimotor Rehabilitation Post-Stroke: The Promise and Current State of the Field. *Current Physical Medicine and Rehabilitation Reports, 1*(1), 9–20.

Frisoli, A., Procopio, C., Chisari, C., Creatini, I., Bonfiglio, L., Bergamasco, M., Rossi, B., & Carboncini, M. C. (2012). Positive effects of robotic exoskeleton training of upper limb reaching movements after stroke. *J Neuroeng Rehabil, 9*, 36.

Goodall, S., Reggia, J. A., Chen, Y., et al. (1997). A computational model of acute focal cortical lesions. *Stroke, 28*(1), 101–109.

Grosse-Wentrup, M., Mattia, D., & Oweiss, K. (2011). Using brain-computer interfaces to induce neural plasticity and restore function. *Journal of neural engineering, 8*(2), 025004.

Han, C. E., Arbib, M. A., & Schweighofer, N. (2008). Stroke rehabilitation reaches a threshold. *PLoS Comput Biol, 4*(8), e1000133.

Hochstenbach-Waelen, A., & Seelen, H. A. (2012). Embracing change: practical and theoretical considerations for successful implementation of technology assisting upper limb training in stroke. *J Neuroeng Rehabil, 9*, 52.

Hu, X. L., Tong, K.-y., Song, R., et al. (2009). A comparison between electromyography-driven robot and passive motion device on wrist rehabilitation for chronic stroke. *Neurorehabilitation and Neural Repair, 23*(8), 837–846.

Iosa, M., Morone, G., Fusco, A., Bragoni, M., Coiro, P., Multari, M., Venturiero, V., De Angelis, D., Pratesi, L., & Paolucci, S. (2012). Seven capital devices for the future of stroke rehabilitation. *Stroke Res Treat, 2012*, 187965.

Jurkiewicz, M. T., Marzolini, S., & Oh, P. (2011). Adherence to a home-based exercise program for individuals after stroke. *Top Stroke Rehabil, 18*(3), 277–284.

Laver, K., George, S., Thomas, S., et al. (2012). Cochrane review: virtual reality for stroke rehabilitation. *Eur J Phys Rehabil Med, 48*(3), 523–530.

Levin, M. F., Heidi Sveistrup, and Sandeep K. Subramanian. (2010). Feedback and virtual environments for motor learning and rehabilitation. *Schedae 1*, 19–36.

Lohse, K. R., Hilderman, C. G., Cheung, K. L., Tatla, S., & Van der Loos, H. F. (2014). Virtual reality therapy for adults post-stroke: a systematic review and meta-analysis exploring virtual environments and commercial games in therapy. *PLoS One, 9*(3), e93318.

Miller, K. J., Schalk, G., Fetz, E. E., et al. (2010). Cortical activity during motor execution, motor imagery, and imagery-based online feedback. *Proceedings of the National Academy of Sciences, 107*(9), 4430–4435.

Murphy, T. H., & Corbett, D. (2009). Plasticity during stroke recovery: from synapse to behaviour. *Nat Rev Neurosci, 10*(12), 861–872.

Page, S. J., Szaflarski, J. P., Eliassen, J. C., et al. (2009). Cortical plasticity following motor skill learning during mental practice in stroke. *Neurorehabil Neural Repair, 23*(4), 382–388.

Peters, D. M., McPherson, A. K., Fletcher, B., et al. (2013). Counting repetitions: an observational study of video game play in people with chronic poststroke hemiparesis. *J Neurol Phys Ther, 37*(3), 105–111.

Pfurtscheller, G., & Neuper, C. (1997). Motor imagery activates primary sensorimotor area in humans. *Neuroscience letters, 239*(2), 65–68.

Reinkensmeyer, D. J., Guigon, E., & Maier, M. A. (2012). A computational model of use-dependent motor recovery following a stroke: optimizing corticospinal activations via reinforcement learning can explain residual capacity and other strength recovery dynamics. *Neural Netw*, 29–30, 60–69.

Renard, Y., Lotte, F., Gibert, G., et al. OpenViBE: an open-source software platform to design, test, and use brain-computer interfaces in real and virtual environments. *Presence: teleoperators and virtual environments, 19*(1), 35–53.

Rizzolatti, G., Fabbri-Destro, M., & Cattaneo, L. (2009). Mirror neurons and their clinical relevance. *Nat Clin Pract Neurol, 5*(1), 24–34.

Shadmehr, R., Smith, M. A., & Krakauer, J. W. (2010). Error correction, sensory prediction, and adaptation in motor control. *Annu Rev Neurosci, 33*, 89–108.

Shin, J. H., Ryu, H., & Jang, S. H. (2014). A task-specific interactive game-based virtual reality rehabilitation system for patients with stroke: a usability test and two clinical experiments. *J Neuroeng Rehabil, 11*, 32.

Steinisch, M., Tana, M. G., & Comani, S. (2013). A post-stroke rehabilitation system integrating robotics, VR and high-resolution EEG imaging. *IEEE Trans Neural Syst Rehabil Eng, 21*(5), 849–859.

Stinear, C. M., Barber, P. A., Petoe, M., et al. (2012). The PREP algorithm predicts potential for upper limb recovery after stroke. *Brain, 135*(Pt 8), 2527–2535.

Takeuchi, N., & Izumi, S. (2013). Rehabilitation with poststroke motor recovery: a review with a focus on neural plasticity. *Stroke Res Treat, 2013*, 128641.

Taylor Ii, R. M., Hudson, T. C., Seeger, A., et al. (2001). *VRPN: a device-independent, network-transparent VR peripheral system.* Paper presented at the Proceedings of the ACM symposium on Virtual reality software and technology.

Tunik, E., Saleh, S., & Adamovich, S. V. (2013). Visuomotor discordance during visually-guided hand movement in virtual reality modulates sensorimotor cortical activity in healthy and hemiparetic subjects. *IEEE Trans Neural Syst Rehabil Eng, 21*(2), 198–207.

Turolla, A., Dam, M., Ventura, L., et al. (2013a). Virtual reality for the rehabilitation of the upper limb motor function after stroke: a prospective controlled trial. *J Neuroeng Rehabil, 10*, 85.

Turolla, A., Daud Albasini, O. A., Oboe, R., Agostini, M., Tonin, P., Paolucci, S., Sandrini, G., Venneri, A., & Piron, L. (2013b). Haptic-based neurorehabilitation in poststroke patients: a feasibility prospective multicentre trial for robotics hand rehabilitation. *Comput Math Methods Med, 2013*, 895492.

Tyryshkin, K., Coderre, A. M., Glasgow, J. I., Herter, T. M., Bagg, S. D., Dukelow, S. P., & Scott, S. H. (2014). A robotic object hitting task to quantify sensorimotor impairments in participants with stroke. *J Neuroeng Rehabil, 11*(1), 47.

Vourvopoulos, A., Faria, A. L., Cameirão, M. S., et al. (2013, October 9–12). *RehabNet: A Distributed Architecture for Motor and Cognitive Neuro-Rehabilitation. Understanding the Human Brain through Virtual Environment Interaction.* Paper presented at the 2013 IEEE 15th International Conference on e-Health Networking, Applications and Services (Healthcom), Lisbon.

Wright, M. (2005). Open Sound Control: an enabling technology for musical networking. *Organised Sound, 10*(03), 193–200.

Wu, C., Trombly, C. A., Lin, K., et al. (2000). A kinematic study of contextual effects on reaching performance in persons with and without stroke: influences of object availability. *Arch Phys Med Rehabil, 81*(1), 95–101.

You, S. H., Jang, S. H., Kim, Y. H., et al. (2005). Virtual reality-induced cortical reorganization and associated locomotor recovery in chronic stroke: an experimenter-blind randomized study. *Stroke, 36*(6), 1166–1171.

Pedro Gamito, Jorge Oliveira, Rodrigo Brito, and Diogo Morais

15 Active Confluence: A Proposal to Integrate Social and Health Support with Technological Tools

Abstract: Ageing demographic structures produce higher rates of physical and cognitive impairments, lack of independence, and social isolation of old people. This poses challenges to general and mental health care. In this chapter, we present a framework for seamlessly integrated, web-based digital systems to enhance active ageing and independent living by unobtrusively monitoring older people's health signs and providing feedback both to them and to important nodes in their social support network.

Keywords: Active Ageing, Confluence, Interaction, Sensing, Symbiosis

15.1 Introduction

The demographic structure of most of the industrialised world and emerging economies, including Europe, North America, and much of Asia, is in an irreversible process of ageing (UN Population Division, 2005). European societies, together with Japan, face particularly marked ageing. As a consequence, they also face growing problems associated with old age, such as cognitive decline, motor impairments and lack of independence (Beard, Biggs, Bloom, et al., 2011). These problems carry additional burdens for families with shrinking younger cohorts and rising financial costs for societies as a whole. Digital technology is currently addressing these impacts of ageing by assisting daily living. Another characteristic of an elderly or impaired population is isolation. Digital media is in some ways fighting back isolation. Best use of digital technology and media requires, however, sufficient technological literacy, and too often technology is not adapted to users' needs. We adopt the view that technology needs to reach the person by being designed to adapt to people's natural behaviours and routines, instead of having people deal with the intricacies of technology. In this chapter, we discuss a conceptual framework advocating personalised services for independent living and active ageing. Our perspective is that digital systems can be unobtrusively incorporated into the daily life activities of communities, e.g. the elderly population, in a seamless, low-cost, immersive way, and we are not alone in this perspective (ICAA, 2014). Smartphones, remote sensors, biofeedback, virtual reality, and intelligent systems can be integrated in a single all-inclusive platform that connects the elderly with their social support networks, providing personalised information and feedback to nodes (people) in the network and acting in a symbiotic fashion. Beyond the practical advantage such a system offers, seamless integration of individuals, technologies, and the social network should be able to reproduce an embodied perception of social belongingness typical of communal groups such as families, thereby making usage intuitive, pleasant, and emotionally rewarding.

15.1.1 An Ageing Society

Europe enjoyed a steady growth in GDP from 1820 to the end of the XXth Century (Gordon, 2002), and an unprecedented rise in standard of living after World War II. However, this growth has slackened since the 1970s, and unemployment has increased (Blanchard, 2005). At the same time, lower fertility rates, driven by social changes, contraception, and the expansion of female participation in the workforce, have slowed demographic growth and contributed to ageing. Although the population of Europe is still growing, the demographic distribution has been changing, with contractions in the youngest cohorts and expansions in the eldest. The number of Europeans aged 65–79 years old increased from c. 60 to 65 million between 2001 and 2011, and that of 80 years or older from less than 17 to almost 25 million in the same period (Pordata, 2013). This new demographic reality, along with the current financial and economic constraints, has sparked policy debates on health care across the EU. At present, most EU countries are unable, unwilling, or discouraged from sustaining their past levels of investment in their national healthcare systems. There is thus a demand for novel, cost-effective solutions that are still able to provide better and broader responses, but at a lower cost.

15.1.2 Ageing and General and Mental Health

Ageing is a process inherent in every living organism; it is an irreversible biological state, with a progressive decrease in functional ability. One of the main reasons for the increased costs in health and personal care of older populations is the escalation of physical diseases coupled with mental disorders, which implies increased impairments in both physical and cognitive capacities and, thus, a decrease in the autonomy and general quality of life among the elderly.

Depression is the most common mental condition in older people and has been increasing in prevalence in developed countries. Its prevalence also increases with age, with an estimated value of 11% to 13% among the elderly of developed countries (Steffens, Fisher, Langa, Potter and Plassman, 2009). Depression is related to a number of health conditions – such as cardiovascular and cerebrovascular diseases – through its influences on health behaviours and exposure to stress; extreme and prolonged episodes of depression can even lead to death.

The main symptoms of depression are a depressed mood, apathy and hopelessness, which are often chronic among the elderly. Depression is related to deregulation of prefrontal circuits of the brain, resulting in cognitive deficits and executive dysfunction (Willner, Scheel-Krüger, & Belzung, 2012). Cognitive deficits are also common in older people with depression, being often associated with poor prognosis and decreased response to treatment (Alexopoulos, Meyers, Young, et al., 2000).

Suicide is also a problem related to the elderly, and suicide rates have been increasing (WHO, 2012). People over 65 years have the highest rates of suicide, reaching 20/100.000 in people older than 85 in the U.S., (Hawton & van Heeringen, 2009) and 148/100.000 for men above 85 in France (Ritchie et al., 2004). Older people have difficulties in coping with the effects of chronic pain (which becomes more frequent with ageing), medications and the consequences of organic diseases, which may contribute to increased incidence of depression in the elderly and eventually on suicide rates.

Declining health and cognitive capacity associated with ageing are currently the focus of much research. Epidemiological studies have shown that prevalence of organic dementias, including Alzheimer's, increases with age, from 5% of people aged 71–79 years to 37.4% for people over 90 years (Plassman et al., 2007). In Europe, a recent meta-analysis of studies carried out during the 1990s suggests that prevalence rates double every 5 years for people aged above 65 years-old. This poses a challenge to older people's ability to live independent and happy lives.

15.1.3 Social Support and General and Mental Health

Humans are an incredibly social species, and extremely sensitive to being included in groups, attached to close others, and cared for. Social support therefore has both direct and indirect effects in tackling disease and impairment. On the one hand, social support can be of direct help in solving practical problems. On the other hand, it enhances individual patients' psychological resilience by tackling loneliness and preventing depression.

However, the potential social support that people receive from others varies immensely according to the social relations that they have with those others. Despite the incredible expansion of online social networks such as Facebook, people still rely mostly on the inner circle of their offline social networks – namely family and close friends – for social support. Indeed, family and close friends provide a completely different kind of psychological (emotional, affective) support from that which can be provided by the broader society, by colleagues and acquaintances, or even by professional caregivers.

This is because these different social relations are guided to varying extents by each of the fundamental cognitive, social-relational models that humans use to produce and sustain sociality: communal sharing, authority ranking, equality matching, and market pricing (Fiske, 1992). Family and close friends are strongly guided by a communal sharing model of relation, in contrast to professional relations or even most friendships (Brito, Waldzus, Sekerdej, & Schubert, 2011). The communal sharing model is defined by closeness, attachment, affection, kindness, and caring for others in the relation, in particular according to their needs (Haslam & Fiske, 1999). This means that it has the double benefit, for the sake of social support, of at the same time being oriented to the satisfaction of actual needs, and of providing emotional support, thus buffering the elderly against psychological stressors that facilitate mental health problems. Conversely, the lack of significant social relationships is the most important trigger for feelings of loneliness in the elderly and, ultimately, depression.

Indeed, the available evidence points not only to the important role of family and close friends in providing social support to the elderly, but also to their direct effect on general and mental health outcomes of those who are supported. For example, a large US study found an important effect of informal support from non-spouse family/friends on lowering depression, and that States supporting Home and Community-Based Services (which substitute informal networks) experienced lower depression rates among seniors with functional declines and low informal support (Muramastu, Yin, & Hedeker, 2010). Recent research in a poor neighbourhood in Brazil also indicated that social support (in mostly unmarried older women) is negatively correlated with depression (Lino, Portela, Camacho, Atie, & Lima, 2013). And, in Canada, another large study (n>1300) found a negative effect of social support on stress, mediated by a sense of self-mastery (Gadalla, 2009).

15.1.4 Ageing and Social Support

Unfortunately, as people get older, they experience an increased likelihood of losing social support and suffering personal loss at the same time through mortality in their network of family (including spouses) and friends. These are ubiquitous events that lead to social isolation and functional problems in older people. The elderly tend to create new friendships, if at all, with people from the same age cohort (Singh & Misra, 2009). But, with advancing age, the opportunity for these new friendships decreases. Other social factors, such as financial difficulty, may also contribute to personal and social dysfunction (Mojtabai and Olfson, 2004).

These problems are compounded by the current demographic dynamics of ageing populations, which are related to smaller family sizes and, thus, to smaller family networks. Greater demographic mobility of the general population also spells greater demographic dispersal of these networks, which means they are spread rather thinly on the ground. Together with the problems that the elderly face in their own mobility, this requires technological support to sustain communication and relational closeness over social support networks.

15.2 Active Confluence: A Case for Usage

To counter the general and mental health problems associated with ageing, as well as social problems associated with an aged demographic structure, policies designed to enhance active ageing have been gaining critical importance across Europe, and are actively supported by the European Commission. Self-managed or home-based exercises and activity programs are a centrepiece of those policies; adherence to and compliance with these programs have been identified as a key factor in the improvement of functional outcomes (Deutscher et al. 2009). In the past few years, technology has been gaining importance in the domain of active ageing, and technological solutions have been suggested and used to promote these outcomes, improving an individual's adherence to self-exercise programmes, and enabling them to engage in simulated activities. However, the gap between the individual and the technology is still too large; technology is still a dark passenger that must be moved from place to place. In order to bridge the gap between users (especially older ones) and technology, symbiotic solutions must be provided.

Until now, technological solutions for monitoring and caregiving have been developed almost exclusively for clinical settings, namely hospitals and other healthcare-oriented facilities, and even there, the results are far from optimal (Olson & Windish, 2010; Uphold, 2012). This means that these solutions require the physical presence and engagement of caregivers. Features such as user-friendliness, ubiquity, and mobility are usually neglected because support is always around. On the other hand, the interaction between user and exercise platform is a mediated one. Pencil, paper, a joystick or a keyboard create a gulf between the individual and the exercise, making the experience far from natural. Considering the need for remote/home solutions for individuals' interaction and monitoring, the criterion of achieving confluent solutions must quickly become a priority in the development of active programs that are concomitantly pervasive and non-intrusive in the elderly's daily lives.

We argue that the way individuals interact within the applications must be similar to the way they interact with the real world. This means that both software and hardware need to be integrated in a seamless fashion so that they can be perceived as a natural complement of individuals' actions, rather than yet another difficult system for individuals to deal with, and this is available in some areas (Sik Lanyi, Brown, Standen, Lewis, & Butkute, 2012). The system also needs to display solutions that are compatible with an individual's physical or psychological status. Seamless devices should feed the system with data so that the status of the user can be inferred and the most appropriate exercise displayed. Thus, the system needs also to be permanently accessible, anytime and anywhere. For this to be possible, it must use off-the-shelf displays and interactive platforms such as tablets, smartphone and TV and mobile sensors, and run over the Internet. Finally, the system should be an integral part of an individual's social world, extending and enhancing the individual's capacity to manage his or her health and daily life.

Here, we describe the most salient aspects of a concept for an integrated technological solution designed to address the needs of active ageing and the shortcomings of current remote/health monitoring systems, based on the symbiotic paradigms of Human-Computer Confluence (HCC) (Viaud-Delmon, Gaggioli, Ferscha, & Dunne, 2012). These paradigms include new forms of improving perception and interaction, on the one hand, and sensing and monitoring, on the other. Our proposal brings these two aspects together and reinforces them with the connection of the system to the social support network of individuals using the solution.

15.2.1 Perception and Interaction

Virtual reality (VR) is probably the best solution for cognitive training to enhance natural perception and interaction. VR provides "close-to-real" experience, allowing users to interact and move around at their will and at their own pace, providing a full and natural perception of the tasks at hand. It can thus be integrated in an engaging and appealing way, much like a realistic game, into users' daily activity.

The 3D perspective enables users a better apprehension of the phenomena under simulation. This is because visual perception processing in the brain relies on different areas in the cortex that are specialized in different aspects of visual information. For example, colour, form and depth are processed in the V1 and V2 occipital areas and motion in the middle temporal cortex. Complete cognitive integration of a real-life four-dimensional phenomena (three spatial – 3D – and one temporal dimension) summons up different areas of the brain. Consequently, cognitive load is distributed. Therefore, the load on cognitive processing can be reduced if the task at hand is performed within a set-up that is perceived as being as close to reality as possible. Gramb, Schweizer & Mühlhausen, (2008) reported higher mental demand and higher perceived workload in a group of participants engaged in a 2D task (controlling a thermohydraulic process of producing particle boards) than in another group engaged in the same task but with a 3D interface.

Once immersed in the virtual world, older people can train and accomplish all the proposed tasks in a similar manner to how they would in the real world. VR has already been applied as a reality surrogate for motor and cognitive exercise purposes. VR settings can be tailored to users' needs (Lange et al., 2012; Ortiz-Calan et al., 2013; Tost et al., 2009), can provide feedback (Sveistrup, 2004), and because they are similar to games (in fact, this type of platform is often associated with Serious Games), they motivate the user in engaging the tasks, facilitating the repetition of the exercises (motivation and repetition are two quintessential requirements for exercise adherence). VR has also been used in combination with Internet wideband in order to provide and support training, as the wideband technology provides mobile and remote application of the 3D virtual environments for tele-rehabilitation (Wang, Kreutzer, Bjärnemoa, & Davies, 2004; Kurillo, Koritnik, Bajd & Bajcsy, 2011).

15.2.2 Sensing

A baseline component of the system we conceive should be a smart, adaptive monitoring system, which aims at assisting the elderly, on a daily basis, in achieving an active life-style and reducing their reliance on the assistance of others. Such a system could help by providing pervasive exercises, meeting the challenging goal of at the same time increasing quality of life and keeping costs low. While implementing the monitoring system, a parallel goal should focus on the integration of the monitoring system within the realm of existing commercial systems (e.g., MediServe[19]) and solutions (e.g., UTS Blood Pressure Monitor Palm OS Software[20]). Existing medical electronic solutions should be employed for acquiring the user's vital signals and converting them into digital data, which could be stored in the monitoring system's local database. The system would be able to display bio-signals' waveforms in real-time, store data locally, or trigger an alert. The system would then transfer these physiological data to a remote workstation in real time (remote monitoring) using an advanced wireless networking platform with ubiquitous access to the database.

Monitoring should be mostly performed by portable devices, wearable devices, smart objects, or devices that are commonly available to the user and that can be accessible anytime and anywhere (i.e. are pervasive) . With a collaborative arrangement of these devices, the system would monitor various metrics related to behaviour and to bodily and brain functions (e.g., activity, sleep, physiological and biochemical parameters). The signals to be collected would include: heart rate, blood pressure, skin temperature, galvanic skin response, and movement (body movement, kinematics, posture, etc.). The GPS data from the smartphone could be used to infer individuals' behaviour. The use of sensors integrated in clothing or weight sensors (integrated in beds) could measure the quality of rest and restlessness during sleep.

The touchstone of the framework would be to provide monitoring and support of older people's active living in a symbiotic fashion. The use of vital signs as data sources would be based on wearable or home-based sensorial devices to gather, process and feed the system with data. The system would become aware of an individual's status through the recognition of vital signs and display the best exercise and care solutions to respond to that status. The services to be provided by such a system would be based on off-the-shelf and-low budget solutions that can be acquired and used by the general public. Devices to be used by the system would consist of an ordinary tablet, smartphone or TV set, with a plugged motion detector (for example, XBOX, Wii or other equivalent product available on the market) and internet connection, which would display an interactive portal where the elderly could work out and

---

19 http://www.mediserve.com/ (accessed 28.10.2013)

20 http://www.qweas.com/downloads/home/other/overview-uts-blood-pressure-for-palm-os.html (accessed 28.10.2013)

interact with others. The exercises to help maintain or reinforce active standards of living would be displayed in a virtual reality world so that the users could freely interact with it. 3D games designed to boost cognitive functioning and to promote physical exercises would be available with different levels of difficulty, customized to each user's ability and needs. One important path to be explored consists of developing intelligent systems to act/react according to a user's needs and condition through psychophysiological monitoring.

Usually, the interaction with VR applications is measured by clinically oriented self-reports. Nevertheless, during VR exercises several researchers have also recorded patients/participants psychophysiological activity (e.g. heart rate, skin conductance resistance [SCR] and respiratory activity). The individual status level could, hence, be inferred through the sensing system such as this, but also through tracking previous individual activity. For example, for monitoring the statistics for patients, calculator software of varying complexity is available. Calculators tend to be focused on either practitioner use (MediKit[21]), or patient use (e.g., Glucose tracker[22], Blood Pressure tracker[23]), but some of them offer combined functionality. Evidence-based calculators also exist, especially for mobile phones or PDAs (InfoRetriever[24]), providing a good tool for feeding the system with data.

15.2.3 Physical and Cognitive Multiplayer Exercises

A multiplayer feature is probably the *sine qua non* condition to motivate older people to keep coming back to the system. The social characteristics of the system would be of paramount importance to the reinforcement of the feelings of social support (Gaggioli, Gorini, & Riva, 2007; Lange, Koenig, Chang, McConnell, Suma, Bolas, & Rizzo, 2012; Maier, Ballester, Duarte, Duff, & Verschure, 2014), in particular by peers of their age group, family members, or close friends involved in the system. In this system, the elderly would interact with a TV set or a tablet using only their gestures; the system would respond based on this input and on the input from data collected by sensors and actuators that are incorporated on daily use devises such as smartphones or digital wrist watches. All the technology to meet this purpose is available on the market and is able to "communicate" with each other in a seamless way, allowing for a symbiotic relation between the system and the individual.

---

21 http://www.medikit.co.jp/english/ (accessed 28.10.2013)

22 http://download.cnet.com/Free-Glucose-Tracker/3000-2129_4-10454535.html (accessed 28.10.2013)

23 http://www.heart.org/HEARTORG/Conditions/HighBloodPressure/HighBloodPressureToolsResources/Blood-Pressure-Trackers_UCM_303465_Article.jsp (accessed 28.10.2013)

24 https://library.mcmaster.ca/news/2484 (accessed 28.10.2013)

15.2.4 Integrated Solutions for Active Ageing: The Vision

What we propose here is a framework for integrated solutions for elderly people who wish to maintain a healthy standard of living, as well as for those whose health is compromised by physical disease or mental disorder or impairment. It is widely accepted that the best way to maintain illness at bay is to exercise both body and mind. Our vision is to offer a comprehensive set of exercises for the elderly to work out and to stimulate their cognitive functions and physical activity, which may serve to either help maintain a healthy status or, for those suffering from disease, slow the progress of disease. Additionally, the selection of exercises would be managed by an automated caregiver function displays alerts on compliance to medication schedules and AI (artificial intelligence) avatars would be devised to answer older people's questions on health issues on demand.

Along with prevention and care facilities, such a system should be designed to promote older people's independence. The proposed platform should thus also nest functions enabling the user to carry out a myriad of real-life activities within the system (e.g. shopping, movies, interacting with friends, focus-groups and volunteering). Such a platform would be presented in the form of a synthetic online world, a TV-based or tablet-based portal gathering the most up-to-date ICT (Information and Communication Technology) services. Internet, multiplayer functions, VR environment, telemedicine, interacting with the system through motion detection, and adjusting the system to an individual's status in a symbiotic fashion would be the central properties of the system. And, because life must not revolve around the disease, an integrated solution for daily life activities such as shopping, socialization and doing "good deeds" should also be included. This platform will enable users to shop online, to get together, to stroll with their friends' avatars in virtual parks, and to engage in online volunteer sites. At this point one should remember that reactive depression is, among the elderly, a common associated condition, which in most of the cases prompted by loneliness reduces the efficacy of treatments (Figure 15.1).

To imagine the possibilities, read our Mrs. Simon and Mrs Garfunkel scenario:

> "Mrs. Simon has just come back from the hospital where she underwent an elbow surgery and spent the subsequent month in rehab. Sitting down on her sofa, she turns on her TV. A rehab app shows up as an alternative to her usual 300-channels choice. Accessing the portal by speaking out her password, a welcome message from her doctor is displayed: "Hi Paula. Everything is going along smoothly. But now you need to attend to your medication – please take a look at the list displayed on the upper right-hand corner of the screen. I know it is a long list. No worries. An alert will be sent to your mobile 5 minutes before you have to take each medicine. And remember, the drugs are not the only thing you need to take! Remember that this app has some juicy menus adapted to your condition for you». After this message, a BOT (digital robot) appears: «Hi Mrs. Simon. How are you today? Ready for some nice elbow exercises?» As the synthetic personal trainer (PT) begins the exercise, the motion sensor attached to the TV is activated and starts detecting Mrs. Simon's movements, reproducing them on the screen. Her wrist device begins to

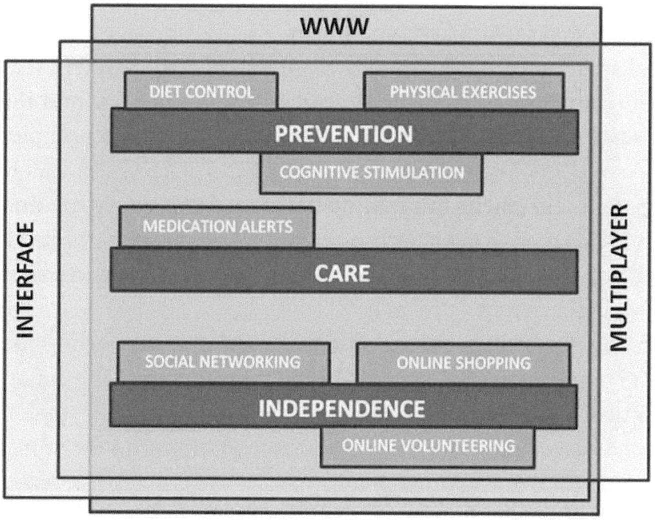

Figure 15.1: The vision: An ICT online platform for preventing and retarding elderly diseases and for promoting older people's autonomy

feed the system with biosignals. As Mrs. Simon is a newbie, the BOT corrects her movements, encouraging and motivating her throughout the exercise, while adapting the exercises to Paula's condition. When the exercises are about to end, a message from Mrs. Simon's friend, Mrs. Garfunkel, pops on the screen: "Hi Paula, can I join you?" Using the voice detector she replies: "Hi, Arthurina. How are you doing? I'm about to finish my exercises. Do you care to join me tomorrow, a bit earlier? Or, how about going shopping together right now? I need to buy something for my nephew's birthday. I've learned that the HippsterMegaStore now has an interactive VR site, where we can shop online». «I'm sorry but I'm not feeling like shopping» – Mrs. Garfunkel replies – «I think that I will log on to Volunteers'R us site and give a hand in raising some funds to the victims of the earthquake in Ramonetii. Bye, now. I'll join you tomorrow for training. By the way, can we change our PT's appearance? I don't particularly like his hair...»"

15.3 Conclusion

As ageing has become an important concern for the European Union and national governments, it has pushed them to design policies to minimize its on society. The importance of active and healthy ageing in Europe is increasing, and this is expressed in the research and development calls of the Framework Program 7 of the EU and even more so in Horizon 2020, its successor programme.

A brief description of active ageing is provided by the WHO (2002), highlighting the importance of promoting physical activity as a way to increase the functional independence of the elderly in daily living activities. The roadmaps of the latest framework programmes for research and innovation in the EU have been focusing on the use of ICT solutions for successful ageing in our societies. However, most of the current technological solutions are based solely on old-fashioned exercises that do not address the social-emotional dimension of ageing. Nor do they address the problem of adherence to technological solutions that are, more often than not, perceived as “difficult”.

Thus, future developments are crucial to a fully operative and integrative solution for monitoring and intervention among the elderly population that meets, at the same time, the principles of an active confluence solution concomitant with pervasiveness, unobtrusiveness, and a socially-friendly approach.

These principles can be met with a service-oriented platform, connecting the elderly, their families, and practitioners, using state-of-the art technology, thus offering innovative and unobtrusive forms of monitoring and exercising.

Closed-loops based on wearable sensors, caregivers’ collaboration and decisions, and elderly interaction could produce autonomous support, enabling a first interaction. There would be multiple benefits for the elderly, who would feel supported by the local loop and become more self-confident and autonomous. Another effect is that the elderly would not need to visit practitioners so often, as feedback can be sent by their local sensorial and processing devices. This would be reflected in reduced costs, and enhanced safety and quality of life.

In short, there is a clear need for the provision of both cost-effective tools for active ageing, disease prevention and retardation, and for independent living services at the point of need to provide the elderly with innovative activities and continuous support, and for an ICT interface that melds these tools with a more global lifestyle management system for independent living. Therefore, pervasive and confluent-solution exercises will improve older people’s quality of life while assisting in reducing the cost of the process. New ICT-based exercises hold the promise of improving the quality of existing care services, enlarging the scope of exercises and prevention services on offer (e.g. adverse events detection), and providing these services to a broader segment of the population than that which is presently reached. However, there are significant challenges that need to be faced, including older people’s adherence to the program. We believe that the most important obstacle to overcome relates to the difficulty of interaction with the available technology. Our concept is a convergent solution that will co-exist symbiotically with the individual.

References

Alexopoulos, G.S., Meyers, B.S., Young, R.C., et al. (2000). Executive dysfunction and longterm outcomes of geriatric depression. *Archives of General Psychiatry, 57*: 285–290. doi:10.1001/archpsyc.57.3.285

Beard, J. R., Biggs, S., Bloom, D. E., et al. (Eds.). (2011). *Global Population Ageing: Peril or Promise.* Geneva, Switzerland: World Economic Forum. Available at http://www.weforum.org/reports/global-population-ageing-peril-or-promise.

Blanchard, O. (2005). *European Unemployment: The Evolution of Facts and Ideas*. MIT Department of Economics Working Paper No. 05–24.

Brito, R., Waldzus, S., Sekerdej, M., & Schubert, T. (2011). The contexts and structures of relating to others: How memberships in different types of groups shape the construction of interpersonal relationships. *Journal of Social and Personal Relationships* 28 (3): 406–431. doi:10.1177/0265407510384420.

Deutscher, D., Horn, S., Dickstein, R., Hart, D., Smout, R., Gutvirtz, M., Ariel, I. (2009).Associations Between Treatment Processes, Patient Characteristics, and Outcomes in Outpatient Physical Therapy Practice. *Archives of Physical Medicine and Rehabilitation, 90* (8): 1349–1363. doi:10.1016/j.apmr.2009.02.005.

Fiske, A. P. (1992). The four elementary forms of sociality: Framework for a unified theory of social relations. *Psychological Review 99*: 689–723.

Gadalla, T. M. (2009). Sense of Mastery, Social Support, and Health in Elderly Canadians. *Journal of Aging and Health 21*, (4): 581–595 DOI: 10.1177/0898264309333318

Gaggioli, A., Gorini, A., & Riva, G. (2007, September). Prospects for the use of multiplayer online games in psychological rehabilitation. In *Virtual Rehabilitation, 2007* (pp. 131–137). IEEE. doi:10.1109/ICVR.2007.4362153

Gordon, R. (2002). *Two Centuries of Economic Growth: Europe Chasing the American Frontier*. Paper prepared for Economic History Workshop, Northwestern University.

Gramb, D., Schweizer, K., & Mühlhausen, S. (2008). Influence of Presence in Three-Dimensional Process Control. In *Proceedings of the 11th Annual International Workshop on Presence, 2008* (pp. 319–325).

Haslam, N., & Fiske, A. P. (1999). Relational models theory: A confirmatory factor analysis. *Personal relationships 6*: 241–250. doi:10.1111/j.1475-6811.1999.tb00190.x.

Hawton, K. & Van Heeringen, K. (2009). Suicide. *The Lancet, 373*: 1372–1381. doi:10.1016/S0140-6736(09)60372-X.

International Council on Active Aging (2014). *The ICAA Model*. Retrieved on May, 2014, from http://www.icaa.cc/activeagingandwellness.htm.

Kurillo, G., Koritnik, T., Bajd, T., and Bajcsy, R. (2011). Real-time 3d avatars for tele-rehabilitation in virtual reality. *Studies in Health Technology Informatics, 163*:290–296.

Lange, B.S., Koenig, S., Chang, C., McConnell, E., Suma, E., Bolas, M. & Rizzo. A. (2012). Designing Informed Game-Based Rehabilitation Tasks Leveraging Advances in Virtual Reality. *Disability and Rehabilitation,* 34 (22): 1863–1870., doi:10.3109/09638288.2012.670029.

Lino, V. T., Portela, M. C., Camacho, L. A., Atie, S., Lima, M. J. (2013). Assessment of social support and its association to depression, self-perceived health and chronic diseases in elderly individuals residing in an area of poverty and social vulnerability in Rio de Janeiro City, Brazil. *Plos One* 8 (8):e71712. doi:10.1371/journal.pone.0071712

Maier, M., Ballester, B. R., Duarte, E., Duff, A., & Verschure, P. F. (2014). Social Integration of Stroke Patients through the Multiplayer Rehabilitation Gaming System. In *Games for Training, Education, Health and Sports* (pp. 100–114). Springer International Publishing.

Mojtabai, R. & Olfson, M. (2004). Major depression in community-dwelling middle-aged and older adults: prevalence and 2- and 4-year follow-up symptoms. *Psychological Medicine, 34*: 623–634. doi:10.1017/S0033291703001764

Muramatsu, N., Yin, H. J., & Hedeker, D. (2010). Functional declines, social support, and mental health in the elderly: Does living in a state supportive of home and community-based services make a difference? *Social Science and Medicine 70*, 70 (7): 1050–1058 doi:10.1016/j.socscimed.2009.12.005

Olson, D. P., & Windish, D. M. (2010). Communication discrepancies between physicians and hospitalized patients. *Archives of internal medicine*, 170 (15): 1302–1307. doi: 10.1001/archinternmed.2010.239.

Ortiz-Catalan, M., Nijenhuis, S., Ambrosh, K., Bovend'Eerdt, T., Koenig, S., & Lange, B. (2013). Virtual Reality. In J. L. Pons & D. Torricelli (Eds.), *Emerging Therapies in Neurorehabilitation, Biosystems & Biorobotics 4*, doi: 10.1007/987-3-642-38556-8_13, Springer-Verlag: Berlin Heidelberg.

Plassman, B.L., Langa, K.M., Fisher, et al. (2007). Prevalence of Dementia in the United States: The Aging, Demographics, and Memory Study. *Neuroepidemiology, 29*: 125–132. doi:10.1159/000109998

PORDATA: Base de Dados Portugal Contemporâneo [Em linha]. Lisboa: FFMS, 2009: URL: http://www.pordata.pt/ (accessed 22.10.2013).

Ritchie, S., Artero, S., Beluche, I., Ancelin, M.L., Mann, A., Dupuy, A.M., Malafosse, A. & Boulenger, J.P. (2004). Prevalence of DSM-IV psychiatric disorder in the French elderly population. *British Journal of Psychiatry, 184*: 147–152. doi:10.1192/bjp.184.2.147.

Sik Lanyi, C., Brown, D., Standen, P., Lewis, J., & Butkute, V. (2012). Results of user interface evaluation of serious games for students with intellectual disability, *Acta Polytechnica Hungarica, 9*, 1, pp 225–245, ISSN: 1785-8860.

Singh, A. & Misra, N. (2009). Loneliness, depression and sociability in old age. *Industrial Psychiatry Journal*, 18 (1):51–55. doi:10.4103/0972-6748.57861.

Steffens, D.C., Fisher, G.G., Langa, K.M., Potter, G.G. & Plassman, B.L. (2009). Prevalence of depression among older Americans: the aging, demographics and memory study. *International Psychogeriatrics, 21*: 879–888. doi:10.1017/S1041610209990044.

Sveistrup, H. (2004). Motor rehabilitation using virtual reality. *Journal of NeuroEngineering and Rehabilitation;1*: 10. doi:10.1186/1743-0003-1-10.

Tost, D., Grau, S., Ferré, M., García, P., Tormos, J. M., García, A., & Roig, T. (2009, June). Previrnec: a cognitive telerehabilitation system based on virtual environments. In *Virtual Rehabilitation International Conference, 2009* (pp. 87–93). IEEE. doi:10.1109/ICVR.2009.5174211

UN Population Division (2005). *Population Challenges and Development Goals*. New York: United Nations.

Uphold, C.R. (2012). Transitional care for older adults: The need for new approaches to support family caregivers. *Gerontology and Geriatrics Research,* 1: e107.

Viaud-Delmon I., Gaggioli A., Ferscha A. & Dunne S. (2012). Human Computer Confluence Applied in Healthcare and Rehabilitation. *Studies in health technology and informatics*, 181: 42–45.

Wang, P., Kreutzer, I.A., Bjärnemoa, R. & Davies, R.C (2004). A Web-based cost-effective training tool with possible application to brain injury rehabilitation. *Computer Methods and Programs in Biomedicine, 74*, 235–243. doi:10.1016/j.cmpb.2003.08.001

Willner, P., Scheel-Krüger, J., & Belzung, C. (2012). The neurobiology of depression and antidepressant action, Neurosclerose and Biobehavioral Reviews 37: 2331–2371.

World Health Organization (2002). Active Ageing: A policy framework. http://whqlibdoc.who.int/hq/2002/WHO_NMH_NPH_02.8.pdf

World Health Organization (2012). *Public Health Action for the Prevention of Suicide: a framework*: http://apps.who.int/iris/bitstream/10665/75166/1/9789241503570_eng.pdf (accessed 28.10.2013).

Georgios Papamakarios, Dimitris Giakoumis, Manolis Vasileiadis, Anastasios Drosou and Dimitrios Tzovaras

16 Human Computer Confluence in the Smart Home Paradigm: Detecting Human States and Behaviours for 24/7 Support of Mild-Cognitive Impairments

Abstract: The research advances of recent years in the area of smart homes highlight the prospect of future homes equipped with sophisticated systems that monitor the resident and cater for her/his needs. A basic prerequisite for this is the development of non-obtrusive methods to detect human states and behaviours at home. Especially in the case of residents with mild cognitive impairments (MCI), such systems should be able to identify abnormal behaviours and trends, supporting independent living and well-being through appropriate interventions. The integration of monitoring and intervention mechanisms within a home needs special attention, given the fact that after a period of time, these will be perceived from the resident as inherent home features, altering the traditional way that the notion of home is perceived by the mind, transforming it into a Human Computer Confluence (HCC) paradigm.

Activity detection and behaviour monitoring in smart homes is typically based on sensors (e.g. on appliances) or computer vision techniques. In this chapter, both approaches are explored and a system that integrates sensors with resident vision-based location tracking is presented. Location tracking is based herein on low-cost depth cameras (Kinect), allowing for privacy preserving, unobtrusive monitoring. The focus is on detecting the MCI resident's Activities of Daily Living (ADLs), as well as extracting parameters, toward identifying abnormalities within her/his behaviour. Preliminary results show that the sole use of user position trajectories has potential toward effective ADL and abnormality detection, whereas the addition of sensors further enhances effectiveness, with increase however in system cost and complexity.

Keywords: Human Computer Confluence, Smart Homes, Mild Cognitive Impairments, Activity Detection, Computer Vision, Multisensorial Networks

16.1 Introduction

Promoting independent living and well-being of people with mild cognitive impairments (MCI) is a significant challenge. Due to increasing life expectancy, the world population is continuously aging. Aging is often accompanied by MCI, leading to functional limitations and impairments in daily life (Ahn, et al., 2009; Wadley, Okonkwo, Crowe, & Ross-Meadows, 2008), degrading the way activities of daily living (ADLs) are performed and the person's capability of effectively catering for her/his own needs. MCI is an intermediate stage between the expected cognitive decline of normal aging and the more serious decline of dementia (Ahn, et al., 2009); it can involve problems with memory, language, thinking and judgment that are greater than normal age-related changes. MCI can thus affect the person's ability to perform ADLs consisting of a series of steps, involving cognitive functions, related for instance to telephone usage, meals preparation, medication, management of belongings etc. (Ahn, et al., 2009). As the patient's cognitive state is reflected on daily activities, the capacity of the patient to perform these activities, or significant changes in the way that they are performed, can provide valuable clues toward the evaluation of MCI and its progression into dementia.

Future smart homes can play a vital role toward promoting independent living and well-being of MCI and dementia residents, by providing sophisticated 24/7 support for both the proper execution of ADLs and the early identification of cognitive decline signs. Following the research and technological advances of recent years in the area of smart homes, future houses are expected to transform into living environments that monitor the behaviour of their residents, adjust over it and allow for resident-home interaction that eases daily life and promotes well-being. A prerequisite for this is the development of non-obtrusive methods to detect human states and behaviours at home. Especially in the case of residents with mild cognitive impairments (MCI), such systems should be able to identify abnormal behaviours and trends, supporting independent living and well-being through appropriate interventions. These interventions may range from stimulating the resident to undertake a forgotten step of a meal preparation process (e.g. turning the oven off) to informing her/him about e.g. a significant increase in the duration of meal preparation or eating activities, decrease in resting activities, pointless movement around the house etc. The integration of monitoring and intervention mechanisms within a home needs however special attention, given that after a period of time, these will be perceived by the resident as inherent home features, altering the traditional way that the notion of home is perceived by the mind, transforming it into a Human Computer Confluence (HCC) paradigm.

In this line, the present chapter examines how in-house activity detection systems can be applied in practice, providing the basis of HCC in the smart home paradigm by enabling the home to sense its resident's behaviour. Typically, ADL detection is either based on ambient sensors that monitor for instance the operational state of appliances, or on vision-based techniques that monitor the resident directly. In this chapter, both approaches are explored; a novel framework for resident location trajectory-based ADL detection, built from a network of Hidden Markov Models (HMMs) and Support Vector Machines (SVMs) is introduced and compared with an ambient-sensor based approach, whereas an ADL monitoring system integrating sensors with resident location tracking is also presented.

16.2 Detecting Human States and Behaviours at Home

The present section overviews the current state of art in activity detection within smart homes. Typically, the goal of relevant systems is to detect whether the resident is engaged in some of the “Basic ADLs”, such as eating (Katz, Ford, Moskowitz, Jackson, & Jaffe, 1963) or “Instrumental ADLs”, e.g. cooking (Lawton & Brody, 1969) and, once an ADL is detected, to monitor its characteristics.

16.2.1 Ambient Sensor-Based Activity Detection

The capability of ambient sensors to capture the monitored person’s state has been extensively exploited toward activity detection (Chen, Hoey, Nugent, Cook, & Zhiwen, 2012). One of the first examples was presented by Tapia, Intille, and Larson (2004), where a wireless network of unobtrusive state-change sensors was deployed at home and the naive Bayes algorithm was used to learn the resident’s ADLs. In a similar fashion, van Kasteren and Krose (2007) experimented with static vs. dynamic Bayesian networks, trying to incorporate temporal information in the detection process. They also studied the effect of the total number of sensors on detection accuracy, concluding that increasing sensor count above some level does not necessarily improve performance, arguing instead in favour of using small sets of strategically located sensors. Van Kasteren, Noulas, Englebienne, and Krose (2008) studied Hidden Markov Models (HMM) and Conditional Random Fields. HMMs were also used by Singla, Cook, and Schmitter-Edgecombe (2008), with state duration explicitly modelled after a Gaussian distribution. Furthermore, van Kasteren, Englebienne, and Kröse (2011) exploited the inherent hierarchical nature of activities via a two-layer hierarchical HMM, where the top layer corresponded to activities and the bottom to unit actions. Discriminative classification was preferred by Fleury, Vacher, and Noury (2010), where a Support Vector Machine (SVM) was trained to automatically discriminate among activities using a multimodal set of sensors.

The fusion of information among heterogeneous sensors is an important practical issue. In this line, Medjahed, Istrate, Boudy, and Dorizzi (2009) used fuzzy logic for information fusion, together with fuzzy rules for activity inference. Liao, Bi, and Nugent (2011) used the Dempster-Shafer theory of evidence, accounting for the relative uncertainty of sensor readings. In a recent approach, Chen, Nugent, and Wang (2012) presented an ontological model of the smart home universe, addressing variability in sensor modalities by sensor abstractions.

16.2.2 Resident Movement-Based Activity Detection

Parallel to sensor-based activity detection are approaches that rely on monitoring the way the resident moves. Le, Di Mascolo, Gouin, and Noury (2008) monitored areas of interest by passive infra-red (PIR) sensors and represented activities as sequences of moving and stationary states. Duong, Phung, Bui, and Venkatesh (2009) used a two-layer Hidden Semi-Markov Model to infer activities solely based on resident location trajectories. Park and Kautz (2008) combined wide-field-of-view cameras with narrow-field-of-view cameras, for coarse- and fine-level activity detection respectively. Similarly, using only a fisheye camera, Zhou et al. (2008) collected activity statistics in a hierarchical manner at multiple levels of detail. Recent advances in depth sensing, resulting to low-cost depth sensors such as Microsoft Kinect (Zhang, 2012), have pushed research in vision-based activity recognition forward. Zhang and Tian (2012) utilized skeleton information. Noting that skeleton extraction methods perform poorly under occlusions or cluttered background, Zao, Liu, Yang, and Cheng (2012) proposed extracting local features from the RGB and depth channels instead.

16.2.3 Applications and Challenges of ADL Detection in Smart Homes

Accurate ADL detection is a necessary condition in order to build truly occupant-aware houses. It allows for extracting ADL-related parameters, toward efficient modelling of resident behaviour. This enables the detection of long-term behavioural trends as well as abnormalities, allowing smart homes to be utilized for elder care and support, as well as for early diagnosis of otherwise unidentifiable symptoms of mental or physical deterioration. To this end, Lotfi, Langensiepen, Mahmoud, and Akhlaghinia (2012) presented a framework for detecting abnormal behaviour of early dementia sufferers, based on deviations from predicted long-term trends. Trustworthy abnormality detection can also enable smart home systems to be more than a sensing device and intervene when necessary, generate alerts, engage the resident in positive action and assist in decision making (Hossain & Ahmed, 2012). Ambient-intelligence context-aware environments are eventually transformed into an HCC paradigm in the service of human support and well-being.

For such a confluence between the smart environment and the resident to be made practically feasible, certain design and implementation issues need to be tackled. It is of vital importance that the smart system be integrated in the home smoothly and transparently, without disrupting normal resident behaviour or compromising the comfort one feels at home. Privacy is an important issue that must be respected and non-obtrusiveness is a strong prerequisite. This holds for both monitoring and intervention mechanisms, whereas the latter should be designed by also having in mind that it is better to assist residents in a way that helps exercising cognitive skills, instead of merely facilitating their everyday life. Another important issue is the ease of installation, as it should interfere as little as possible with the resident.

Following the above, the present work examines whether ADL detection can be effectively conducted in practice using only a limited set of low-cost depth cameras installed in a house, tracking only the person's location, compared to a more typical ambient-sensor based approach that requires a large amount of sensors installed throughout the house. However, given that ambient sensors can provide further resident behavioural information (e.g. appliances usage statistics), we further explore the potential of integrating the above two approaches toward a more effective ADL monitoring schema.

16.3 A Behaviour Monitoring System for 24/7 Support of MCI

In the present section, the system which has been developed in the present study is described, for monitoring six typical ADLs, namely cooking, eating, dishwashing, visiting the bathroom, sleeping and watching TV, on the basis of the two modalities under examination, i.e. resident trajectories and sensor-based features.

16.3.1 Activity Detection Based on Resident Trajectories

Our novel framework for ADL detection through resident trajectories is introduced herein. In order to record location trajectories we used a camera network consisting of a small set of Kinect[25] depth sensors. Normally three or four cameras are enough to cover a small apartment, as the one of Figure 16.1. The cameras are calibrated with respect to the house, that is, each camera knows its 3D position and orientation inside the house, the latter serving as a common frame of reference. Each camera maintains a depth image of the house background. The resident, not being part of the background, is detected by comparing all incoming video frames with the stored background image. The difference of the two images is the depth image of the resident at a particular time, from which the relative location of the resident to the camera can be calculated. This procedure is simultaneously performed by all cameras to which the resident is visible at any time. Since for each camera, we know its location in the house and the relative location of the resident with respect to the camera, the exact location of the resident in the house can be computed. This location is continuously tracked by the system, producing a stream of 2D locations. As a last step, this stream of locations is processed to remove possible measurement noise and thus a highly accurate estimate of the resident's 2D trajectory in the house is extracted.

---

25 http://www.xbox.com/en-US/xbox360/accessories/kinect

We hypothesize that 2D location trajectories as the ones of Figure 16.1 can be a sufficient indicator of the activity being performed. Our goal is therefore to model trajectories which are typically generated when a person performs a certain activity. Figure 16.1 suggests that this is possible, since different activities produce undoubtedly distinct trajectories. The trajectory of a resident is sequential and probabilistic in nature. As such, we consider HMMs (Rabiner, 1989) as appropriate for modelling it, using one HMM per activity. The HMM's states correspond intuitively to general regions in space, whereas the observed variables correspond to successive points of the 2D trajectory. Each HMM is trained using only trajectories of its respective activity found in the train set, using the Baum-Welch algorithm (Rabiner, 1989).

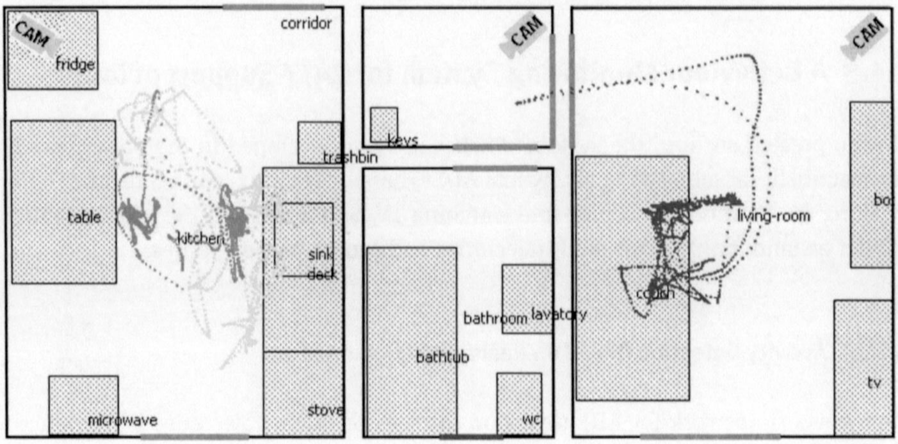

Figure 16.1: Trajectories corresponding to various activities: cooking (green), dishwashing (red), eating (magenta), watching TV (blue)

Eventually, our framework (Figure 16.2) consists of an array of HMMs calculating the resemblance between the resident's movement and respective patterns related to the target ADLs. These HMMs provide input to binary SVMs, one per activity, which recognize in turn whether the HMM-based input trajectories resemblance to ADL patterns justifies the occurrence of any of the target ADLs within a given time period. Our novel use of these binary SVMs after the HMMs layer in trajectory-based ADL detection, allows detecting both the simultaneous occurrence of multiple activities in the same interval and no target ADL occurrence.

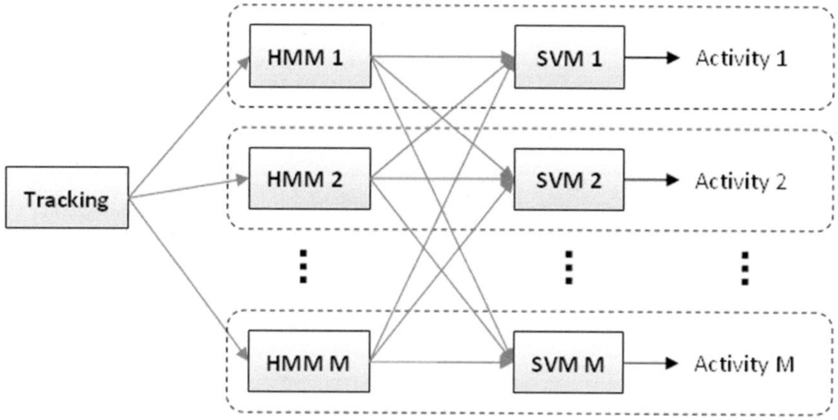

Figure 16.2: Overview of tracking-based activity detection

During activity monitoring, suppose the input data consist of a 2D trajectory $r(t)=[x(t) + y(t)]^T$ describing the resident's movement, where $t \in (t_1, t_2) \subset \mathbb{R}$, and there are M activities to be detected. We use M HMMs, each trained to model the trajectories of one target activity and M Radial Basis Function (RBF) kernel SVMs, each trained through 10-fold cross validation on the train set. During monitoring, our method proceeds as follows:

1. For each activity, time is segmented in consecutive intervals of length $T_i = aT_i^{avg}$, where T_i^{avg} is the average duration of activity i in the train set and $0 < a \leq 1$. In our experiments we have set $a = 0.1$, after a trade-off analysis between high availability of training samples (small a) and increased information content per interval (large a).
2. For each decision interval t, the resident's trajectory is evaluated against all HMMs, producing a feature vector $S_t^i = [S_t^{i,1} \quad S_t^{i,2} \quad \cdots \quad S_t^{i,M}] \in \mathbb{R}^M$, where $S_t^{i,j}$ is the log-likelihood score against HMM j, denoting the probability that $r(t)$ is produced by HMM j.
3. For each activity i, the feature vector S_t^i is fed to an SVM, in order to determine whether activity i was being performed during interval t.

16.3.2 Ambient Sensor-Based Activity Detection

Our approach for ambient sensor-based activity detection is based on a multimodal set of Phidget sensors (www.phidgets.com), strategically located in the house (Table 16.1). Sensor selection was driven by three factors: The monitoring system should be unobtrusive and able to integrate naturally in the home, as if it were part of it, without compromising the resident's privacy. The sensors should provide rich information relevant to the target ADLs. Last, the system should be cost-effective and easy to install.

Table 16.1: Set of sensors used for ADL detection

Sensor type	Position	Measurement	Most relevant ADL(s)
Temperature	Near stove	Local ambient temperature	Cooking
Humidity	Inside bathroom	Local ambient relevant humidity	Bathroom
Light (I)	Inside each room, near the lamp	Ambient luminance	All
Light (II)	On TV screen	Luminance of the TV screen	Watching TV
AC current	On stove's supply cord	RMS value of the stove's AC current	Cooking
Pressure	Under the bed's mattress	Pressure on the bed	Sleeping
Proximity (I)	On cupboard doors	Cupboard state (open/close)	Cooking, dishwashing, eating
Proximity (II)	On tap handles	Tap state (open/close)	Dishwashing, bathroom, cooking
IR receiver	Next to TV	IR TV codes sent by the remote	Watching TV

Assume again a set of *M* activities. In our approach, for each activity $i \in \{1,2,...M\}$, in each decision interval *t*, a feature $F_t^{i,j}$ is calculated for each sensor *j*, as the proportion of time, or probability, that sensor *j* is activated during *t*, that is:

$$F_t^{i,j} = \frac{T_{on}}{T_i}$$

where $0 \leq T_{on} \leq T_i$ is the total amount of time that sensor *j* is activated during interval *t*, the latter having a total duration of T_i. To accommodate the heterogeneity of sensors, we use a separate activation criterion for each sensor type, as shown in Table 16.2.

Table 16.2: Activation criteria for each sensor type

Sensor type	Activation criterion
Temperature sensor	Temperature first derivative is above a small positive threshold (that is, temperature is rising)
Humidity sensor	Relative humidity first derivative is above a small positive threshold (that is, relative humidity is rising)
Light sensor (I)	Luminance is above a threshold
Light sensor (II)	Luminance variance is above a threshold (since the luminance of the TV screen is highly agitated when the TV is on)
AC current sensor	RMS AC current is above a threshold
Pressure sensor	Pressure is above a threshold

An exception to the above rule was made for proximity sensors on cupboards and the IR receiver. Since activation of those sensors is typically instantaneous and therefore $T_{on}/T_i \cong 0$, the number of activations was used as feature instead (i.e. number of opening/closing for cupboards and number of detected IR codes for the TV).

Figure 16.3 depicts our methodology for ambient sensor-based ADL detection. Assume a set of *N* sensor units providing input data and *M* activities. The method proceeds as follows:

1. For each activity $i \in \{1,2, \ldots M\}$ time is discretized in non-overlapping consecutive intervals of equal per-activitv duration $T_i = aT_i^{avg}$, by setting again *a*=*0.1*.
2. For each interval *t*, a feature $F_t^{i,j} \in \mathbb{R}$ is extracted for each sensor $j \in \{1,2, \ldots N\}$ and the feature vector $F_t^i = [F_t^{i,1} \quad F_t^{i,2} \quad \cdots \quad F_t^{i,N}] \in \mathbb{R}^N$ is formed. The different per-activity extractor components of Figure 16.3 denote that feature extraction is conducted on time intervals of different per-activity duration.
3. Each feature vector F_t^i is classified with a binary RBF SVM (trained with 10-fold cross validation) to determine whether activity *i* occurred during interval *t*.

Activities are detected again independently, allowing detecting occasions where two or more activities occur at the same time, or no target activity is taking place.

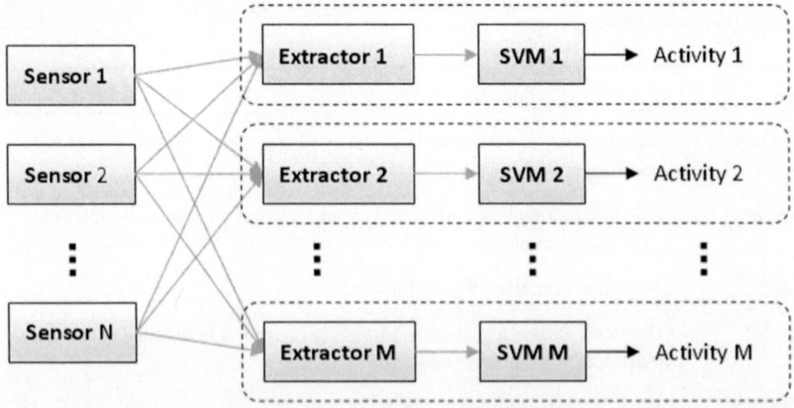

Figure 16.3: Overview of sensor-based activity detection

16.3.3 Activity Detection Based on Both Sensors and Trajectories

The above two methodologies focus on (a) resident trajectories and (b) sensor readings alone. In this section we move a step forward, combining the two approaches into an integrated and flexible framework, in order to simultaneously exploit information from both modalities. Noting that in essence, both trajectory-based and sensor-based features describe probabilities, and thus the two modalities can be fused by feature concatenation, forming the feature vector:

$$C_t^i = \left[\left(F_t^i\right)^T \quad \left(S_t^i\right)^T\right]^T = \left[F_t^{i,1} \quad F_t^{i,2} \quad \cdots \quad F_t^{i,N} \quad S_t^{i,1} \quad S_t^{i,2} \quad \cdots \quad S_t^{i,M}\right]^T$$

which is used to train and evaluate the final array of SVMs (Figure 16.4). This integrated framework is essentially a generalization of the afore-described two, since the absence of a certain modality easily produces the framework for the other one.

16.4 Experimental Evaluation

16.4.1 Data Collection

In order to evaluate our proposed ADL detection framework, two experiments were performed, a small-scale one held in a kitchen using only resident trajectories and a larger-scale one held in a real apartment, using both trajectories and sensor-based features.

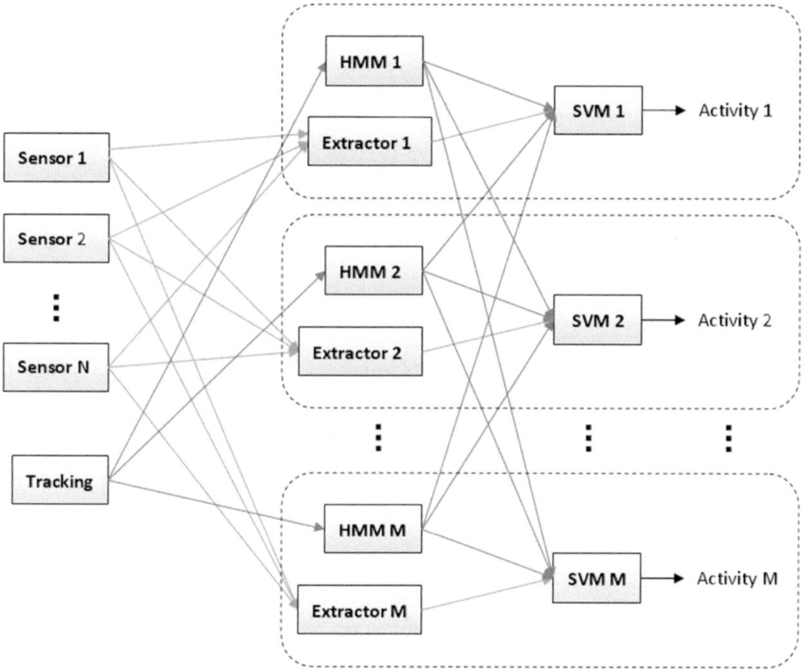

Figure 16.4: Overview of the generic framework, fusing sensor readings with trajectories

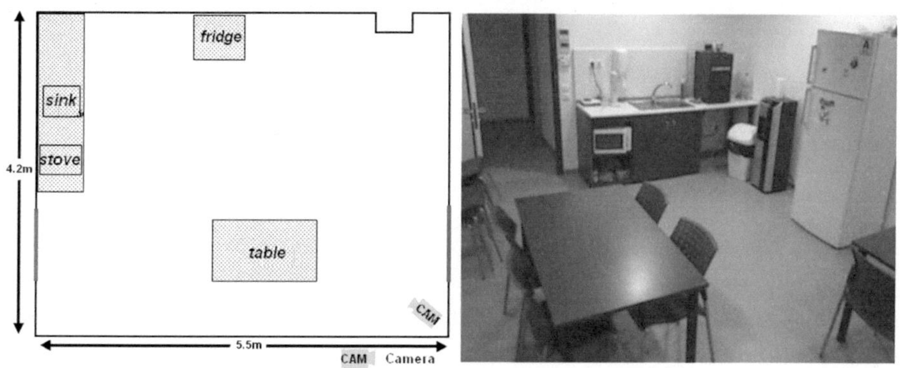

Figure 16.5: Sensor setup for the kitchen experiment (left), camera view (right)

In the kitchen experiment, a single Kinect camera was used to record occupant trajectories (Figure 16.5). Three kitchen activities were involved: cooking, eating and dishwashing. Nine sessions were recorded in total from two subjects, each session consisting of a single person entering the room, performing the three activities once and leaving. Four sessions were used for system training and the remaining five for evaluation.

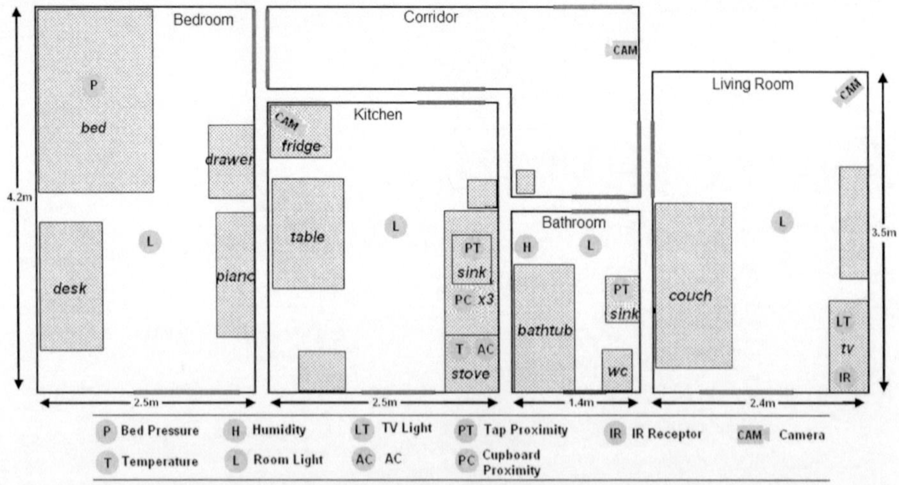

Figure 16.6: Sensors setup for the apartment experiment

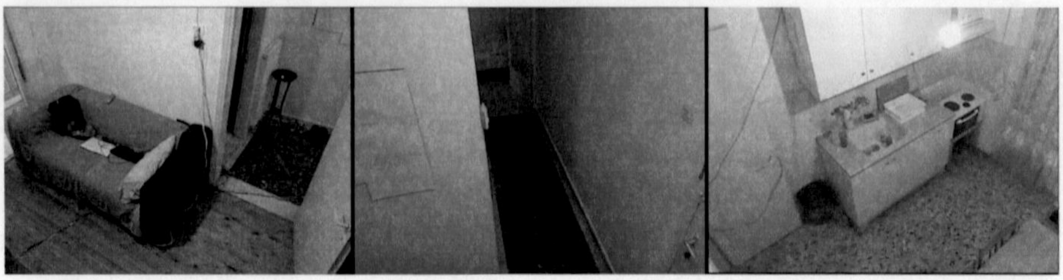

Figure 16.7: Camera views in the apartment experiment. Living-room (left), corridor (center), kitchen (right)

The apartment experiment focused on both trajectory and sensor-based detection. A wireless sensor network of environmental sensors was deployed as described in Table 16.1 and shown in Figure 16.6, together with a network of three Kinect cameras, covering the living-room, the corridor and the kitchen (Figure 16.7). For privacy reasons, the bedroom and bathroom were not covered by cameras. Six activities were involved herein: cooking, eating, dishwashing, visiting the bathroom and watching TV. Three full days of annotated data were recorded, two of which were used for training and one for evaluation.

16.4.2 Experimental Results

In both experiments, our system's detection performance was evaluated by calculating the precision Pr=TP/(TP+FP) and recall Re=TP/(TP+FN) of the detection of each activity. TP is the total number of seconds where the activity was correctly detected. FP is the total number of seconds where the activity was being detected without happening. FN is the total number of seconds where the activity was happening without being detected.

16.4.2.1 Kitchen Experiment

The results of trajectory-based activity detection in the kitchen experiment are presented in Table 16.3. Furthermore, Figure 16.8 shows a temporal comparison between the actual activities and the detected ones.

Table 16.3: Activity detection performance results for the kitchen experiment

		Cooking	Eating	Dishwashing	Average
Session 1	Precision (%)	97.10	72.73	87.50	85.78
	Recall (%)	76.40	80.00	70.00	75.47
Session 2	Precision (%)	100.00	99.57	91.67	97.08
	Recall (%)	81.51	95.10	100.00	92.20
Session 3	Precision (%)	99.59	92.86	85.47	92.64
	Recall (%)	93.25	90.00	100.00	94.42
Session 4	Precision (%)	100.00	90.91	91.92	94.28
	Recall (%)	51.97	100.00	100.00	83.99
Session 5	Precision (%)	100.00	87.50	95.06	94.19
	Recall (%)	77.60	81.29	88.00	82.30
Average	Precision (%)	99.34	88.71	90.32	92.79
	Recall (%)	76.15	89.28	91.60	85.67

The results show considerably high detection accuracy, with precision/recall rates often above 90% and all activity instances successfully detected with no false positives. All errors were in fact observed near the start or the end of activities, where it is natural for activities to appear ambiguous even to a human observer.

16.4.2.2 Apartment Experiment

Table 16.4 and Figure 16.9 present the ADL detection results for the apartment experiment, using (a) sensor-based features, (b) resident trajectories and (c) fusion of both modalities. Since the bathroom and bedroom were excluded from the

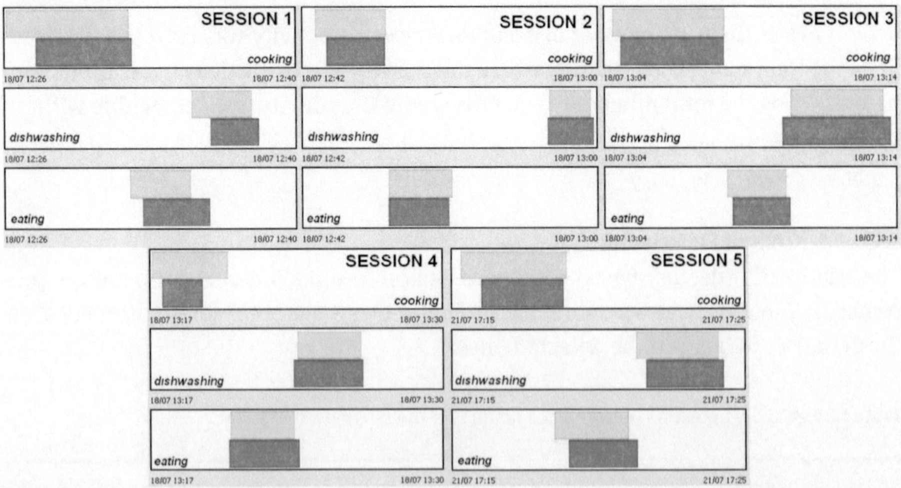

Figure 16.8: Graphical representation of the detection accuracy in the kitchen experiment. Actual activities (green–top), detected activities (red–bottom)

trajectory-recording process, the bathroom and sleeping activities are excluded from the trajectory-only evaluation.

Table 16.4: Activity detection performance results for the apartment experiment

		Sensor-based	Trajectory-based	Fusion
Bathroom	Precision (%)	100.00	-	100.00
	Recall (%)	87.40	-	87.40
Cooking	Precision (%)	100.00	66.07	66.07
	Recall (%)	90.00	92.50	92.50
Dishwashing	Precision (%)	75.00	100.00	90.00
	Recall (%)	60.00	90.00	90.00
Eating	Precision (%)	55.56	100.00	100.00
	Recall (%)	100.00	45.00	45.00
Sleeping	Precision (%)	100.00	-	100.00
	Recall (%)	99.47	-	99.47
Watching TV	Precision (%)	92.73	92.73	100.00
	Recall (%)	100.00	100.00	88.24
Average	Precision (%)	87.22	89.70	92.68
	Recall (%)	89.48	81.88	83.77

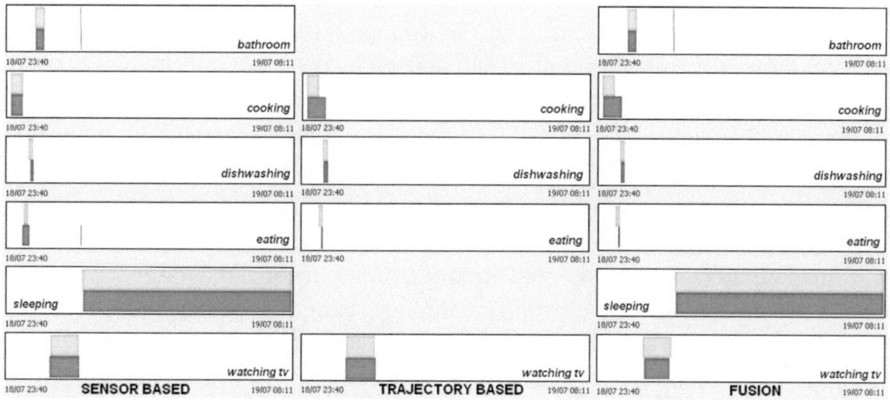

Figure 16.9: Graphical representation of the activity detection accuracy in the apartment experiment. Actual activities (green – top), detected activities (red – bottom)

From the above results, it is evident that both modalities demonstrated significant ADL detection potential. When examining each modality alone, average precision and recall rates above 80% were found. Both modalities exhibited comparable performance to each other, with the trajectory-based approach having slightly lower recall. The sensor-based method performed worse for the eating activity, demonstrating precision of only 55.56% as well as a falsely detected instance. This can be explained by the fact that no sensors existed that monitored directly this activity; instead, the detection method inferred the eating activity from the pattern formed by all sensors in general. On the other hand, the trajectory-based method removed the eating false positive, albeit not improving the recall rate. The best performance was achieved by fusing the two modalities, where the average precision exceeded 90% and no false positives or false negatives occurred. Note that most erroneous detection appeared again near the start and end of activities.

16.5 Toward Behavioural Modelling and Abnormality Detection

Following ADL detection, our system records a set of parameters for each detected activity, such as its duration and time of occurrence. In case location trajectories are involved, they allow keeping track of locations that the resident visited during an activity and the time s/he spent at each of them. Moreover, the use of ambient sensors allows monitoring the state of house devices during activities. The locations visited or the devices operating during a detected activity can be directly or indirectly associated with it (e.g. state of kitchen stove during cooking or during watching TV respectively).

The set of recorded parameters is then used to model the resident's ADL-specific behaviour, allowing for long-term trend and abnormality detection. For instance, trends related to constant increase in the average duration of daily routine ADLs (e.g. cooking), or even resignation from them can be detected. Indicative detectable abnormalities refer to cases of pointless movement around the house (movement not associated with any specific ADL), or even potentially dangerous situations that call for immediate intervention, such as going to sleep without turning off the stove. Apparently, the joint use of the trajectory and sensor modalities broadens the range of detectable abnormalities. As a further example, through the IR sensor that monitors the TV remote control usage, the resident's difficulties in understanding TV programs can be inferred, by detecting constant continuous changes in TV programs.

The possibility for accurate abnormality detection enhances a smart home with the ability to intervene when necessary. Such intervention can be either handled by the smart home itself (e.g. automatically turn off the stove when the resident is not cooking or urge the resident to do so) or by automatically calling for external help when deemed necessary (e.g. inform the doctor upon detecting restlessness/lack of sleep).

16.6 Conclusion

The prospect of future smart homes capable of sensing their residents, adapting to their behaviour and catering for their needs, gives rise to a new form of interaction that is expected to emerge, altering the traditional way that the notion of home is perceived by the mind, transforming it into an HCC paradigm. The present chapter focused on the resident monitoring part of this interaction cycle, a basic prerequisite for HCC within smart homes, whose significance is further highlighted when considering MCI residents. Persons with MCI and dementia often face difficulties in conducting ADLs composed of a series of steps and cognitive tasks, whereas their capability of successfully performing them can be considered as an indicator of their cognitive state. Thus, systems monitoring MCI residents' behaviour and abnormalities can have a significant two-fold impact in their daily life; they will allow (a) interventions facilitating the proper execution of ADLs to take place and (b) assessment of the person's cognitive state to be conducted on the basis of how ADLs are being performed within the person's daily life.

In the present work, ambient sensor-based and vision-based monitoring approaches were examined toward future effective, yet unobtrusive, in-house activity monitoring systems. This resulted in the development of a system, capable of detecting ADLs through the use of a depth-based camera network installed in the house, the use of sensors, or the fusion of the two modalities. Our developed vision-based modality, due to the small number of low-cost cameras needed, allows for low installation costs, both financially and in human effort. Moreover, it utilizes solely streams of depth images, which are significantly less obtrusive than RGB, as they do not capture facial or other identifying characteristics of the resident. Although vision-based, this specific modality can be regarded as less obtrusive also than the sensors modality, since it does not require a large amount of sensors to be installed throughout the house, whereas the only information it processes regards the resident's location. Experimental results showed that the sole use of user location trajectories detected through the vision modality has potential toward effective ADL and abnormality detection, whereas the addition of sensors can further enhance effectiveness and provide further details regarding the resident's behaviour, with an increase however in system cost and complexity.

The present chapter focused on a highly important topic of the HCC field, that of unobtrusive methods to detect human states and behaviours in naturalistic contexts. Providing computer systems with such sensing capabilities can be considered as an important step toward establishing new forms of natural interactions; interactions that will build upon advanced knowledge of the user's state and behaviour, bringing the computer system closer to the human user and advancing their confluence. Herein, emphasis was paid on in-home monitoring of MCI persons' activities, taking into account both the importance of human-computer coexistence in the context of smart homes and the potential HCC applications in the health domain. Unobtrusive sensing of resident activities and behaviour will allow future homes to facilitate on their own, the establishment of daily activities and also cognitive skills monitoring, providing support that will be properly adapted to user needs which evolve over time. Nevertheless, it should be noted that this side of research can have strong impact on the overall HCC field as well, providing the latter with a basic prerequisite; that of advanced context-awareness through user state and behaviour sensing, driving adaptation of system properties to the current situational context of users, toward optimal personalized, adaptive, proactive and invisible interaction.

Acknowledgments: This work was supported by the Greek, nationally funded research project En-NOISIS.

References

Ahn, I. S., Kim, J. H., Kim, S., Chung, J. W., Kim, H., Kang, H. S., & Kim, D. K. (2009). Impairment of instrumental activities of daily living in patients with mild cognitive impairment. *Psychiatry investigation*, *6*(3), 180–184.

Chen, L., Hoey, J., Nugent, C. D., Cook, D. J., & Yu, Z. (2012). Sensor-based activity recognition. *Systems, Man, and Cybernetics, Part C: Applications and Reviews, IEEE Transactions on*, *42*(6), 790–808.

Chen, L., Nugent, C. D., & Wang, H. (2012). A knowledge-driven approach to activity recognition in smart homes. *Knowledge and Data Engineering, IEEE Transactions on*, *24*(6), 961–974.

Duong, T., Phung, D., Bui, H., & Venkatesh, S. (2009). Efficient duration and hierarchical modeling for human activity recognition. *Artificial Intelligence*, *173*(7), 830–856.

Fleury, A., Vacher, M., & Noury, N. (2010). SVM-based multimodal classification of activities of daily living in health smart homes: sensors, algorithms, and first experimental results. *Information Technology in Biomedicine, IEEE Transactions on*, *14*(2), 274–283.

Hossain, M. A., & Ahmed, D. T. (2012). Virtual caregiver: an ambient-aware elderly monitoring system. *Information Technology in Biomedicine, IEEE Transactions on*, *16*(6), 1024–1031.

Katz, S., Ford, A. B., Moskowitz, R. W., Jackson, B. A., & Jaffe, M. W. (1963). Studies of illness in the aged: the Index of ADL: A standardized measure of biological and psychosocial function. *Jama*, *185*(12), 914–919.

Lawton, M. P., & Brody, E. M. (1969). Assessment of older people: self-maintaining and instrumental activities of daily living. *Nursing Research*, *19*(3), 278.

Le, X. H. B., Di Mascolo, M., Gouin, A., & Noury, N. (2008, August). Health smart home for elders – a tool for automatic recognition of activities of daily living. In *Engineering in Medicine and Biology Society, 2008. EMBS 2008. 30th Annual International Conference of the IEEE* (pp. 3316–3319). IEEE.

Liao, J., Bi, Y., & Nugent, C. (2011). Using the Dempster-Shafer theory of evidence with a revised lattice structure for activity recognition. *Information Technology in Biomedicine, IEEE Transactions on*, *15*(1), 74–82.

Lotfi, A., Langensiepen, C., Mahmoud, S. M., & Akhlaghinia, M. J. (2012). Smart homes for the elderly dementia sufferers: identification and prediction of abnormal behaviour. *Journal of Ambient Intelligence and Humanized Computing*, *3*(3), 205–218.

Medjahed, H., Istrate, D., Boudy, J., & Dorizzi, B. (2009, August). Human activities of daily living recognition using fuzzy logic for elderly home monitoring. In *Fuzzy Systems, 2009. FUZZ-IEEE 2009. IEEE International Conference on* (pp. 2001–2006). IEEE.

Park, S., & Kautz, H. (2008, July). Hierarchical recognition of activities of daily living using multi-scale, multi-perspective vision and RFID. In *Intelligent Environments, 2008 IET 4th International Conference on* (pp. 1–4). IET.

Rabiner, L. R. (1989). A Tutorial on Hidden Markov-Models and Selected Applications in Speech Recognition. *Proceedings of the IEEE*, *77*(2), 257–286.

Singla, G., Cook, D. J., & Schmitter-Edgecombe, M. (2008, July). Incorporating temporal reasoning into activity recognition for smart home residents. In *Proceedings of the AAAI workshop on spatial and temporal reasoning* (pp. 53–61).

Tapia, E. M., Intille, S. S., & Larson, K. (2004). Activity recognition in the home using simple and ubiquitous sensors. *Pervasive Computing, Proceedings*, *3001*, 158–175.

Van Kasteren, T., & Krose, B. (2007). *Bayesian activity recognition in residence for elders*. Paper presented at the 3rd International Conference on Intelligent Environments, 2007. IE 07.

Van Kasteren, T., Englebienne, G., & Kröse, B. A. (2011). Hierarchical activity recognition using automatically clustered actions. In D. Keyson, M. Maher, N. Streitz, A. Cheok, J. Augusto, R. Wichert, G. Englebienne, H. Aghajan & B. A. Kröse (Eds.), *Ambient Intelligence* (Vol. 7040, pp. 82–91): Springer Berlin Heidelberg.

Van Kasteren, T., Noulas, A., Englebienne, G., & Kröse, B. (2008, September). Accurate activity recognition in a home setting. In *Proceedings of the 10th international conference on Ubiquitous computing* (pp. 1–9). ACM.

Wadley, V. G., Okonkwo, O., Crowe, M., & Ross-Meadows, L. A. (2008). Mild cognitive impairment and everyday function: evidence of reduced speed in performing instrumental activities of daily living. *The American Journal of Geriatric Psychiatry*, *16*(5), 416–424.

Zhang, C., & Tian, Y. (2012). Rgb-d camera-based daily living activity recognition. *Journal of Computer Vision and Image Processing*, *2*(4), 12.

Zhang, Z. (2012). Microsoft kinect sensor and its effect. *MultiMedia, IEEE*, *19*(2), 4–10.

Zhao, Y., Liu, Z., Yang, L., & Cheng, H. (2012, December). Combing rgb and depth map features for human activity recognition. In *Signal & Information Processing Association Annual Summit and Conference (APSIPA ASC), 2012 Asia-Pacific* (pp. 1–4). IEEE.

Zhou, Z., Chen, X., Chung, Y. C., He, Z., Han, T. X., & Keller, J. M. (2008). Activity analysis, summarization, and visualization for indoor human activity monitoring. *Circuits and Systems for Video Technology, IEEE Transactions on, 18*(11), 1489–1498.

Andreas Riener, Myounghoon Jeon and Alois Ferscha

17 Human-Car Confluence: "Socially-Inspired Driving Mechanisms"

Abstract: With self-driving vehicles announced for the 2020s, today's challenges in Intelligent Transportation Systems (ITS) lie in problems related to negotiation and decision making in (spontaneously formed) car collectives. Due to the close coupling and interconnectedness of the involved driver-vehicle entities, effects on the local level induced by cognitive capacities, behavioral patterns, and the social context of drivers, would directly cause changes on the macro scale. To illustrate, a driver's fatigue or emotion can influence a local driver-vehicle feedback loop, which is directly translated into his or her driving style, and, in turn, can affect driving styles of all nearby drivers. These transitional, yet collective driver state and driving style changes raise global traffic phenomena like jams, collective aggressiveness, etc. To allow harmonic coexistence of autonomous and self-driven vehicles, we investigate in this chapter the effects of socially-inspired driving and discuss the potential and beneficial effects its application should have on collective traffic.

Keywords: Socially-behaving Vehicles, Collective Driving Mechanisms, Driver-vehicle Confluence, Social Actions

17.1 Introduction

Motivated by the expected need for solutions to solve problems related to the coexistence of autonomous and manual-driven cars, this chapter aims at discussing the vision of driver-vehicle symbiosis and its potential applications such as collective information sharing, ride negotiation, traffic flow and safety improvements, etc. Critical variables such as driving performance and workload are the motivational forces to include human factors in future information and communication technologies to reflect the singularity of a user. This calls for an interdisciplinary approach and this chapter tries to outline how this could be implemented.

After a brief review of the psychological view about the driver-car relationship and its transition in Section 2, the rest of this chapter discusses the status quo of social aspects of driving and proposes how socially acting vehicles and socially-inspired traffic can contribute to road traffic to make it safer, more efficient, and more convenient. Section 3 describes driver-car entanglement (i.e., the relationship between individual drivers and ITS or ETS) and Section 4 delineates social traffic and collective, adaptive systems (i.e., the relationship between a driver and another driver, and the higher network relationship among drivers, cars, and infrastructure). Also in Section

4, a sample scenario of the symbiosis between drivers using a collective awareness system is provided, followed by a conclusion with a future outlook in Section 5.

17.2 Psychology of Driving and Car Use

So far, vehicles have been ignorant of (or not able to be aware of) social aspects; it has been mainly the individual drivers with their desires, intentions, preferences, or usage patterns that are responsible for unpredictable social behaviors and, thus, need to be represented by a driver-vehicle related research model (Ferscha & Riener, 2009). With regard to sustainability, it is important to mention that the willingness to reduce traveling by car or to change over to alternative modes of transport highly depends on the social status and attitude of a person. In other words, altruistic population groups are more willing to change usage behavior as opposed to egoistic, anti social persons (Gatersleben, 2012). The awareness of the first group that their car use causes environmental problems seems to induce guilt, which leads to a sense of obligation to use, for example, a more environmentally friendly means of transportation (Bamberg, Hunecke, & Blöbaum, 2007). This social awareness seems to be absent or just ignored in the second group.

17.2.1 From Car Ownership to Car Sharing

First, even though a car does not express anything for itself, many individuals feel that their car has a strong symbolic appeal (Joshi & Rao, 2013). The type of car one drives could be an indication of the person's personality and the decision for buying a car is often made by the social value ('status symbol') of the new car. There is evidence that "cool cars" reinforce the self-confidence of drivers and a recent study shows that females find males driving a luxury car more attractive than those driving a compact car (Dunne2010). The social value of vehicles is also represented in the latest sales figures in 2013: US car makers established a new sales record of (heavy) pick-up trucks and German premium brands Audi and Porsche also set new sales records (Zeit Online, 2013). On the other side, this might also be a warning bell to make people rethink if it really makes sense to use a fuel wasting truck for commuting, in particular with confirmed car occupancy rates (in Europe and US) of 1–1.5 persons/car (European Environment Agency (EEA), 2010). Moreover, the relationship drivers currently have with their cars has to be reconsidered, as in the long term they will most likely have to give up to reflect their status symbol by their car due to economical, ecological, or other reasons.

Two trends are foreseeable. First, self-driving vehicles will emerge on the road and in that case fewer people will (have to) own a private car. However, according to a recent study by the carmaker Ford (Falk & Mundolf, 2013), 7 out of 10 people aged 35 or below would like to use technology and social services to adopt the car to their life style and 58% of the same group would like to precisely configure the "look & feel" of their car – customization will be the success criteria. Second, rural depopulation will result in more and more people living in the cities, and as a consequence most of the trips will be short distance. Nowadays, about 40% of British people already state that they can use the bike, bus, or walk for many journeys instead of riding a car (Gatersleben, 2012).

Fortunately, a turnaround in vehicle use and value are noticeable today. A series of studies still confirm that a considerable number of young drivers insist that their own cars express their personality (plus Marktforschung, 2011), but recent statistics show that lot of people from this group do not have an emotional relationship with their car any more. Asked about what personal things are the most important ones, the Smarthpone, an own apartment and a (mountain) bike are top-ranked while the former 'status symbol' car has in the past 10 years lost much ground (Schulz-Braunschmidt, 2012). In addition, more and more young people do not even own a driving license – between 2000 and 2008 the rate of German driving license holders (age group 18 to 26) decreased from 90.5% to 75.5%, and further decreased between 2007 and 2010 by more than 10 percent (Grass, 2011). (E-)bikes and public transport are the preferred way of travelling around (Bratzel, 2011). This could be seen as an ideal prerequisite to improve the future of mobility using "connected technology" to provide sustainable car-rental, -sharing, -pooling services and optimization services for intermodal transport.

17.2.2 Intelligent Services to Support the Next Generation Traffic

Self-owning and individual use of vehicles will likely be increasingly replaced by intelligently organized mobility services that are easy to use and provide intuitive user interfaces. The shift in values requires sophisticated cooperation strategies between all traffic participants, communication technologies, and road infrastructure to fulfil all the diverse transportation requirements with a different means of transportation. Therefore, the next generation of Intelligent Transportation Systems (ITS) is challenged by the complex interactions of technological advancements and the social nature of individuals using these technologies. Traffic in the future will not be determined by individual drivers' selfish desires and intentions, but by the negotiation between the collection of cars and utilization requests of drivers (Figure 17.1). According to a recent study (Kalmbach, Bernhart, Kleimann, & Hoffmann, 2011, p. 63), if used interurban, one shared vehicle could replace up to 38 cars! – a strong motivation toward the development of novel vehicular services and self-driving mechanisms.

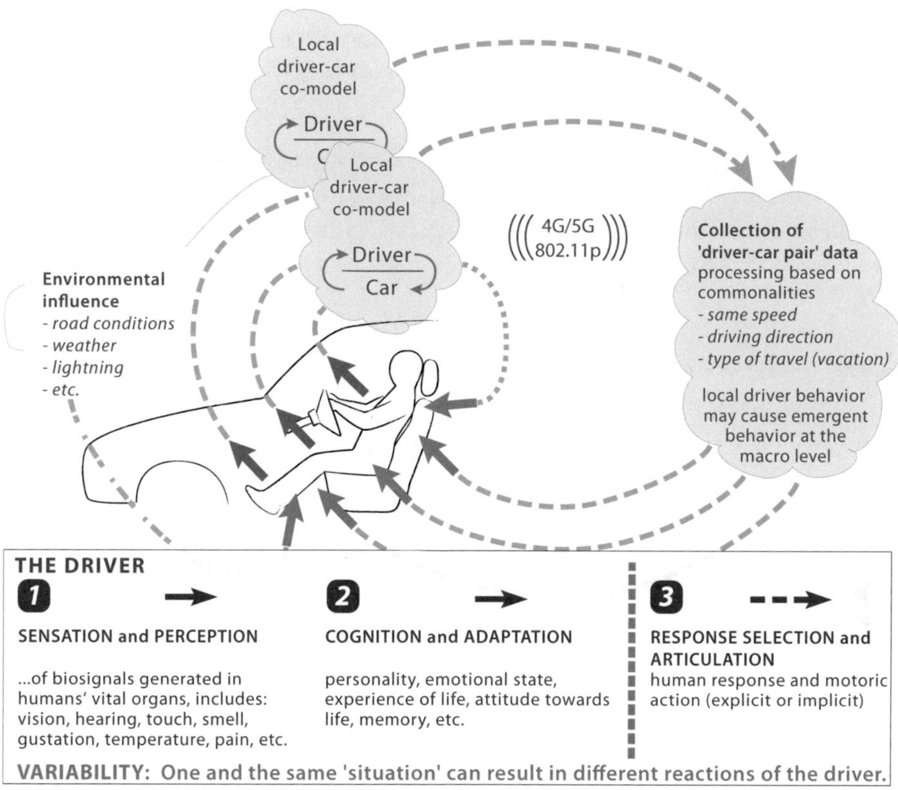

Figure 17.1: Overview of the Human-Car confluence concept (based on (Ferscha & Riener, 2009))

Research in the field has shown considerations and issues related to driver behavior models or the information/knowledge flow in such a highly connected setting. To illustrate, (Lee, Lee, & Salvucci, 2012) showed computational models of driver behavior and (Schroeter, Rakotonirainy, & Foth, 2012) discussed the challenges and opportunities that place- and time-specific digital information may offer to road users. The concept of driver-vehicle confluence discussed by (Riener, 2012) goes one step further, by aiming at understanding the symbiosis between drivers, cars, and (road) infrastructure by including reasoning about driver states and social or emotional interaction. Also the calls of national and international funding agencies further reflect that both researchers and practitioners have serious interests in developing the research field of socially-inspired cars.

17.3 Human-Car Entanglement: Driver-Centered Technology and Interaction

Researchers and practitioners have realized that efforts should be put on 'drivers' to improve driver-vehicle interaction and thus, drivers can be released from subsidiary activities and can concentrate on the primary task. To this end, it is necessary to understand human capability and limitation and apply those principles to system design.

17.3.1 Intelligent Transportation Systems (ITS)

To design human-centered driver assistance systems, a number of research groups have explored ITS based on a multidisciplinary approach, e.g., (Doshi, Tran, Wilder, Mozer, & Trivedi, 2012). For example, to capture the "complete vehicle context", researchers at the University of California, San Diego (UCSD) have used a combination of computer vision and behavioral data analysis. Further, they have tried to forecast the trajectory of the vehicle in real-time, by predicting a driver's behaviors (Doshi & Trivedi, 2011). Such a system can allow the ITS to compensate for risky circumstances, such as lane change departures (Salvucci, 2004) or rear end collisions. Researchers have also applied a vision-based approach to analyze the foot movement before, during, and after the pedal operation to gather information about driver behaviors, states, and styles (Tran, Doshi, & Trivedi, 2012). This is similar to the prediction of steering behavior based on body posture and movement (Riener, Ferscha, & Matscheko, 2008). In addition, the possibility of using haptic feedback has been tested to support the driver in reallocating his or her attention to critical situations and thereby, enhance their situation awareness (Mulder, Abbink, & van Paassen, 2011). The HumanFIRST Program in Minnesota employs psychology and human factors engineering to investigate the distraction potential associated with in-vehicle signing information and analyze drivers' opinions about mileage-based road usage fees (Creaser & Manser, 2012). The National Advanced Driving Simulator (NADS) Center in Iowa has worked on data reduction and safety systems to detect where the driver looks at (e.g., instrument panel or mirrors) (Schwarz, He, & Veit, 2011). In addition, they have contributed to the development of systems that take over the vehicle control and safety policies (e.g., by studying alcohol impairment sensitivity (Brown, Fiorentino, Salisbury, Lee, & Moeckli, 2009)). The University of Michigan Transportation Research Institute (UMTRI) has addressed the problem of older drivers on the road and suggested launching separate vehicles for older drivers (Eby & Molnar, 2012). Nowadays, they also conduct research on connected vehicles on the road. Even though many more researchers are working on ITS, there remains a research gap between research settings and actual settings that needs to be further

bridged. Our conceptualization also includes the individual driver's states and their connection to external information streams (e.g., car to backbone).
Emotional Transportation Systems (ETS)

Given that humans have affective, cognitive, and behavioral elements, driver-centered technology should consider all of the three elements to be truly intelligent. Whereas driver cognition and behavior have been continuously addressed, emotions and affect have not been focused on in driving research until recently. In a dynamic driving context, information processing might interact with a driver's emotional state in a more complicated way. From this background, to achieve more natural and social interactions between a driver and a car, a car needs to detect a driver's affective states and appropriately respond to the driver and this necessity of research on driver emotions has appeared fairly recently, e.g., (Eyben et al., 2010). Research has shown that not just the driver arousal level, but also specific emotional states influence driving performance differently (e.g., anger (Dula, Martin, Fox, & Leonard, 2011), nervousness (Li & Ji, 2005), sadness (Jeon & Zhang, 2013), frustration (Y. Lee, 2010), etc.). Diverse emotion detection methods for the driving context have been suggested including physiological sensors (e.g., (Riener, 2009, Ferscha, & Aly, 2009)), speech recognition systems (e.g., (Eyben et al., 2010)), or the combinations of more than two methods (e.g., facial detection + speech detection (Jeon & Walker, 2011)). However, all of these attempts are still in an early stage and research is still needed to develop a more robust, but unobtrusive means to detect a driver's emotional states. A more critical issue is how the emotional transportation systems can intervene in a driver's emotional context after detecting it. Harris (e.g., cognitive reappraisal (Harris & Nass, 2011)) and Jeon (e.g., attention deployment (Jeon, 2012)) have tried to apply a psychological emotion regulation model (Gross, 2002) to driving situations using speech-based systems. Further, other modalities/methods could also be explored and developed such as a type of emotional gauge (just like a speedometer), a certain piece of music, or specific haptic feedback.

17.3.2 Recommendations

Time has come to change the long tradition of system-centered design, and to move over to systems, applications, and devices that focus on new forms of sensing, perceiving, interpreting, and reacting in the junction of 'man and machine'. To implement this in a car, new forms of interaction and communication emerging at the confluence between human and systems need to be incorporated by integrating real world contexts, socio-cultural aspects, and multi-faceted functions. Interaction concepts have to take care of the facts that (i) driving is almost a pure visual task with viewing direction toward the street, (ii) a driver has limited cognitive abilities and attentional resources, (iii) configuring an instrument cluster and displays in the car compete with limited attentional resources of the driver, and (iv) a full range of apps and cloud computing services can enable the driver to work in the car in a similar way than to those in the office or at home. The adoption of human factors for the next-generation (dynamic and ubiquitous) vehicular environment raises crucial challenges within the field of ITS/automotive ICT. Those challenges include (i) implementing sensors, actuators, and communication interfaces for drivers, (ii) analyzing driver behavior data from those embedded sensors, (iii) reacting proactively based on those data, (iv) predicting collective system behaviors, and (v) solving ethical issues regarding all of these processes.

Dealing with all these issues calls for a novel driver state model, including full-fledged knowledge of the state transitions and the relationship between diverse emotions and cognitive processes. Drivers’ cognitive and affective mental states alter dynamically and have a deep impact on how to perceive a task or an interface. Thus, these should be considered critically in future vehicular user interfaces. In addition to detecting drivers’ state, the system should infer their intention and accordingly react in problematic situations. Here, we also need to identify a means to inform or stimulate the driver in an unobtrusive way. Note that this approach should be carefully taken, given that user freedom and controllability is generally a critical issue in HCI (Molich & Nielsen, 1990).

Many drivers still think that cars are a vehicle of personal freedom, and they do not want to relinquish vehicle control (O’Dell, 2012). More precisely, at least two kinds of driving need to be differentiated: (i) if drivers enjoy driving (“driving per se is fun”), they will insist on manual control and (ii) if drivers only want to commute efficiently, then they will use an autonomous car and enjoy reading the paper or relaxing. All these aspects are directly influential for human-centered intelligent driver assistance systems research, but so far research has been only focusing on improvements of the individual driver (driver-car pair). Thinking one step further, to achieve improvements in road throughput, avoid traffic jams, or reduce CO_2 emissions on a larger scale, driver-vehicle pairs should be connected to a sort of vehicular backbone, and information from this network should be used to optimize traffic on the macro scale. For example, intentions/reservations of all the individual drivers within a certain area or with a common goal could be collected and forwarded to a cloud service featuring data aggregation, common decision making, etc. to finally attain global changes in traffic behavior. We will have a look into this “collective driving” paradigm in the next section.

17.4 Socially-Inspired Traffic and Collective-Aware Systems

The Safe Intelligent Mobility – Test Field Germany (simTD) project gives a foretaste of possibilities of collective approaches in future traffic. It aims to help drivers select the best routes, detect obstacles before they see them, or reduce emissions through energy-efficient driving. To achieve these goals, a fleet of 120 networked cars using car-to-car and car-to-x communication is running on highways, country roads, and city streets. (Results from the large-scale field operational trial are expected to appear in 2014). While innovative, this project also focuses on the 'traditional' problems, and does not really bring up novel ideas in the field of collective adaptive or socially-inspired systems. In the end, it is not provocative enough to force the required paradigm change.

Successful applications of socially-inspired driving mechanisms (Figure 17.2) require to understand how the driver-vehicle pairs could make use of their (i.e., the drivers) social habitus, composed from (past and present) driving and mobility behaviors, social interactions with passengers, pedestrians, bicyclists, other vehicles, infrastructure, and last but not least, drivers' vital states when exposed to other road participants in live traffic. It further requires to define what social behavior in this context is. We agree on the definition of the US National Center for Biotechnology Information (NCBI), which states that social behavior is "any behavior caused by or affecting another individual, usually of the same species" (National Center for Biotechnology Information (NCBI), 2014). In addition, social behavior refers to interaction and communication (e.g., provoke a response, or change in behavior, without acting directly on the receiver) and includes terms, such as aggression, altruism, (self-)deception, mass (or collective) behavior, and social adjustment. Social behavior, as used in sociology, is followed by social actions directed at other people and designed to induce a response. Transferring this definition into the automotive domain, social behavior could be understood as the behavior of drivers, vehicles, pedestrians, and other road participants affecting each other.

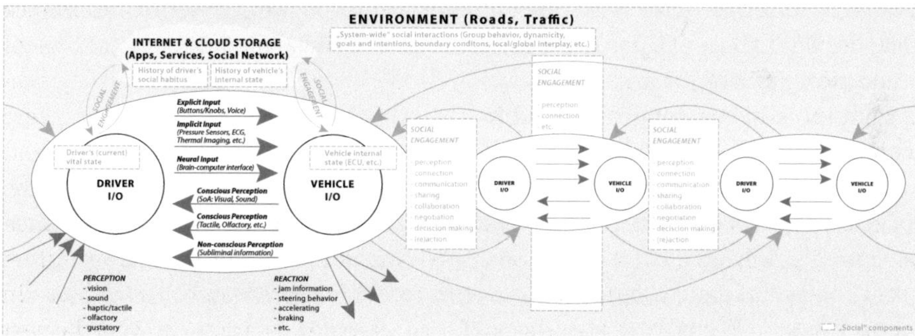

Figure 17.2: Social engagement in a collective traffic system. Successful application requires a) reliable and accurate data sources (driver, vehicle), b) authentic models to predict driver behavior and vehicle state, c) intelligent cloud services, d) non-distracting (driver) notification channels

17.4.1 The Driver: Unpredictable Behavior

Each and every driver has his/her own personality and the internal state of the driver may change by different reasons from one moment to the next. This is, of course, a source of unpredictable and unsafe behavior. Legislatory regulations and traffic control can prevent danger caused by alcohol, drugs, fatigue, but there are other sources that (temporarily) influence the normal competence of a driver (for example, stress, anger, or rage). In the meantime, advances in sensor technology have enabled the detection of drivers’ mental/physiological or emotional states, but the detection accuracy and reliability is still far from being applied in widespread networks of self-organizing cars to influence decision making and negotiation processes.

Another factor that plays a significant role in the dynamicity of traffic is social forgivingness (Aarts, 2012). Traffic is a social system in which road users interact with each other and it is important in terms of safety that drivers steer their cars with anticipation. That is, drivers prepare themselves to detect another driver’s potentially unsafe action early enough so that they can react appropriately and prevent, or at least, minimize negative consequences (Houtenbos, 2010). In addition, more competent road users could allow, for example, the less competent road users to commit errors without any serious consequences (Aarts, 2010). In order for a (willing) driver to be capable of acting with social forgivingness he/she must (i) have the correct expectations of the situations he/she is in, (ii) be capable of assessing the intentions of other road users correctly, and (iii) have the capacity to adapt his/her own behavior. The willingness to act in a socially forgiving manner is often influenced by external factors. For example, if the traffic light on a busy junction turns green for only a short time, the willingness of a particular driver to act with social forgivingness (i.e., yield) would most probably be low.

Advances in communication and in-car technology, together with the growing complexity and interdependence (Giannotti et al., 2012) of modern societies and economies, have been the main motivation for the emergence of approaches such as collective awareness, collective judgment, and collective action or behavior change (Mulgan & Leadbeater, 2013). Based on virtual communities for social change linked to environmental monitoring systems to enhance their awareness, collective systems can be used to effectively guide drivers in their everyday decisions (travelled route, departure time, etc.) and optimize traffic behavior based on efficiency (road throughput) and ecological (CO_2 emission) impacts (Sestini, 2012). Trust in technology (e.g., in semi-autonomous vehicles) or information presented on a display serves as a substantial success factor for services operating in large (self-organizing) systems. There is evidence that people in this human-technology intermix have a “fundamental bias to trust one’s own abilities over those of the system” (de Vries, Midden, & Bouwhuis, 2003). It is also important to understand to what extent a person is willing to get out of his/her fundamental bias by adopting (and trusting) an ICT system. However, there already exist networks of people helping each other (e.g., forums), and people joining these networks and empowering each other on their own. According to a recent survey, more than two thirds of people (68%) say that they trust what (other people in) the network tells them more than what companies or the state says; just 5 percent disagrees (Perrin, 2013), which indicates a high possibility of the successful application of collective services.

17.4.2 The Car: Socially Ignorant

Cars have recently become "smart" and they have nowadays an increasing perception of what is going on on the road and in the environment (e.g., road and weather condition, traffic density and flow, emerging jams, accidents, etc.), but, as of now, they are mindless and need to be controlled by an individual. The first step toward social intelligence in traffic was made by equipping all (newly sold) cars with wireless Internet, and the next step toward socially-inspired behavior was enabled by social services, already available in the car and used there to share sort of social driving information (experience, traffic situation) amongst other vehicles via social networking services (SNS) such as Facebook or Twitter. An online survey recently conducted in three different countries (Jeon, Riener, Lee, Schuett, & Walker, 2012) revealed that about 70% of people are active social network service users (61.9% Austrians, 84.6% US citizens, 85% Koreans), and about 20% of them are using these services while in the car. More interesting is that drivers not only track (44%) the status of a friend or a driver with the same commuting pattern, but also comment on the statuses of others (27%) or tweet traffic updates (26%) while operating the car.

However, still neither vehicles nor all the embedded (assistance) systems integrated into vehicles can act socially. Instead, it is drivers that socially act based on emotions or mood, situation, experience, or learned behavior. For instance, they stop their car on the curbside, wave their hand, let another car back out, and use the headlight flasher to inform upcoming traffic about dangerous situations. However, with the emergence of self driving or (semi-) autonomous vehicles, the communications between computer-controlled and manually-controlled vehicles (c.f., social driver-vehicle units or "the driver-car" (Dant, 2004)) and other road participants (pedestrians and bicyclists) need to be improved to allow efficient coexistence without severe danger of the involved parties. The next generation ITS has to include the essence of social intelligence to improve efficiency and safety by enabling cars to interact in a similar way humans communicate and interact one with another. The car should, for example, relieve drivers by taking over their tasks and accomplishing them as efficiently as the human driver by applying sort of social intelligence. Socially behaving cars should create true value (Riener, 2012) for the road participants, and not just post the social status or feelings of a driver or provide status information of the car (and collect "Like's") as Facebook does. This requires to embed social skills to consider social interaction, collective negotiation, and concerted (re)action between all the entities.

17.4.3 Networks of Drivers and Cars: Socially-Aware?

Social interaction in the car was previously offered only on an individual level, i.e., between one driver and another or between a driver and his or her vehicle. However, recent technological advances have led to a stronger interrelationship between the entities (Riener & Ferscha, 2013) and allowed for spontaneous formation of cooperative car crowds. Going one step further, social awareness has to deal with both individual and group behaviors and goals (Serbedzja, 2010), and such a system is basically comprised of many local actors (driver-car pairs) with (i) individual information (habits, customs, character, daily routine, personality, emotions, cognitions, physical states, intrinsic and extrinsic behaviors, restricted perception of their environment, and a limited capacity of action, etc.) as well as (ii) collective information (social grouping, long and short term social behaviors, social practice, both prejudices and tolerance, fashion, tradition, social etiquette, etc.).

With regard to individual information, (social) criteria characterizing human behavior and/or reputation need to be validated. Attributes to be considered include the ability to communicate and interact, willingness to negotiate, cognitive abilities, self-managing behavior history, reputation, ability to assert oneself, forget/forgive, rapid assessment and decision making, and learning/adaptation capabilities. For collective information, cars are socializing to achieve a global optimum goal based on a cost (fitness) function that concerns the environment of the problem in its totality. The difficulties in traffic include (i) that different time scales are evident (driving action: seconds, emergence of a jam: minutes to hours; change of weather: hours to days; legal regulations: month to years), (ii) that driving is a highly dynamic task (negotiation, re-distribution of the decision to local actors, or behavior adaption, etc. is often not possible by the due time), (iii) that there are many (local) actors with individual behavior, restricted perception of their environment, and a limited capacity of action involved, and (iv) that the context and its boundary conditions are continuously changing (traffic situation, jams/accidents, driver state (e.g., sleepy driver), infrastructure failures (e.g., no traffic lights), weather conditions (dry to snow storm), etc.) (Bersini, 2010; Bersini & Philemotte, 2007). Furthermore, to provide more stable solutions (interplay of individual and collective levels), it is required to perfectly understand the reality to be faced, i.e., the contexts and its boundary conditions in which the scenario is embedded into. Last but not least, the aspect of ethics needs to be integrated in solutions to provide ethical sensitivity to each of the above aspects.

17.4.4 Recommendations

Traffic density and likelihood/duration of jams have considerably increased in the past decades and with it more and more drivers feel increased stress and anger from traffic; finally a number of people cancel or postpone planned trips due to anticipated high traffic. These problems cannot be solved by just adding another lane to the highway, building new roads, or pushing public transportation. A sustainable solution requires a holistic approach including new ways of traveling (platooning, car- and bike-sharing, active mobility), concerted coordination, and proactive traffic management. This can be already achieved by the current technology, and by further applying concepts such as incentivization, driver behaviors can be changed specifically. Moreover, a socially-enabled car requires a social environment (for example, intelligent roads with dynamically changing lanes; road signs adapting to the driver, etc.) and social cars should have social capabilities, such as (i) "learning" (a car automatically recommends alternative routes if having learned that there is a traffic jam every workday in that region at a certain time; such a behavior would be relevant for drivers using a rental car in an unknown area), (ii) "remembering" (a vehicle remembers from one winter to the next, that driving at or near the speed limit is not wise on temperatures below zero degrees or snow coverage on the road), or (iii) "forgetting" (a car moves more carefully after having been involved in an accident; however, the incident is forgotten after some time and avoids that the car is fearful and drives too slow in the long term), etc. To give a concrete example to force safety, ITS could take over the control of a car moving inappropriately in convoy (e.g., a driver ignoring a road situation or reacting too slowly) by applying the brakes, changing the steering angle, or accelerating the vehicle. It needs to be argued, however, whether drivers are able to prohibit a broad application of this auto pilot-like safety system as they would not be willing to accept restrictions in their personal liberty. Traffic fully under control of computer systems and network communications also poses potential for criminal activities (central control can be (mis)used to induce mass collisions or to generate gridlocks from everywhere).

By merging all the information from drivers, cars, and infrastructure into a common database, the basis for an improved interaction between the involved parties could be established. This implies more than developing new interfaces or driving assistance systems. To implement it, looking into similarities in biology can be a good starting point. For example, driving is in some aspects similar to ants moving on a trail, and they use pheromones to share information about the environment (e.g., food sources (Karlson & Lüscher, 1959). Likewise, other drivers' signal can cause short-term changes in the driving behavior (i. e,. hormones (Huber & Gregor, 2005) or neurotransmitters). Other examples from biology include stigmergy (a concept to store states in the environment that can be easily retrieved by specialized sensors) or superorganisms (in our sense a collection of agents which can act in orchestration to produce phenomena governed by the collective (Kelly, 1994)).

17.4.5 Experience Sharing: A Steering Recommender System

One example scenario accentuating the potential of the symbiosis between drivers with different knowledge is the steering recommender system. The idea behind is, that drivers familiar with a certain route (e.g. daily commuting on that road, living in the area for a long time, etc.) have detailed, intuitive, and implicit knowledge about how to drive as efficient as possible. They know the optimum points of braking before and accelerating in/after a curve, they know the sections where overtaking is possible, and they know potential points of danger (bus stop, cars backing out, blind head, sharp turn, etc.). Collecting and processing the information from all experienced drivers (using CAN bus information and GPS data to keep track of parameters, such as steering (wheel) angle, when (and how often) the brake pedal is pushed, which gear is engaged, and when the gear is changed up/down, etc.) could be used in a service providing steering recommendations to other, unfamiliar drivers (new drivers and/or on holiday trip). By using this service (Figure 17.3), traffic flow should be more homogeneous as vehicles would then drive with similar optimal conditions where appropriate. Further, this system could be used as a warning service to notify vehicles about upcoming hazards detected implicitly by many drivers ahead. Based on it, road safety will increase and also the average fuel consumption should be minimized.

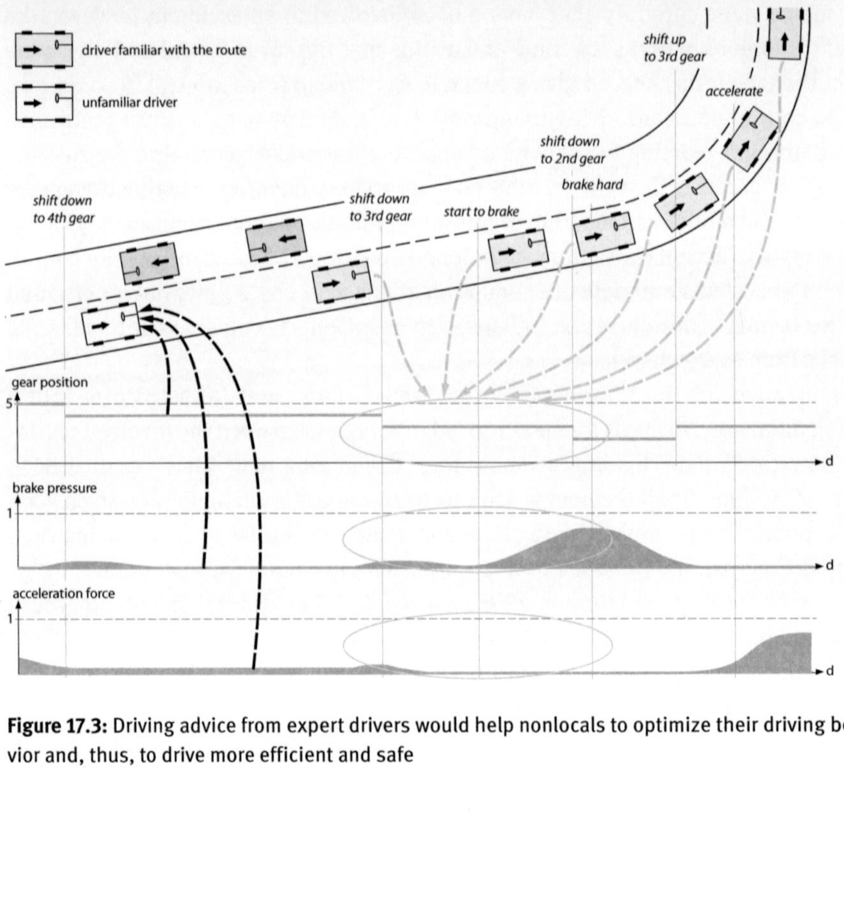

Figure 17.3: Driving advice from expert drivers would help nonlocals to optimize their driving behavior and, thus, to drive more efficient and safe

17.5 Conclusion

In this chapter we have discussed the potential that a collective understanding of the traffic situation together with a concerted behavior modification by socially-acting vehicles have for future traffic. We expect that this allows to automatically resolve conflicts in mass traffic, negotiate with each other, behave as a collective to optimize characteristics such as driving time or efficiency, address the topic of environmental protection, raise safety on the road by monitoring other cars' behavior in the vicinity, and enhancing driving experience, satisfaction, and pleasure.

Based on an analogy with biology, such a system could be implemented as a type of a "collective brain" gathering neural inputs from all the drivers in a common area of interest and featuring common decision making and negotiation on the route or lane taken by each individual driver within the collective, by adopting paradigms known as pheromones, stigmergy, or superorganisms.

Our concept should be understood as a specific instantiation of human-computer confluence working towards the goal of full understanding of the symbiosis between drivers, cars, and infrastructure. It covers not only sharing of information about an oil spill on the road, but also reasoning about driver states and social/emotional interaction. This ultimate goal can be achieved by modeling driver behaviors, conducting simulations and empirical driving studies, investigating distributed negotiation processes, and relating these results to observations in real world.

References

Aarts, L. T. (2010, February). *Sustainable Safety: principles, misconceptions, and relations with other visions* (SWOV Fact sheet). SWOV, Leidschendam, the Netherlands. (pp. 5)

Arts, L. T. (2012, November). *Background of the five Sustainable Safety principles* (SWOV Fact sheet). SWOV Institute for Road Safety Research, Leidschendam, the Netherlands. (pp. 5)

Bamberg, S., Hunecke, M., & Blöbaum, A. (2007). *Social context, personal norms and the use of public transportation: Two field studies*. Journal of Environmental Psychology, 27 (3), 190–203. Retrieved from http://www.sciencedirect.com/science/article/pii/ S0272494407000357 doi: http://dx.doi.org/10.1016/j.jenvp.2007.04.001

Bersini, H. (2010, January). *My vision on "fundamentals of collective adaptive systems"*. Universite Libre de Bruxelles (IRIDIA), 2.

Bersini, H., & Philemotte, C. (2007). *Emergent phenomena only belong to biology*. In Proceedings of the 9th european conference on advances in artificial life (pp. 53–62). Springer. Retrieved from http://dl.acm.org/citation.cfm?id=1771390.1771398

Bratzel, S. (2011). i-Car: *Die junge Generation und das vernetzte Auto* (AutomotiveMARKETS 2011). Center of Automotive Management Bergisch Gladbach.

Brown, T., Fiorentino, D., Salisbury, S. E., Lee, J., & Moeckli, J. (2009, February). *Advanced vehicle-based countermeasures for alcohol-related crashes* (Final Task 1 letter report No. N2009-004). National Advanced Driving Simulator, Iowa City.

Creaser, J., & Manser, M. (2012, March). *Connected vehicles program: Driver performance and distraction evaluation for in-vehicle signing* (Technical report No. CTS 12-05). HumanFIRST Program, University of Minnesota.

Dant, T. (2004). The driver-car. Theory, *Culture and Society – Special issue on Automobilities*, 21 (4), 61–79. (ISSN: 0263-2764)

de Vries, P., Midden, C., & Bouwhuis, D. (2003). *The effects of errors on system trust, self-confidence, and the allocation of control in route planning*. International Journal of Human-Computer Studies, 58 (6), 719–735.

Doshi, A., Tran, C., Wilder, M. H., Mozer, M. C., & Trivedi, M. M. (2012). *Sequential dependencies in driving*. Cognitive Science, 36 (5), 948–963.

Doshi, A., & Trivedi, M. (2011, October). *Tactical driver behavior prediction and intent inference: A review*. In 14th conference on intelligent transportation systems (ITSC) (pp. 1892–1897). doi: 10.1109/ITSC.2011.6083128

Dula, C. S., Martin, B. A., Fox, R. T., & Leonard, R. L. (2011). *Differing types of cellular phone conversations and dangerous driving* [Journal Article]. Accident Analysis and Prevention, 43 , 187–193.

Dunne, M. J., & Searle, R. (2010). *Effect of manipulated prestige-car ownership on both sex attractiveness ratings*. British Journal of Psychology, 101 (1), 69–80. doi: 10.1348/000712609X417319

Eby, D. W., & Molnar, L. J. (2012, February). *Has the time come for an older driver vehicle?* (Techical report No. UMTRI-2012-5). University of Michigan. (pp. 68)

European Environment Agency (EEA). (2010, July). *Occupancy rates of passenger vehicles (Assessment)*. European Union. (http://www.eea.europa.eu/data-and-maps/figures/ term29-occupancy-rates-in-passenger-transport-1)

Eyben, F., Wollmer, M., Poitschke, T., Schuller, B., Blaschke, C., Farber, B., & Nguyen-Thien, N. (2010). Emo*tion on the road – necessity, acceptance, and feasibility of affective computing in the car* [Journal Article]. Advances in Human-Computer Interaction, 1–17.

Falk, B., & Mundolf, U. (2013, September). *Ford Zeitgeist Studie: Das Auto als Schnittstelle sozialer Interaktionen* (Press information). [online]. (http://217.110.41.59/, retrieved June 16, 2014.)

Ferscha, A., & Riener, A. (2009, April). *Pervasive Adaptation in Car Crowds*. In Workshop on user-centric pervasive adaptation (UCPA) at Mobilware (p. 6). Springer.

Gatersleben, B. (2012, September). *The psychology of sustainable transport*. The Psychologist, 25 (9), 676–679.

Giannotti, F., Pedreschi, D., Pentland, A., Lukowicz, P., Kossmann, D., Crowley, J., & Helbing, D. (2012). *A planetary nervous system for social mining and collective awareness*. The European Physical Journal Special Topics, 214 (1), 49–75. Retrieved from http://dx.doi .org/10.1140/epjst/e2012-01688-9 doi: 10.1140/epjst/e2012-01688-9

Grass, K. (2011, October 1). *Ohne Lappen geht's doch auch*. [online]. (http://www.taz.de/!79169/, retrieved June 16, 2014.)

Gross, J. J. (2002). *Emotion regulation: Affective, cognitive, and social consequences* [Journal Article]. Psychophysiology, 39 , 281–291.

Harris, H., & Nass, K. (2011). *Emotion regulation for frustrating driving contexts* [Conference Paper]. ACM Press.

Houtenbos, M. (2010). *Social forgivingness and vulnerable road users*. In Proc. of 11th international conference on walking and liveable communities, the hague (p. 7).

Huber, J., & Gregor, E. (2005). *Die Kraft der Hormone*. Droemer/Knaur. (ISBN: 3-426-66974-9)

Jeon, M. (2012). *Effects of affective states on driver situation awareness and adaptive mitigation interfaces: Focused on anger*. Doctoral Dissertation. Georgia Institute of Technology, Atlanta, GA.

Jeon, M., Riener, A., Lee, J.-H., Schuett, J., & Walker, B. (2012, October). *Cross-Cultural Differences in the Use of In-vehicle Technologies and Vehicle Area Network Services: Austria, USA, and South Korea*. In Proceedings of AutomotiveUI '12 (p. 8). ACM.

Jeon, M., & Walker, B. N. (2011). *Emotion detection and regulation interface for drivers with traumatic brain injury*, ACM SIGCHI Conference on Human Factors in Computing Systems (CHI'11), Vancouver, BC, Canada, May 7–12, 2011.

Jeon, M., & Zhang, W. (2013, September). *Sadder but wiser? Effects of negative emotions on risk perception, driving performance, and perceived workload.* In Proc. of the human factors and ergonomics society annual meeting (HFES 2013) (Vol. 57, pp. 1849–1853).

Joshi, N., & Rao, P. S. (2013). *Environment friendly car: Challenges ahead in India.* Global Journal of Management And Business Research, 13 (4), 9.

Kalmbach, R., Bernhart, W., Kleimann, P. G., & Hoffmann, M. (2011, March). *Automotive Landscape 2025: Opportunities and Challenges Ahead* (Tech. Rep.). Roland Berger Strategy Consultants. (pp. 88)

Karlson, P., & Lüscher, M. (1959). *Pheromones: a new term for a class of biologically active substances.* Nature, 183 (4653), 55–56.

Kelly, K. (1994). Out *of control: the new biology of machines, social systems and the economic world.* Boston: Addison-Wesley. (ISBN: 0-201-48340-8)

Lee, J., Lee, J. D., & Salvucci, D. D. (2012, October). *Evaluating the distraction potential of connected vehicles.* In Proceedings of AutomotiveUI '12 (pp. 33–40). ACM.

Lee, Y. (2010). Mea*suring drivers' frustration in a driving simulator* [Conference Proceedings]. In Proc. of the human factors and ergonomics society annual meeting (HFES 2010).

Li, X., & Ji, Q. (2005). *Active affective state detection and user assistance with dynamic bayesian networks* [Journal Article]. IEEE Transactions on Systems, Man, and Cybernetics, Part A, 35 (1), 93–105.

Molich, R., & Nielsen, J. (1990, March). *Improving a human-computer dialogue: What designers know about traditional interfacce design.* Communications of the ACM , 33 (3).

Mulder, M., Abbink, D., & van Paassen, M. (2011, March). *Design of a Haptic Gas Pedal for Active Car-Following Support.* IEEE Transactions on Intelligent Transportation Systems, 12 (1), 268–279. doi: 10.1109/TITS.2010.2091407

Mulgan, G., & Leadbeater, C. (2013, January). *Systems innovation (Discussion paper).* Nesta, UK.

National Center for Biotechnology Information (NCBI). (2014, June). Medical Subject Headings (MeSH): *Social Behavior.* [online], (http://www.ncbi.nlm.nih.gov/mesh/ 68012919, retrieved 2014, June 16)

O'Dell, J. (2012, August 30). *Here Come Self-Driving Cars. The Technology Is Nearly Ready, but Are We?*, pp. 5 (http://www.edmunds.com/car-technology/here-come-self-driving-cars.html)

Perrin, W. (2013, April). *The importance of largescale communications (Nesta discussion series on systemic innovation).* Director of Talk about Local. (pp. 37–38).

plus Marktforschung. (2011, October 11). *Autos zum Ausdruck der Persönlichkeit.* [online]. (http://de.auto.de/magazin/showArticle/article/61291, retrieved June 16, 2014.)

Riener, A. (2012, October). *Driver-vehicle confluence or How to control your car in future?* In Proceedings of AutomotiveUI '12 (p. 8). ACM.

Riener, A., & Ferscha, A. (2013, May). *Enhancing future mass ict with social capabilities. In Co-evolution of intelligent socio-technical systems* (pp. 141–184). Springer. Retrieved from http://link.springer.com/chapter/10.1007%2F978-3-642-36614-7 7.

Riener, A., Ferscha, A., & Aly, M. (2009, September). *Heart on the Road: HRV Analysis for Monitoring a Driver's Affective State.* In Proceedings of AutomotiveUI '09 (pp. 99–106). ACM. Retrieved from http://doi.acm.org/10.1145/1620509.1620529 doi: 10.1145/1620509.1620529.

Riener, A., Ferscha, A., & Matscheko, M. (2008, February). *Intelligent Vehicle Handling: Steering and Body Postures while Cornering*. In Conference on architecture of computing systems (arcs 2008) (Vol. 4934, p. 14). Springer.

Salvucci, D. D. (2004). *Inferring driver intent: A case study in lane-change detection*. Proceedings of the Human Factors and Ergonomics Society Annual Meeting, 48 (19), 2228–2231. Retrieved from http://pro.sagepub.com/content/48/19/2228.abstract doi: 10.1177/154193120404801905.

Schroeter, R., Rakotonirainy, A., & Foth, M. (2012). *The social car: new interactive vehicular applications derived from social media and urban informatics*. In Proceedings of AutomotiveUI '12 (pp. 107–110). ACM.

Schulz-Braunschmidt, W. (2012, August 29). *Die Jugend verzichtet auf das eigene Auto*. [online]. (http://www.stuttgarter-zeitung.de/inhalt.strassenverkehr-die-jugend -verzichtet-auf-das-eigene-auto.ddbd6af7-c500-4c13-8abf-9d494a03811a.html, retrieved June 16, 2014.).

Schwarz, C., He, Y., & Veit, A. (2011, June). *Eye Tracking in a COTS PC-based Driving Simulator: Implementation and Applications*. In Proceedings of Image 2011 conference (p. 8).

Serbedzja, N. (2010, September 20–27). *Privacy in Emerging Pervasive Systems* [The 3rd International PERADA-ASSYST Summer School on Adaptive Socio-Technical Pervasive Systems, Budapest]. In The 3rd international perada-assyst summer school on adaptive socio-technical pervasive systems, Budapest.

Sestini, F. (2012, April). *Brave New World – or Collective Awareness Platforms as an Engine for Sustainability and Ethics* (Tech. Rep.). European Commission, DG Information Society and Media. (pp. 17).

Tran, C., Doshi, A., & Trivedi, M. M. (2012). *Modeling and prediction of driver behavior by foot gesture analysis. Computer Vision and Image Understanding*, 116 (3), 435–445. Retrieved from http://www.sciencedirect.com/science/article/pii/S1077314211002086 doi: 10 .1016/j.cviu.2011.09.008.

Zeit Online. (2013, August 1). *US-Autokonzerne knüpfen an Glanzzeiten vor Krise an*. [online]. (http://www.zeit.de/wirtschaft/2013-08/usa-wirtschaftskrise-autobauer, retrieved June 16, 2014.).

List of Figures

List of Tables